Economic, Legal and Policy Studies on Health

Pelin Varol İyidoğan / Burcu G. Özcan Büyüktanır /
Ahu Sumbas (eds.)

Economic, Legal and Policy Studies on Health

A Social Science Perspective to Health Studies in Turkey

PETER LANG

**Bibliographic Information published by the
Deutsche Nationalbibliothek**
The Deutsche Nationalbibliothek lists this publication in the Deutsche
Nationalbibliografie; detailed bibliographic data is available online at
http://dnb.d-nb.de.

Library of Congress Cataloging-in-Publication Data
A CIP catalog record for this book has been applied for at the
Library of Congress.

ISBN 978-3-631-85248-4 (Print)
E-ISBN 978-3-631-85305-4 (E-PDF)
E-ISBN 978-3-631-86855-3 (EPUB)
10.3726/b19116

© Peter Lang GmbH
Internationaler Verlag der Wissenschaften
Berlin 2021
All rights reserved.

Peter Lang – Berlin · Bern · Bruxelles · Istanbul · New York · Oxford · Warszawa · Wien

This publication has been peer reviewed.

www.peterlang.com

6 Contents

Part III Gender in Health Policies and Law

Part IV Legal and Public Policy Perspective to Vaccination Application

Part V Reflections of Covid-19 in Law and Economics

Contents

Part I Economic and Public Policy Perspective in the Health Sector

Part II The Impact of Europeanization in Health Law and Policy

Contents 7

Part VI Current Thematic Discussions in Health Studies

Part VII Noticeable Issues in Health Law

Contributors

Çetin Arslan
Professor Criminal and Criminal Procedure Law Department, Faculty of Law, Hacettepe University, Ankara/Turkey
Orcid: 0000-0001-7930-3781; cetinarslan@hacettepe.edu.tr.

Eda Yeşil Balıkçıoğlu
Assistant Professor, Department of Public Finance, Kırıkkale University, Kırıkkale/Turkey
Orcid: 0000-0002-2525-6745; edabalikcioglu@kku.edu.tr

Ayşe Nur Songür Bozdağ
Research Assistant, Department of Nutrition and Dietetics, Faculty of Health Sciences, İzmir Katip Çelebi University, İzmir/Turkey
Orcid: 0000-0001-6412-8650; aysenur.songur.bozdag@ikcu.edu.tr

Kıvılcım Ceren Büken
Ph.D. Student, Department of Public Law, Faculty of Law, Hacettepe University, Ankara/Turkey
Orcid: 0000-0002-1431-556X; kivilcimbuken@hacettepe.edu.tr

Nüket Örnek Büken
Professor, Faculty of Medicine, Hacettepe University, Ankara/Turkey
Orcid: 0000-0001-9166-6569; buken@hacettepe.edu.tr

Burcu G. Özcan Büyüktanır
Associate Professor, Department of Civil Law, Faculty of Law, Hacettepe University, Ankara/Turkey
Orcid: 000-0003-3638-1637; bgozcan@hacettepe.edu.tr

Funda Pınar Çakıroğlu
Professor, Department of Nutrition and Dietetics, Faculty of Health Sciences, Ankara University, Ankara/Turkey
Orcid: 0000-0003-2324-6874; scakir64@hotmail.com

Oytun Canyaş
Associate Professor, Faculty of Law, Hacettepe University, Ankara/Turkey
Orcid: 0000-0003-1991-5641; oytuncanyas@gmail.com

Eylül Erdem
Research Assistant, Criminal and Criminal Procedure Law Department, Faculty
of Law, Hacettepe University, Ankara/Turkey
Orcid: 0000-0003-2616-6853; eylulerdem@hacettepe.edu.tr

Ezgi Aygün Eşitli
Associate Professor, Criminal and Criminal Procedure Law Department, Faculty
of Law, Başkent University Ankara/Turkey
Orcid: https: 0000-0002-5413-2485; aygun.ezgi@gmail.com

Fatma Didem Sevgili Gencay
Associate Professor, Department of Public Law, Faculty of Law, Hacettepe
University Hacettepe University, Ankara/Turkey
Orcid: 0000-0001-8927-8874; didemsevgili@hacettepe.edu.tr

Yiğit İltaş
Ph.D., Criminal and Criminal Procedure Law Department, Faculty of Law,
Cukurova University, Adana/Turkey
Orcid: https://orcid.org/0000-0001-5728-0902; yigitiltas@gmail.com

Pelin Varol İyidoğan
Professor, Department of Public Finance, Faculty of Economics and
Administrative Sciences, Hacettepe University, Ankara/Turkey
Orcid: 0000-0002-4632-9130; pelinv@hacettepe.edu.tr

Orhan Emre Konuralp
Assistant Professor, Department of Civil Procedure, Enforcement and Insolvency
Law, Faculty of Law, Istanbul Aydin University, Istanbul/Turkey
Orchid: 0000-0002-0376-0692; orhanemrekonuralp@aydin.edu.tr

Sezgin Mercan
Assistant Professor, Department of Political Science and International Relations;
Baskent University, Ankara/Turkey
Orcid: 0000-0001-9847-4922; mercan@baskent.edu.tr

Selin Özden Merhaci
Ph.D. Lecturer, Department of Comparative Law, Faculty of Law, Ankara
University, Ankara/Turkey
Orcid: 0000-0002-8233-1166; sozden@law.ankara.edu.tr

Necati Nurcalı
Ph.D. Student, Assistant Specialist, General Directorate of Post and Telegraph
Organization, Ankara/Turkey
Orcid: 0000-0003-1939-1235; n.nurcali@gmail.com

Dila Okyar
Ph.D., Research Assistant, Department of Civil Law, Faculty of Law, Hacettepe
University, Ankara/Turkey
Orcid: 0000-0002-7829-2133; dila.okyar.law@gmail.com

Deniz Odabaş
Professor, Medical Doctor, Public Health Specialist, Department of Public
Health, Faculty of Medicine, Ankara University, Ankara/Turkey
Orcid: 0000-0002-4877-0122; caliskan@medicine.ankara.edu.tr

Sibel Özcan
Ph.D., Research Assistant, Department of Public Finance, Faculty of Economics
and Administrative Sciences, Hacettepe University, Ankara/Turkey
Orcid: 0000-0003-3565-4525; sibel.ozcan@hacettepe.edu.tr

Ezgi Sevinçhan
Research Assistant, Department of Fiscal Law, Faculty of Law, Hacettepe
University, Ankara/Turkey
sevinchanezgi@gmail.com

Azer Sumbas
Research Assistant, Department of Public Law, Faculty of Law, Hacettepe
University, Ankara, Turkey
Orcid: 0000-0002-3024-7499; asumbas@ucdavis.edu, azersumbas@hacettepe.
edu.tr

Ahu Sumbas
Associate Professor, Department of Political Science and Public Administration,
Faculty of Economics and Administrative Sciences, Hacettepe University,
Ankara/Turkey
Orcid: 0000-0003-0944-4751; ahusumbas@yahoo.com

Gamze Yorgancıoğlu Tarcan
Associate Professor, Department of Health Management, Faculty of Economics and Administrative Sciences, Hacettepe University, Ankara/Turkey
Orcid: 0000-0002-5710-9547; gamze@hacettepe.edu.tr

Nazmiye Tekdemir
Research Assistant, Department of Public Finance, Faculty of Economics and Administrative Sciences, Hacettepe University, Ankara/Turkey

Ayşe Nil Tosun
Associate Professor, Department of Public Finance, Faculty of Economics and Administrative Sciences, Hacettepe University, Ankara/Turkey
Orcid: 0000-0001-5161-1037; nilt@hacettepe.edu.tr

Taner Turan
Professor, Department of Economics, Faculty of Economics and Administrative Sciences, Çukurova University, Adana/Turkey
Orcid: 0000-0003-3012-340X; tturan@cu.edu.tr

Sinem Yalçın
Ph.D., Principal Auditor, Turkish Court of Accounts, Ankara/Turkey
Orcid: 0000-0002-8970-771X; sinemyalcin@sayistay.gov.tr

Ayça Zorluoğlu Yılmaz
Ph.D., Research Assistant, Civil Law Department, Faculty of Law, Hacettepe University, Ankara/Turkey
Orcid: 0000-0001-7250-4097; azorluoglu@hacettepe.edu.tr, aycazorluoglu@gmail.com

H. Hakan Yılmaz
Professor, Department of Public Finance, Ankara University, Ankara/Turkey
Orcid: 0000-0003-3046-3236; hhyilmaz@politics.ankara.edu.tr

E. Neval YILMAZ
MD, PhD, LLM, Lawyer, Ankara Bar Association, General and Vascular Surgeon
Orcid: 0000-0003-2310-0269, info@nevalyilmaz.av.tr

Mehmet Onur Yurdakul
Ph.D., Treasury and Finance Expert, International Relations Department, Financial Crimes Investigation Board of Turkey, Ankara/Turkey
Orcid: 0000-0002-8343-5602; moyurdakul@gmail.com

Ahu Sumbas

Pelin Varol İyidoğan

Burcu G. Özcan Büyüktanır

An Introduction: Economic, Legal and Policy Studies on Health: A Social Science Perspective to Health Studies in Turkey

Over the last decades, our understanding of the relationship between social/ human sciences and natural sciences has been transformed by illustrating that they are relational and interrelated areas rather than separated realms of knowledge. It is therefore we believe that this attempt of combining health studies with the perspectives of socials sciences provides an overview of this dynamic and growing field.

Health is considered one of the fundamental human rights. The current global pandemic, Covid-19, explicitly reminds us of the fact that this right cannot be separated from the economic, legal, and political developments and policies. Indeed, the protection of the right to health induces some notable economic and political impacts both at the individual and social levels. In this regard, this book moves from the idea that a comprehensive approach to health studies should have a multi-dimensional and multi-disciplinary perspective. Moreover, it is argued that a critical approach to health studies with an eye of social sciences, particularly benefited from the fields of economics, law, and politics, contributes to the literature on health studies. Thus, this edited book is organized under seven thematic parts as "Economic and Public Policy Perspective in the Health Sector", "The Impact of Europeanization in Health Law and Policy", "Gender in Health Policies and Law", "Legal and Public Policy Perspective to Vaccination Application", "Reflections of Covid-19 in Law and Economics", "Current Thematic Discussions in Health Studies", and "Noticeable Issues in Health Law". In this introduction chapter, we present a brief introduction of each part of this book and how each chapter in a part engages in dialogue with others.

Each chapter in these parts aims to address the current critical debates in the literature of health studies regarding the issues in Turkey. The chapters, therefore, focus on the reflections of Covid-19 in law and economics, the efficiency and effectiveness of health sectors, the impacts of gender equality policies and gender-sensitive taxation to improve women's health, the role of the market, and other political actors in shaping health policies, the impacts of legal regulations and policy implementation on health outcomes as well as the studies examining the existing laws and their impacts on society and existing health system. The chapters also do not claim to be comprehensive, partly because there is not the space to include everything and partly because the interaction of social sciences and health studies is still being rediscovered. It is also important to remember that the aim of this book is to contribute to the literature by illustrating discussions and cases from Turkey.

Following an introductory part, the next four chapters in Part I focus on the issues in the health sector from an economic and public policy perspective. The study of Taner Turan entitled, "A Re-examination of Health Expenditure-Income Nexus in OECD Countries: With a Brief Evaluation for Turkey" leads this part. His empirical work questions the relationship between health expenditures and income, in terms of gross domestic product by employing panel cointegration and causality analysis for OECD countries with a special attention to Turkish experience. The following chapter of Sinem Yalçın is "Health Expenditures and the Fiscal Sustainability of Social Security System: An Investigation for Turkey". In her study, Sinem Yalçın mentions the fiscal sustainability issue for social security organizations, which play important roles in the public financing of health expenditures. Furthemore, she assesses the fiscal sustainability of the Social Security Institution (SSI) in Turkey. In the third chapter of this part, that is "Corruption and Money Laundering in the Health Sector", Mehmet Onur Yurdakul provides the theoretical discussion and literature review on the leading factors and impacts of corruption in health sector, the sector's vulnerability to money laundering, which is a less studied field. The final chapter of this part, entitled "Diabetes in Turkey: A Review of Economic Burden and Medical Nutrition Therapy of the Disease" is written by Ayşe Nur Songür Bozdağ & Funda Pınar Çakıroğlu. They evaluate the current state of diabetes in Turkey, its economic burden and nutritional therapy used to treat this non-communicable disease.

Two chapters in Part II then provide the analysis of the Europeanization and its policy impacts during the pandemic Covid-19 and on Turkey. "Rethinking Health Law and Politics in Turkey: A Dynamic Perspective from the Implementation of the EU Acquis" is written by Azer Sumbas. Sumbas considers Europeanization in the context of applying the Acquis in the Member States and candidate states focusing particularly on Turkey. By doing this, she intends to provide an alternative discussion on health law and politics in Turkey via focusing on how Turkey fulfils its responsibilities by underlining the European Commission Reports, EU Health Policy papers, Turkey's Health Transformation Programme, and National Action Plan. In the second chapter, entitled "Europeanization of Health Policies after Covid-19: Politicization, Governance and Coordination", Sezgin Mercan focuses on the impact of Covid-19 pandemic on the EU and Turkey-EU relations by referring to Europeanization, governance, politicization and coordination. Mercan states that Covid-19 caused a necessity for burden-sharing at the EU level which triggered Europeanization and politicization effect as well as disagreements on a subject result in producing high politicization. In this framework, he concludes that high politicization of health to Covid-19 has increased EU level cooperation and Europeanization of it.

Part III introduces three chapters under the theme of "Gender in Health Policies and Law" which aim to provide an analysis of more concrete issues in Turkish political and legal contexts. This part begins with the chapter of Ahu Sumbas, entitled "Veiled Impact of Gender Equality Policies on Gender Disparities in Self-Rated Health: The Case of Turkey". In this research paper, Sumbas discusses the role of gender equality policies on the elimination of gender disparities in self-rated health in Turkey based on the analysis of the 2019 Turkey Health Interview Survey. She concludes that the adoption of a gender equality approach in formulating family and care policies as well as family and work reconciliation policies at the labour market are critical to improve women's SRH status in Turkey. The second chapter of this part is "Fiscal Justice for Women: Suggestions for Turkey on Menstrual Hygiene Products Taxation" written by Ezgi Sevinçhan. Sevinçhan introduces the popular issue of pink taxes in the field of taxation law. Within this context, she particularly focuses on the implementation of menstrual hygiene products taxation to eliminate gender discrimination in individual earnings and taxation while she is questioning gender blind taxation policies of states including Turkey. The last chapter of Part III belongs to Ayça Zorluoğlu Yılmaz, entitled "Surrogate Motherhood in Turkey". Zorluoğlu Yılmaz presents one of the controversial topics on reproductive rights and technologies from a legal perspective. While she is explaining the issue of surrogacy, she also addresses the advantages and disadvantages of surrogacy for couples and governments by introducing different cases from different countries and legal systems. Benefiting from such framework, she explains the regulation of surrogate motherhood in Turkey and offers the adoption of altruistic or gestational surrogacy as a reproductive technique in the Turkish legal system to give a chance for infertile couples to have a baby.

Three chapters in Part IV discuss the issue of vaccination from legal and public policy perspectives. The leading chapter, entitled "To Be Vaccinated or Not? An Assessment on the Vaccination Attitude Profile in Turkey" is written by Nazmiye Tekdemir & Pelin Varol İyidoğan. Tekdemir & Varol İyidoğan conduct a survey with 838 people including different stakeholders in 12 NUTS regions to reflect different characteristics and dynamics. According to the findings from Independent Groups T-test and one-way analysis of variance (ANOVA) procedure, they conclude that age and education level have a significant effect on attitude to vaccination in the study group. On the other hand, they find no evidence supporting a significant gender effect. In the following chapter, entitled "Compulsory Vaccination Application in Turkish Legal System", Yiğit İltaş discusses the relationship between preventive health services and vaccination. İltaş explains compulsory vaccination practices and the perspective of Turkish Legal System. Last chapter of the Part IV is "Informed Consent in Pandemic Processes Within the Scope of the Crime of Experimentation and Trial on Human Being" which is authored by Ezgi Aygün Eşitli. While Eşitli is explaining the terms of informed consent, criminal experimentation, and trial, she tries to approach the issue of the informed consent in pandemic process in order to provide an analysis of problemed areas in the time of pandemic. In this context, she scrunitizes the possibilities of using off-label drugs on the patient without a duly received consent during pandemic. She also discusses whether the public health precedes the patient's consent according to General Public Health Law.

Part V consists of four chapters which aim to exhibit the reflections of Covid-19 in the fields of law and economics. The first chapter of the part is "The Effect of Health Programs and Expenditures on Credit Rating under Pandemic Era" which belongs to Eda Yeşil Balıkçıoğlu & H. Hakan Yılmaz. They aim to empirically examine the impact of health expenditures together with other determinants on credit scores within a comparative framework for Covid-19 process. According to the findings from ordered probit model, Yeşil Balıkçıoğlu & Yılmaz conclude that public health expenditure has a significant effect on the credit ratings while the impact of Covid-19 period has not appeared yet. They also provide a brief evaluation on Turkey's public health expenditures and debts due to the pandemic process. Çetin Arslan & Eylül Erdem's study, that is "The Evaluation of the Measures Taken Within the Scope of the Covid-19 Pandemic in Turkey in terms of Misdemeanor and Ciriminal Law", is the second chapter of this part. Arslan & Erdem examine the legal framework of the measures taken within the scope of combating the COVID-19 epidemic in Turkish criminal law. They evaluate the consequences of not complying with the measures taken in combating the Covid-19 epidemic in terms of criminal law and misdemeanor law provisions since they consider this field of study as a sub-discipline of criminal law. The third chapter in Part V, entitled "A Comparatie Analysis of Taxation Practices during the Covid-19 Pandemic in Turkey and Selected OECD Countries" is written by Ayşe Nil Tosun, Oytun Canyaş & Necati Nurcalı. Their study comparatively investigates how taxation policies were used in Turkey and selected OECD countries to overcome the COVID-19 pandemic with minimum damage. They point out that Turkey has provided important conveniences to taxpayers regarding tax policies during the pandemic process. On the other hand, they identify the deficiencies in Turkey's tax dimensional struggle in the Covid -19 pandemic, that are the avoidance of practices requiring cash flow towards taxpayers and its tendency toward practices that may disrupt the principle of tax equality. Fatma Didem Sevgili Gencay scrunitizes the physicians' working conditions before and during the pandemic regarding the the continuity principle of public service in the chapter of "Continuity Principle of Public Service and the Working Conditions of Physicians in Turkey (before and during pandemic)". Sevgili Gencay demostrates that healthcare workers have worked in difficult and dangerous conditions in Covid-19 pandemic illegally imposed by the administration (such as the restrictions on leave, resigning, and retirement rights of healthcare workers) who showed a blatant disregard of their rights. In this sense, she points out that the administration should be held liable for not taking the necessary precautions to preserve and protect the health of these employees.

Part VI intents to portray current thematic discussions in health studies addressing the issues of telemedicine, health tourism and ethicolegal aspects of the right to health. In this context, the first chapter, entitled "Ethicolegal Aspects of the Right to Health and Bioethics" is presented by Kıvılcım Ceren Büken & Nüket Örnek Büken. As Büken & Örnek Büken introduce the right to health and bioethics, they aim at underlying how the right to health, medical ethics and bioethics are already intertwined and have a lot to gain from the influence of one another. Another thematic discussion of Part VI belongs to Gamze Yorgancıoğlu Tarcan which is titled as "Electronic Knowledge Technologies: Using of Telemedicine and Mobile Health in Turkey". Yorgancıoğlu Tarcan asserts the importance of Telemedicine and Mobile Health, which forms the basis for knowledge sharing between health care providers and health care recipients. Tarcan Yorgancıoğlu underlines the importance of collaboration between hospital and health software supplier regarding the national electronic knowledge systems. Sibel Özcan presents a conceptual framework on health tourism and free zones by embodying Turkish experience in the third chapter of this part, namely "Health Tourism and Free Healthcare Zones". In the final part of her study, Özcan develops notable evaluation and suggestions. She asserts that any support provided in order to improve the technological and scientific infrastructure, contribute to mitigating the burden of pandemic on countries. As one of this attempts, establishment of healthcare free zones as well as the health valley and healthcare technology development zones provide an advantage in terms of the competition in the health tourism area.

The last part of the book, Part VII, consists of three chapters which seek to present "Noticeable Issues in Health Law". In this context, Burcu G. Özcan Büyüktanır's chapter, titled "Clinical Drug Trials in Children", introduces clinical drug procedure. In this paper, Özcan Büyüktanır states that best interests of children are the main requirement of the clinical trials in children. Following her contribution, Dila Okyar & Orhan Emre Konuralp discuss the consumer status of the patient from the legal perspective in the second chapter, entitled "The Critical Analysis of the Consumer Status of Patients under Turkish Law". The study aims to bring a critical legal perspective to the appropriateness of the consumer status of the patients regarding the cases on the medical malpractice at the consumer disputes. The last chapter of the part and the book is "Medical Malpractice in Comparative Law: A Swot Analysis" authored by Neval Yılmaz, Selin Özden Merhacı & Deniz Odabaş. Their work aims to discuss the ideal system of medical malpractice for Turkey by using a SWOT analysis based on the comparision of different systems. By the help of this analysis, they conclude that health courts should be established in the evaluation of malpractice claims and the judges serving in these courts undergo a special training to prevent contradictory decisions and long durations of the trials.

As the editors of this book, we are very pleased and honoured to host these fellow academics and present their research in this collection. We also greatly appreciate the voluntary contribution that each reviewer gives to the chapters. Last, we are grateful to the members of Hacettepe University Research Center of Health Law who contribute to the work since the book is the second publication of the book series of the Hacettepe University Research Center of Health Law.

Part I Economic and Public Policy Perspective in the Health Sector

Taner Turan

A Re-examination of Health Expenditure-Income Nexus in OECD Countries: With a Brief Evaluation for Turkey

Introduction

Although the relationship between the income and health expenditures has drawn attention for a long time, it has risen to prominence recently. On the one hand, a higher income allows economic agents to allocate and consume more resources for the health (Preston, 1975; Pritchett & Summers, 1996). For example, the health care expenditures are greater in high-income countries than in low- and middle-income countries in not only levels but also as a share of GDP. As of 2016, the current health expenditures are 12.6 % of GDP in high and 5.4 % of GDP in middle- and low-income countries (WDI, 2019). This is also true among OECD countries. The share of health expenditures in GDP in many high-income OECD countries is around 10 % while it is about 5–6 % in some lower income OECD countries (OECD, 2019).

On the other hand, after the recognition of the importance of human capital, many studies suggest that health expenditures, regarded as an input to health capital, would also affect the income (Grossman, 1972; Gyimah-Brempong & Wilson, 2004). Additionally, it is possible to argue that health expenditures mainly impact the income through health status. This implies that both direct and indirect channels, including productivity, capital stock, labour supply, saving and investment decisions, and also demographic changes, would be important in explaining the possible income effects of health expenditures (see, among others, Fogel, 1994; Bloom & Canning, 2000; Bhargava et al., 2001; Lorentzen et al., 2008).

It seems that a bilateral relationship between the health expenditures and income is possible on purely theoretical grounds. However, the empirical literature does not uniformly point to a robust relationship. There is no doubt that both income and health are multidimensional concepts, suggesting that they could be independently determined from each other. It is possible to have a higher growth rate or income level without an increase in health indicators or vice versa (Cutler et al., 2006; Pritchett & Summers, 1996).

Why does this relationship matter? Why should we care about it? Revealing this relationship has some important policy implications. For example, despite having a better health itself is a vital goal for nations, if a better health causes a higher income level, then it is easier to get political and public support to increase the health expenditures. On the other hand, if an increase in the health expenditures leads to a negative effect on the income, then a more complex situation arises. To boost the income, it would be necessary to cut the health expenditures or question its efficiency from an economic point of view. However, cutting health expenditures would have some undesired effects from a non-economic perspective.

Examining the relationship between the health expenditures and income in OECD countries, this study aims to contribute to the existing literature in some important respects. First, we deal with cross-sectional dependence, a crucial but often neglected issue in the literature. Second, to obtain more robust results, we employ relatively new econometric methods including Westerlund (2007) panel cointegration and Dumitrescu & Hurlin (2012) panel causality tests. Third, since the theory makes it clear that there would be a bilateral relationship between the income and health expenditures, we model them both as dependent and independent variables when investigating the cointegration and causality rather than imposing a unidirectional form, which might render some previous results doubtful or invalid. Our empirical findings clearly lend a strong evidence for the argument that income would have a significant impact on health expenditures rather than vice versa. However, we don't detect a Granger causality between our variables in the short run.

We review the literature in the Section 1, give an overview of the health expenditures and income in sample countries in the Section 2, explain data and models in the Section 3, present and discuss the empirical results in Section 4, and finally conclude in Section 5.

I. Literature Review

Although the literature posits a complex and somewhat mysterious relationship between the health and income, Weil (2015) succinctly explains this relationship in a simple but intuitive way by distinguishing between "health view" and "income view". "Health view" suggests that countries have different levels of income due to differences in health environments. More precisely, better health environments lead to a higher per capita income, if all other things are equal. On the other hand, "income view" points to the differences arising from factors which are unrelated to health. At a given health level, one country would have a higher level of per capita income than another one, because of a higher technology or capital accumulation. Since these two alternative or competing views would be valid on theoretical perspectives, an increasing number of studies empirically trying to determine which view is more consistent with the data or reality.

When countries or people get richer, they could and do allocate more resources for health care services. Many studies report that income is a robust determinant of the health spending (Hitiris & Posnett, 1992; Baltagi & Moscone, 2010; Kumar, 2013). Moreover, some studies aim to estimate the income elasticity of health care expenditures and shed light on the issue whether the health care is a luxury or necessity. On the other hand, some researchers indicate that other developments, such as technological inventions in medical sector and their relatively fast and low-cost transfer around the world, are more significant than income in explaining the convergence in observed health indicators (Becker et al., 2005; Cutler et al., 2006; Aghion et al., 2011).

As for the income or growth effects of health, the Solow model predicts that changes in population growth or saving rates have a level but not a permanent growth effect in terms of per capita income. In other words, a rise (decline) in saving (population growth) rates leads to a temporary and positive effect on the economic growth during the transition period. Since the health is closely related to changes in population growth or saving rates, it would make a substantial contribution to the per capita income level in the Solow model. More importantly, original Solow model includes physical but not human capital in explaining the economic growth. Although the recognition of human capital formation, including health, for economic growth is not new (Schultz, 1961; Mushkin, 1962), its explicit inclusion to the growth models is relatively and surprisingly late. Moreover, 1980s witnessed the emergence of influential endogenous growth theories, in which human capital plays a decisive role, pioneered by Romer (1986) and Lucas (1988). Now it is largely accepted that the health status is among the most robust determinants of economic growth (Sala-i Martin et al., 2004).

What are the transmission mechanisms of the health expenditures on income? In principle, as health expenditures can be viewed as investments or inputs to the stock of health capital (Grossman, 1972; Gyimah-Brempong & Wilson, 2004; Atilgan et al., 2017), the effects of health expenditures on the income would mainly operate through this channel. Moreover, there is a close association between health expenditures and different indicators for health status, including life expectancy, mortality, and survival rates (OECD, 2019). Healthy people would be both physically and mentally more productive and supply of more labour (Fogel, 1994; Cole & Neumayer, 2006; Suhrcke & Urban, 2010), tend to better adopt and invent new technologies (Aghion et al., 2011), acquire and develop human capital in the form of education or training (Swift, 2011; Weil, 2014), save and invest more (Zhang & Zhang, 2005; Lorentzen et al., 2008).

On the other hand, it is impossible to argue that the health necessarily exerts a positive effect on the income (van Zon & Muysken, 2001; Acemoglu & Johnson, 2007; Swift, 2011; Bloom et al., 2018). When people live longer, the share of non-working population could increase, implying a growth retarding change in the age structure. Additionally, if health improvements mostly benefit the older people or inactive population, then there is no reason to expect for a positive growth effect via direct labour productivity or other incentive effects. Furthermore, to finance the needs and entitlements of an ageing population, governments could raise the tax rates and also change the size and mix of public expenditures. Finally, if the health sector is more inefficient or creating fewer positive spillover or externality effects than competing sectors then another harmful effect on income is possible (van Zon & Muysken, 2001).

More related to our study, a large literature empirically investigates the relationship between the health expenditures and income or growth in OECD countries. Table 1 gives a summary of selected studies. It seems that there is some evidence for different views on the income-health expenditures nexus. Some studies report a positive health expenditure (income) effect of income (health expenditures), while others point to a bidirectional relationship.

II. An Overview of Health Expenditures and Income in Sample OECD Countries

Per capita health expenditures, the sum of per capita government and household health expenditures, in our sample OECD countries have increased more than twice from 1990 to 2018. There is a considerable variation in countries, nonetheless. For example, the total health expenditures in South Korea has increased more than five times from 1990 to 2018 while in Italy the increase is well below two times. During this period, although both the government and household health expenditures per capita follow an increasing path, former rises more. This might be explained by the change in health care policies and scope of coverage of government health services. Almost three quarters of health expenditures are financed by government schemes or compulsory insurance (OECD, 2019). Among our sample countries, the per capita health expenditure is the highest in the US and lowest in Turkey in both 1990 and 2018.

Tab. 1: A summary of the empirical studies on the relationship between the health expenditures and income in OECD countries

Study	Period	Methodology	Main Findings
Hansen and King (1996)	1960–1987	Engle-Granger test	No cointegration for most countries.
Rivera and Currais (1999)	1960–1990	OLS and IV	Although health has a positive impact on the income, a relationship exists in both directions.
Devlin and Hansen (2001)	1960–1987	Granger causality test	In some countries, health care expenditures Granger cause GDP while in some others the opposite occurs.
Heshmati (2001)	1970–1992	Panel data models	Health care expenditure has a positive effect on the growth rate. Health care expenditures cause GDP but GDP does not cause HCE.
Rivera and Currais (2003)	1960–2000	OLS and IV	Health has a positive impact on income growth.
Gyimah-Brempong and Wilson (2004)	1961–1995	Panel data methods (Dynamic GMM)	Stock of and investment in human capital positively affect the growth rate
Sen (2005)	1990–1998	OLS, GLS and IV	Income has a significant and positive effect on health care expenditures
Dreger and Reimers (2005)	1975–2001	Panel cointegration	Income exerts an impact on health care expenditures

(continued on next page)

Tab. 1: Continued

Study	Period	Methodology	Main Findings
Chakroun (2009)	1975–2003	Panel smooth transition model	Income affects health care expenditures.
Beraldo et al. (2009)	1971–1998	Panel methods (REM, LSDV, GMM)	Health expenditure positively impacts the growth rate. Public health expenditures affect the growth rate more strongly than private expenditures.
Baltagi and Moscone (2010)	1971–2004	Panel data methods	Income has a significant and positive effect on health care expenditures.
Pradhan (2010)	1961–2007	Panel cointegration and causality	Cointegration and bidirectional causality are found.
Mehrara et al. (2010)	1993–2007	Panel Smooth Transition Regression	Income affects the health care expenditures
Yerdelen Tatoğlu (2011)	1975–2005	Panel error correction model	Health care expenditures positively influence the growth.
Amiri and Ventolou (2012)	1975–2003	Granger causality (Toda-Yamamoto approach)	Bidirectional causality exists.
Kumar (2013)	1960–2007	System GMM and Panel causality	Bi-directional relationship exists between GDP and health spending.
Amiri and Linden (2016)	1970–2012	Granger causality	Bilateral relationship is common in sample countries.

Ye and Zang (2018)	1971–2015	Linear and Non-linear Granger causality tests	Unidirectional and bidirectional causality found for some countries while no causality for some others.
Wang et al. (2019)	1975–2017	Bootsrap ARDL and Granger causality	Bi-directional and unidirectional relationship exist.

Source: Compiled by the author.

There is a reduction in the growth rate of health expenditures during and aftermath the last global financial crisis. However, this reduction did not last long. Recently, an increase in the growth rate of health expenditures is observed. Health expenditures grew at 1 (2.4) % from 2008 (2013) to 2013 (2018) in OECD countries (OECD, 2019). We should note that growth in health expenditures outpaced the growth of GDP per capita in 1990s and 2000s. Therefore, the health expenditure in relation to GDP significantly increased in these decades. However, the share of health expenditures in GDP has been stable since 2013. The health expenditures as a percent of GDP are 8.8 in OECD countries, highest in the US with 17 and lowest in Turkey with 4.2. There is a remarkable increase in the share of health expenditures in GDP in South Korea after the second half of 2000s, while a considerable reduction experienced in some countries including Hungary and Ireland after 2010 (OECD, 2019). The share of health expenditures does not show a significant variation in many OECD countries, among others Austria, Canada, Belgium, Germany and France, in recent years.

Average GDP per capita increased by almost 70 % in our sample countries during the period examined. Except for the last global crisis period, we see a stable increase in GDP per capita with some variation across countries. For example, the last financial crisis hit some countries hard with a long-lasting effect, such as Greece, Ireland, and Spain. On the other hand, some countries, including the US, South Korea and Turkey, escaped relatively fast. Additionally, especially after 2014 the growth rate seems to gain momentum again in many countries. As of 2018, Norway (Turkey) has the highest (lowest) per capita GDP in our sample countries. Moreover, the growth rates in some countries, such as Turkey and South Korea, lend some evidence for the convergence hypothesis.

III. Data and Empirical Methods

This study aims to examine the relationship between the per capita health expenditure and GDP for 18 OECD countries[1] over the period 1990–2018. We use the logs of GDP per capita and health expenditure (the sum of government and household health expenditures) per capita in constant US $ (PPPs), obtained from OECD health statistics (2019). Since there might be a two-way relationship we use both variables as dependent and independent. In other words, we

---

1   The sample OECD countires, which are selected with regard to data availability are Australia, Canada, Czech Republic, Denmark, Finland, France, Germany, Hungary, Iceland, Ireland, Italy, Korea, New Zealand, Norway, Poland, Turkey, the UK and the US.

think that it is possible that the income and health expenditure would affect each other. Our empirical methods include the cross-sectional dependence, unit root, cointegration and causality tests. We should firs test the presence of cross-sectional dependence as it is important to decide which unit root, cointegration and causality tests would be more appropriate. To examine the presence of cross-sectional dependency we employ Pesaran (2004), which provides more appropriate testing framework when which time dimension (T) is large compared to cross-sectional dimension (N) as in our panel. To examine the stationarity properties of the series we employ the cross-sectionally augmented Im-Pesaran-Shin (CIPS) panel unit root test of Pesaran (2007). We use a relatively new cointegration test developed by Westerlund (2007), which accommodates the dependence of cross-sectional units and does not impose any common factor restriction. Westerlund (2007) suggests four different statistics to test panel cointegration. Two of those are the panel tests, namely P_t and P_a which have the alternative hypothesis that the whole panel is cointegrated. On the other hand, the other two tests are group-mean tests, denoted by G_t and G_a which have the alternative hypothesis that cointegration exists for at least one cross-section unit. Moreover, the methodology gives *p-values* which are robust against cross-sectional dependency by bootstrapping.

Finally, we apply Granger-causality test of Dumitrescu & Hurlin (2012) which is proposed for heterogeneous panels and preferably used in the presence of cross-sectional dependence to evaluate short-run dynamics. To implement this test, we take the first difference of the series to eliminate the unit root characteristic.[2] Dumitrescu & Hurlin (2012) assume a potential presence of Granger-causality for a number of individuals rather than all. Thus, they propose a procedure, which tests the null of no homogeneous Granger-causality against the existence of causality for at least one cross-sectional unit. This approach is based on the cross-sectional average of the individual Wald-statistics.

IV. Empirical Results and Discussion

Based on the results in Tab. 2, we reject the null of no cross-sectional dependence both for series and panels under fixed effect specification.

---

2   As emphasized by Liddle and Messinis (2013); while the approach of Dumitrescu & Hurlin does not explicitly address cross-sectional dependence, it is important to note that, after first differencing the variables, either cross-sectional independence cannot be rejected or any remaining cross-sectional correlation has been highly mitigated.

Tab. 2: Test of cross-sectional dependence

Test of Cross-Sectional Dependence for the Series		
	Pesaran CD_{LM}	p-value
Income	61.565	0.00
Total	62.453	0.00
Test of Cross-Sectional Dependence for the Panel Models		
Dep. Var: Income	8.622	0.00
Dep. Var. Health exp.	14.886	0.00

Due the the existence of cross-sectional depence we employ the cross-sectionally augmented Im-Pesaran-Shin (CIPS) panel unit root test of Pesaran (2007) to examine the stationarity properties of the series. The CIPS test statistics, that are the sample averages of the individual cross-sectionally augmented Dickey-Fuller (CADF) statistics for the panel are given in Tab. 3. The CIPS panel unit root test results, which fail to reject the null of unit root indicate that our series are non-stationary.

Tab. 3: Panel unit root tests

Series	Statistics	*p*-value
Income	2.4673	0.9932
Health expenditure	2.5041	0.9939

Note: The results are for no time trend specification.

The results of panel cointegration tests are presented in Tab. 4. We obtain evidence of long-run relationship with regard to group-mean or panel tests with the income variable is the regressor to explain health expenditures since we cannot reject the null of no cointegration. The robust p-values which consider cross-sectional dependency provide same results. On the other hand, we fail to find any evidence for a cointegrating relationship between our variables when we use the income as the dependent variable.

Tab. 4: Cointegration test results

	Value	p-value	p^b-value
Dep: Var: Income	1.290	1.00	1.00
Gt	0.950	1.00	1.00
Gp	2.614	1.00	0.800
Pt	0.466	0.986	0.730
Pa			
Dep. Var: Health exp.	-1.431	0.032	0.090
Gt	-2.865	0.809	0.410
Gp	-6.031	0.001	0.050
Pt	-2.443	0.019	0.050
Pa			

Notes: Optimal lag/lead length determined by Akaike Information Criterion with a maximum lag/lead length of 3. Width of Bartlett-kernel window set to 3. Number of bootstraps to obtain bootstrapped p-values (p^b-value) which are robust against cross-sectional dependencies set to 100.

Dumitrescu & Hurlin (2012) causality test results reported in Tab. 5 don't provide any evidence for a causal relationship between the income and health expenditure in the short term. In other words, we fail to reject the null hypothesis of no causality between our variables.

Tab. 5: Causality test results

	Statistics	p-value	% 95 critical values
Health exp.⇨ Income	−1.1538 (1)	0.3520	2.91
Income ⇨Health exp.	6.7423 (7)	0.1780	10.35

Notes: p-values are computed by using 500 bootstrap replications. The optimal lag lengths are determined with regard to AIC criterion and reported in the parantheses. The p-values are associated with $\bar{Z}$ test statistics.

V. A Brief Evaluation of Health Expenditures and Income in Turkey

Like many other OECD member countries there is a clear increase in both per capita income and health expenditures in Turkey over time. It seems that per capita health expenditures have a stronger upward trend especially from 1995 to 2007. During this period, per capita health expenditures almost tripled.

However, note that the health expenditures do not rise much from 2008 to 2012. Then, we observe another sharp increase after 2013.

In Turkey per capita income rises in 1990s with a stagnation during the late 1990s. More precisely there is no remarkable change in per capita income from 1997 to 2000 while per capita health expenditures continue to increase. Turkish economy experiences a higher average growth rate in 2000s compared to the 1990s. On the other hand, during the last 3 years, namely 2017, 2018 and 2019, there is no significant rise in per capita income while the per capita health expenditure is on the rise. It seems that per capita income is affected by internal and international economic crises during the period examined. As a result, we observe a reduction in per capita income in 1994, 2001 and 2009. Somewhat interestingly, we don't see a decline in per capita health expenditure during the 2001 crisis. Finally, during the period examined the health expenditures have a significantly higher average growth rate than the per capita income. More concretely, per capita health expenditure (income) is about four (two) times more in 2019 than what it was in 1990. Our analysis suggests that there might be a close even casual relationship between these two variables in Turkey. However, we need a more robust econometric analysis to test and establish the existence of a causal relationship.[3]

Conclusion

This study empirically examines the relationship between the health expenditures and income in 18 OECD countries over the period 1990–2018 employing Westerlund (2007) cointegration and Dumitrescu & Hurlin (2012) causality tests. Our empirical results indicate that when we model the per capita income as the dependent and health expenditure as a regressor, we fail find a cointegrating relationship. In other words, there is no evidence for the income effect of health expenditures. However, when the health expenditure is used as the dependent and the income as the independent variable, a cointegration is found. However, there is no evidence for a causal relationship in the short term.

We should note some important points. First, since there is a strong evidence for the existence of cross-sectional dependence, it is necessary to deal with this

---

3   For this purpose, we employ Toda-Yamamoto Granger non-causality test using Turkish data from 1975 to 2019 and find that a unidirectional causal relationship going from the per capita health expenditure to per capita income, consistent with the results reported in Turan (2020). We don't report these causality tests because of space considerations, they are available from the author.

issue to obtain robust and reliable econometric results. Second, our results cast doubts on some previous studies which ignore or neglect the possibility that the income rather than health expenditures should be the explanatory or exogenous variable, implying a crucial misspecification in this context. Third, another implication of our findings is that the arguments for allocation of more resources for health expenditures should be based on non-economic reasoning. In other words, our empirical findings make it difficult to justify the argument that an increase in health expenditures leads to an increase in the income or growth rate. Finally, we think that it would be interesting and illuminating to examine the relationship between the health expenditures and health outcomes in detail. As the health expenditures have significantly increased recently it would be more important to focus on the efficiency of health expenditures in improving the health status and indicators. Moreover, considering the impact of other variables such as technology or demographic characteristics on health spending and efficiency would be a worthwhile effort.

References

Acemoglu, D., & Johnson, S. (2007). Disease and development: The effect of life expectancy on economic growth. *Journal of Political Economy*, 115(6), 925–985.

Aghion, P., Howitt, P., & Murtin, F. (2011). The relationship between health and growth: When Lucas meets Nelson-Phelps. *Review of Economics and Institutions*, 2, 1–24.

Amiri, A., & Linden, M. (2016). Income and total expenditure on health in OECD countries: Evidence from panel data and Hsiao's version of Granger non-causality tests. *Economics and Business Letters*, 51, 1–9.

Amiri, A., & Ventelou, B. (2012). Granger causality between total expenditure on health and GDP in OECD: Evidence from the Toda–Yamamoto approach. *Economics Letters*, 116(3), 541–544.

Atılgan, E., Kılıc, D., & Ertugrul, H. M. (2017). The dynamic relationship between health expenditure and economic growth: Is the health led-growth hypothesis valid for Turkey. *The European Journal of Health Economics*, 18, 567–574.

Baltagi, B., & Moscone, F. (2010). Health care expenditure and income in the OECD reconsidered: Evidence from panel data. *Economic Modelling*, 27(4), 804–811.

Becker, G. S., Philipson, T. J., & Soares, R. R. (2005). The quantity and quality of life and the evolution of world inequality. *American Economic Review*, 95, 277–291.

Beraldo, S., Montolio, D., & Turati, G. (2009). Healthy, educated and wealthy: A primer on the impact of public and private welfare expenditures on economic growth. *The Journal of Socio-Economics*, 38, 946–956.

Bhargava, A., Jamison, D. T., Lau, L., & Murray, C. J. (2001). Modeling the effects of health on economic growth. *Journal of Health Economics*, 20(3), 423–440.

Bloom, D. E., & Canning, D. (2000). The health and wealth of nations. *Science*, 287, 1207–1209 (2000).

Bloom, D. E., Kuhn, M., & Prettner, K. (2018). Health and economic growth. *IZA Institute of Labor Economics, Discussion Paper Series No. 11939.*

Cole, M. A., & Neumayer, E. (2006). The impact of poor health on total factor productivity. *The Journal of Development Studies*, 42(6), 918–938.

Chakroun, M. (2009). Health care expenditure and GDP: An international panel smooth transition approach. *MPRA, No. 17493.*

Cutler, D. M, Deaton, A., & Lleras-Muney, A. (2006). The determinants of mortality. NBER Working Paper 11963.

Devlin, N., & Hansen, P. (2001). Health care spending and economic output: Granger causality. *Applied Economics Letters*, 8(8), 561–564. DOI: 10.1080/13504850010017357.

Dreger, C., & Reimers, H. E. (2005). Health care expenditures in OECD countries: A panel unit root and cointegration analysis. *International Journal of Applied Econometrics and Quantitative Studies*, 2(2), 1–21.

Dumitrescu, E. I., & Hurlin, C. (2012). Testing for Granger non-causality in heterogeneous panels. *Economic Modelling*, 29(4), 1450–1460.

Fogel, W. (1994). Economic growth, population theory, and physiology: The bearing of longterm processes on the making of economic policy. *The American Economic Review*, 84(3), 369–395.

Grossman, M. (1972). On the concept of health capital and the demand for health. *The Journal of Political Economy*, 80(2), 223–255.

Gyimah-Brempong, K., & Wilson, M. (2004). Health human capital and economic growth in Sub-Saharan African and OECD countries. *The Quarterly Review of Economics and Finance*, 44, 296–320.

Hansen, P., & King, P. (1996). The determinants of health care expenditure: A cointegration approach. *Journal of Health Economics*, 15(1), 127–137.

Heshmati, A. (2001). On the causality between GDP and health care expenditure in augmented Solow growth model. *SSE/EFI Working Paper Series in Economics and Finance, No. 423, Stockholm School of Economics, The Economic Research Institute (EFI).*

Hitiris, T., & Posnett, J. (1992). The determinants and effects of health expenditure in developed Countries. *Journal of Health Economics*, 11 (2), 173–181.

Kumar, S. (2013). Systems GMM estimates of the health care spending and GDP relationship: A note. *European Journal of Health Economics*, 14, 503–506.

Liddle B., & Messinis G. (2013). Which comes first- urbanization or economic growth? Evidence from heterogeneous panel causality test. *MPRA Papers, No. 53983*.

Lorentzen, P., McMillan, J., & Wacziarg, R. (2008). Death and development. Journal of Economic Growth, 13, 81–124.

Lucas, R. (1988). On the mechanics of economic development. *Journal of Monetary Economics*, 22(1), 3–42.

Mehrara, M., Musai, M., & Amiri, H.(2010). The relationship between health expenditure and GDP in OECD countries using PSTR. *European Journal of Economics, Finance and Administrative Sciences*, 24, 50–58.

Mushkin, S. J. (1962). Health as an investment. *Journal of Political Economy*, 70(5), 129–157.

Pesaran M. H. (2004). General diagnostic tests for cross section dependence in panels. *IZA Discussion Paper Series, No. 1240*.

Pesaran M. H. (2007). A simple panel unit root test in the presence of cross-section dependence. *Journal of Applied Econometrics*, 22, 265–312.

Pradhan, R. P. (2010). The long run relation between health spending and economic growth in 11 OECD countries: Evidence from panel cointegration. *International Journal of Economic Perspectives*, 4(2), 427–438.

Preston, S. (1975). The changing relation between mortality and level of economic development. *Population Studies*, 29(2), 231–248.

Pritchett, L., & Summers L. H. (1996). Wealthier is healthier. *The Journal of Human Resources*, 31(4), 841–868.

Rivera, B., & Currais, L. (1999). Income variation and health expenditure: Evidence for OECD countries. *Review of Development Economics*, 3(3), 258–267.

Rivera, B., & Currais, L. (2003). The effect of health investment on growth: A causality analysis. *International Advances in Economic Research*, 9(4), 312–323.

Romer, P. M. (1986). Increasing returns and long-run growth. *Journal of Political Economy*, 94, 1002–1037.

Sala-I-Martin, X., Doppelhofer, G., & Miller, R. I. (2004). Determinants of long-term growth: A Bayesian Averaging of Classical Estimates (BACE) approach. *American Economic Review*, 94(4), 813–835.

Schultz, T. W. (1961). Investment in human capital. *The American Economic Review*, 51(1), 1–17.

Sen, A. (2005). Is health care a luxury? New evidence from OECD data. *International Journal of Health Care Finance and Economics*, 5, 147–164.

Suhrcke, M., & Urban, D. (2010). Are cardiovascular diseases bad for economic growth? *Health Economics*, 19(12), 1478–1496.

Swift, R. (2011). The relationship between health and GDP in OECD countries in the very long run. *Health Economics*, 20, 306–322.

The Organization for Economic Co-operation and Development (OECD) (2019). Health at a glance 2019: Indicators.

The World Bank (2019). *World Development Indicators*. Washington, DC: World Bank.

Turan, T. (2020). Bounds testing approach to the relationship between health and economic growth in Turkey. *Finance, Politics & Economic Reviews*, 652, 911–112.

van Zon, A., & Muysken, J. (2001). Health and endogenous growth. *Journal of Health Economics*, 20(2), 169–185.

Wang, C-M, H-P, H., Li, F., & Wu, C-F (2019). Bootstrap ARDL on health expenditure, CO2 emissions, and GDP growth relationship for 18 OECD countries. *Frontiers in Public Health*, 7, 324, 1–9.

Weil, D. N. (2014). Health and economic growth. *Handbook of Economic Growth*, Volume 2B, 623–683.

Weil, D. N. (2015). *Economic Growth*. Third Edition, 175–178, Essex, London: Pearson Education Limited:.

Westerlund, J. (2007). Testing for error correction in panel data. *Oxford Bulletin of Economics and Statistics* 69, 709–748.

Ye, L., & Zhang, X. (2018). Nonlinear Granger causality between health care expenditure and economic growth in the OECD and major developing countries. *International Journal of Environmental Research and Public Health*, 15, 1953.

Yerdelen Tatoğlu, F. (2011). The relationships between human capital investment and economic growth: A panel error correction model. *Journal of Economic and Social Research*, 13(1), 75–88.

Zhang, J., & Zhang, J. (2005). The effect of life expectancy on fertility, saving, schooling and economic growth: Theory and evidence. *Scandinavian Journal of Economics*, 107(1), 45–66.

Sinem Yalçın

Health Expenditures and the Fiscal Sustainability of Social Security System: An Investigation for Turkey

Introduction

The concept of human capital, which is the main source of economic growth, is used to express concepts such as knowledge, skills, abilities, health status, social status, and education level of a person or society. According to the theory of human capital, when a person improves his knowledge and skills, his productivity in economic activities naturally increases. Educated and healthy people are needed for developing human capital. Therefore, education alone is not enough for developing human capital; people should also be healthy to be able to get education and engage in economic activity.

Good health, which is an essential element of human capital and one of the basic requirements of increasing social well-being, has also been important for the United Nations (UN). Health is the overall purpose of the third goal "Good Health and Well-Being" of the Sustainable Development Goals adopted by the UN. According to this, states should guarantee the right to health, which is the right to access and use the necessary facilities and conditions to achieve the goal of attaining healthy people and healthy society.

In this scope, financing should be provided to increase the health expenditures required for a healthy society. Health expenditures and the resources needed for their financing are mostly provided by social security institutions in the public sector. This makes the issue of the fiscal sustainability of the social security system important.

This study focuses on the importance of health expenditures, which is one of the keystones of human capital and enables the more effective use of production factors necessary for economic growth and development. Then, it discusses per capita health expenditures in OECD countries and Turkey, comparatively. After that reviews the studies in literature on the fiscal sustainability of social security organizations, which play important roles in the public financing of health expenditures. Finally, it assesses the fiscal sustainability of the Social Security Institution (SSI) in Turkey.

Sinem Yalçın

I. Economic Significance of Health Expenditures and Its Course in the World

A. Economic Significance of Health Expenditures

There is a close and reciprocal relationship of causality between the health level of a society and its level of economic development. Today, developed countries allocate more resources each year to improve the quality of their healthcare services with the aim of investing in manpower (Selim et al., 2014).

There are many studies arguing that, as the society's health level increases, the workforce is used more efficiently and this positively affects the total output and the development of a country. Health has a direct effect on the society's income and welfare, labour productivity, labour engagement, saving and investment rates, demographic factors, and other human capital factors (Ak, 2012). This, in turn, increases the economic development levels of the countries.

Figure 1 below shows the effects of increasing the health level of the society on education, demographic factors, and economic development.

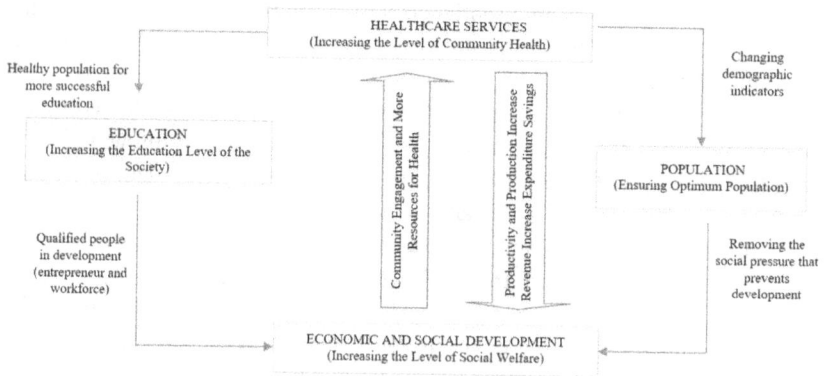

Fig. 1: Effects of Increasing the Health Level of the Society on Education, Demographic Factors, and Economic Development

Source: Mazgit, 1998.

For a country to have a healthy society, its economy should be strong, economic growth should be ensured and sustained, and healthcare services should be provided to meet the needs of the society. (Giray & Çimen, 2018). All expenditures made to provide healthcare services are referred to as "health expenditures". This covers the expenditures made for regaining health in the event of loss of health, as well as preventive health expenditures and investment expenditures in the field of health (Akın, 2007).

The increase in health expenditures positively affects economic growth with a multiplier effect, and thanks to the higher quality of human capital, the determining dynamics of economic growth can start interacting. Ensuring economic growth increases the share allocated to health expenditures and enables more health expenditures (Akıncı & Tuncer, 2016). Increased health expenditures also increase the physical investments in the relevant sector. Increased physical investments accelerate technological development, and scientific and technological advancements ultimately stimulate economic growth (Akar, 2014). Moreover, healthcare services can act as a driver of economic development by playing an important role in reducing problems such as social inequality and poverty.

B. Course of Health Expenditures in the World

Since the 1970s, the effect of health expenditures on the economic growth and development of countries has gradually increased. For this reason, the high rate of health expenditures, and per capita health expenditures in particular, is included in the criteria of social development and welfare (Demir & Tanyıldızı, 2017).

The generally accepted economic indicator used in studying the relationships between health and growth and comparing health expenditures is the per capita health expenditures. Table 1 shows the amount of per capita health expenditure in OECD and non-OECD countries.

Sinem Yalçın

Tab. 1: Per Capita Health Expenditures (US $)

	Countries	2010	2011	2012	2013	2014	2015	2016	2017	2018
OECD	Canada	5.048,3	5.355,7	5.460,0	5.409,8	5.189,8	4.615,6	4.610,9	4.845,6	4.994,9
	Australia	4.945,0	5.861,7	6.025,3	5.814,0	5.607,9	4.860,4	4.971,6	5.308,8	5.425,3
	France	4.598,3	4.939,3	4.651,1	4.901,9	4.998,7	4.208,4	4.268,2	4.424,5	4.690,1
	Germany	4.611,8	5.036,5	4.762,8	5.096,8	5.304,3	4.622,2	4.742,0	5.052,7	5.472,2
	Hungary	983,1	1.063,4	961,1	990,6	1.006,2	870,5	914,2	981,0	1.081,8
	Japan	4.060,5	5.087,4	5.212,2	4.336,1	4.099,3	3.733,4	4.174,4	4.121,0	4.266,6
	Korea	1.366,4	1.512,5	1.566,1	1.701,2	1.898,9	1.918,7	2.034,4	2.258,7	2.542,8
	Poland	809,2	866,1	815,1	878,1	911,3	804,0	813,5	909,6	P978,7
	Spain	2.789,5	2.909,1	2.591,0	2.629,6	2.679,8	2.349,2	2.376,7	2.522,6	2.736,3
	Turkey	**539,3**	**531,4**	**524,3**	**551,4**	**525,8**	**453,1**	**466,8**	**442,6**	**389,9**
	United Kingdom	3.955,5	4.208,4	4.282,0	4.350,3	4.740,9	4.472,5	4.066,1	3.978,6	4.315,4
	United States	7.930,2	8.130,8	8.399,2	8.599,5	9.023,6	9.491,1	9.877,9	10.209,6	10.623,8
Non-OECD	Greece	2.564,4	2.338,9	1.948,2	1.813,9	1.705,1	1.452,1	1.488,2	1.505,9	1.566,9
	Indonesia	92,5	107,7	107,2	107,3	108,8	99,7	109,9	110,0	111,7
	New Zealand	3.216,2	3.625,8	3.806,0	3.954,7	4.143,8	3.582,3	3.746,5	3.940,4	4.037,5

Source: World Health Organization (Downloaded on 19.04.2021)

Table 1 indicates that per capita health expenditures among OECD countries are over 4500 USD in Canada, Australia, France, and Germany, whereas it is below 1000 USD in Turkey and Poland. Moreover, per capita health expenditures in Turkey increased between 2010 and 2013 but decreased between 2014 and 2018. Along with this decrease, the country with the lowest per capita health expenditures among OECD countries is Turkey with 390 USD in 2018.

Table 2 shows the shares allocated to health from the national revenues of countries.

Tab. 2: Ratio of Total Health Expenditure to Gross Domestic Product (%)

OECD	Countries	2010	2011	2012	2013	2014	2015	2016	2017	2018	2019
	Canada	10,7	10,3	10,4	10,3	10,3	10,7	11	10,8	10,8	10,8
	Australia	8,4	8,5	8,7	8,8	9	9,3	9,2	9,2	9,3	9,3
	France	11,2	11,2	11,3	11,4	11,6	11,5	11,5	11,4	11,3	11,2
	Germany	11,1	10,8	10,8	11	11	11,2	11,2	11,4	11,5	11,7
	Hungary	7,5	7,5	7,4	7,2	7,1	6,9	7	6,8	6,7	6,4
	Japan	9,2	10,6	10,8	10,8	10,8	10,9	10,8	10,8	11	11,1
	Korea	5,9	6,0	6,1	6,2	6,5	6,7	6,9	7,1	7,6	8,0
	Poland	6,4	6,2	6,2	6,4	6,2	6,4	6,5	6,6	6,3	6,2
	Spain	9,1	9,2	9,2	9,1	9,1	9,1	9,0	8,9	9,0	9,0
	Turkey	5,1	4,7	4,5	4,4	4,3	4,1	4,3	4,2	4,2	4,4
	United Kingdom	10,0	10,0	10,1	10,0	10,0	9,9	9,9	9,8	10,0	10,3
	United States	16,3	16,3	16,3	16,2	16,4	16,7	17,0	17,0	16,9	17,0
Non-OECD	Brazil	7,9	7,8	7,7	8,0	8,4	8,9	9,2	9,4	..	..
	Russia	5,0	4,8	4,9	5,1	5,3	5,3	5,3	5,4	5,3	..
	India	3,0	3,0	2,9	3,0	3,1	3,0	3,1	3,0	..	..

Source: OECD Statistics, 2020 (downloaded on 19.04.2021)

According to this table, the country that allocates the least share from GDP to health expenditures among OECD countries is Turkey.

In general, healthcare services are provided by public and private sector institutions. The next section focuses on the financing sources of health expenditures in Turkey.

II. Financing of Health Expenditures in Turkey

Numerous international documents, in particular the UN Universal Declaration of Human Rights, acknowledge that social security is one of the basic and universal human rights and that it must be fulfilled by states (Directorate of Presidential Strategy and Budget, 2018).

Although healthcare services primarily provide individual benefits, their social benefit is also an undeniable public service. At this point, the functioning and efficiency of the health systems of countries are very important for preventing and fighting against diseases to protect the people living in that country (Kekeç et al., 2018).

In Turkey, health expenditures are mainly financed by the public and private sectors. Table 3 shows the financing rates of health expenditures by public and private sectors separately:

Tab. 3: Financing of Health Expenditures in Turkey (2018–2019)

	2018		2019	
	Total amount (million TL)	Pay (%)	Total amount (million TL)	Pay (%)
Total Health Expenditure	165.234	100,0	201.131	100
General Government	**128.021**	**77,5**	**156.819**	**78**
-Central Government	40.461	24,5	51.492	25,6
Local Government	1.439	0,9	1.373	0,7
-Social Security Institution	86.121	52,1	103.954	51,7
Private Sector	**37.213**	**22,5**	**44.212**	**22**
-Households	28.655	17,3	33.626	16,7
-Insurance Institutions	4.625	2,8	5.801	2,9
-Other	3.933	2,4	4.785	2,4

Source: Turkish Statistical Institute, Health Expenditure Statistics, 2019. (Downloaded on 20.04.2021.)

Table 3 indicates that the majority of Turkey's total health expenditure is made by the public sector. In 2019, 78 % of the total health expenditure was financed by the state and 22 % by the private sector. 51.7 % of the health expenditures financed by the state were met by the SSI. Therefore, it is very important to ensure the actuarial balance of the SSI.

The next section looks into studies in literature on the financial difficulties faced by the social security system.

III. Literature Review

The financial burden of social security institutions has increased especially in European countries due to the increase in health expenditures and pensions as a result of the ageing of the society. This has made the issue of fiscal sustainability of social security institutions vital, and several studies have been made on the need for reform in social security systems.

The study by Blanco-Encomienda & Ruiz-Garcia (2017) explains that the social security system in Spain is experiencing financial difficulties with the ageing of the society and underlines the need for reform in the social security system.

The report titled *"Sustainability of Social Security System"* prepared by the Directorate of Presidential Strategy and Budget (2018) states that the fiscal sustainability of the social security system in Turkey should be analysed continuously. The report states that interventions, which disrupt the actuarial balances on the public social security system, may place the system in a financial impasse, and at this point, it draws attention to the importance of increasing premium collections.

The report titled "*10 Global Challenges for Social Security*" prepared by the International Social Security Association (2019) mentions the importance of the public in financing the increasing health expenditures especially in the fight against epidemics with the increase of globalization and mobility. In this context, the report emphasizes the importance of having sufficient technical and financial capacity for the social security systems of countries.

The next section evaluates the fiscal sustainability of the social security system, which has an extremely important share in the financing of health expenditures in Turkey.

IV. Assessment of the Fiscal Sustainability of Social Security System in Turkey

Social security can be defined as a financial program that includes the rules and practices providing assurance to all individuals in the society against social risks and ultimately aims to eliminate future concerns in the society (Blanco-Encomienda & Ruiz-Garcia, 2017).

According to the health system in Turkey, hospital expenditures, other medical health expenditures, and pension payments are financed by the social security system. Therefore, regular collection of social security premiums, which have a significant share in financing health expenditures, and ensuring the fiscal sustainability of the social security system are among the key policy priorities of all countries.

In our country, the task of managing the social security system belongs to the SSI. The main purpose of the SSI is to be able to cover the pension and health payments with premium revenue. In this respect, the income-expense balance of the SSI is important.

Tab. 4: SSI's Income-Expense Balance between 2008–2020 (Million TL)

Years	Premium Revenues	State Contribution	Other Revenues	Total Revenues	Expenditures	Deficit	Deficit Financing	Compensation Rate (%)
2008	54.546	1.719	10.993	67.258	93.159	-25.901	25.689	72,2
2009	54.579	10.879	12.614	78.072	106.775	-28.703	29.368	73,1
2010	66.913	15.170	13.190	95.273	121.997	-26.724	27.069	78,1
2011	89.561	21.176	13.743	124.480	140.715	-16.235	16.509	88,46
2012	99.359	23.537	20.032	142.928	160.223	-17.295	17.250	89,21
2013	118.729	27.471	16.814	163.014	182.689	-19.675	20.348	89,23
2014	135.239	30.512	18.578	184.329	204.400	-20.071	21.269	90,18
2015	159.480	37.526	23.096	220.102	231.546	-11.444	11.947	95,06
2016	184.446	46.457	24.977	255.880	276.536	-20.656	20.244	92,53
2017	208.064	51.767	28.728	288.559	312.735	-24.176	25.019	92,27
2018	255.619	57.560	56.032	369.211	384.962	-15.751	16.261	95,91
2019	293.828	71.222	59.178	424.228	464.173	-39.945	41.481	91,4
2020*	323.181.066	85.070.016	64.374.826	472.625.908	540.095.250	-67.469.343	71.980	87,5

Source: Republic of Turkey Social Security Institution, Statistical Bulletins. (2020). (downloaded on: 15.04.2021)

Table 4 indicates that the ratio of the total revenues of the SSI between 2008 and 2020 to total expenditures is in the range of 73–96 %. However, the item included in SSI revenues under "State contribution" except for premium revenues shows the contribution made by the State to the SSI at the rate of one-fourth of the invalidity, old-age and death insurances, and the Universal Health Insurance premiums collected monthly by the SSI according to Article 81 of the Social Security and Universal Health Insurance Law No. 5510. In other words, one-fourth of the premium revenues collected monthly by the SSI is calculated under "state contribution", and this amount is transferred to the SSI budget by the Treasury within 15 days following the request date. In this way, in addition to the year-end deficit financing, appropriations are transferred from the state budget to SSI accounts every month. Therefore, it is necessary to subtract the state contribution from the total income to calculate the income-expense balance regarding the activities of the SSI.

Tab. 5: Ratio of Premium revenue to Retirement Pensions and Health Payments between 2008–2020 (Except for State Contribution) (Million TL)

Years	Premium Revenue (Except for State Contribution)	Pension Payments Total (B)	Health Payments(C)	Total Payments (D = B+C)	Compensation Rate of Pension and Health Payments by Premium Revenue (%) (A/D)
2008	54.546	59.137	25.346	84.483	64,6
2009	54.579	68.604	28.811	97.415	56,0
2010	66.912	78.957	32.509	111.466	60,0
2011	89.561	91.615	36.500	128.115	69,9
2012	99.359	105.294	44.111	149.405	66,5
2013	118.729	119.162	49.889	169.051	70,2
2014	135.239	134.392	54.551	188.943	71,6
2015	159.480	151.990	59.356	211.346	75,5
2016	184.446	185.158	67.993	253.151	72,9
2017	208.064	209.546	77.632	287.178	72,5
2018	255.619	245.106	91.512	336.618	75,9
2019	293.828	298.615	110.697	409.312	71,8
2020	323.181	343.045	135.674	478.719	67,5

Source: SSI statistics (05.04.2020)

Table 5 indicates that, excluding state contribution, the ratio of SSI's operating income (premium revenue) to its expenses was in the range of 62–80 % between 2008 and 2020. In other words, excluding state contribution, social security premium revenues can cover 62–80 % of pension payments and health expenditures. The negative difference between revenues and expenditures is covered by the state budget. From a macroeconomic point of view, the negative difference in the budget of the SSI is borrowed by the Treasury, and it creates a burden on economic indicators.

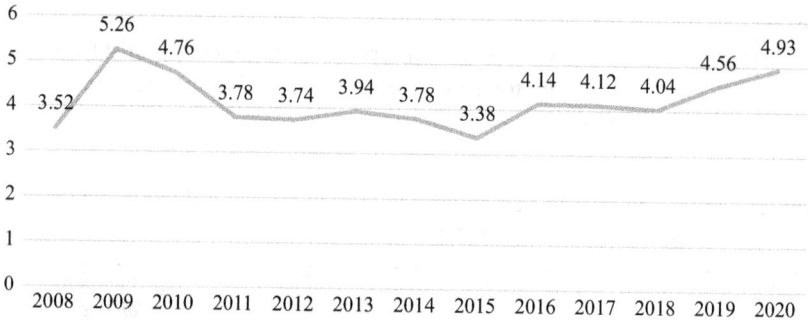

Graph 1: Budget Transfers to SSI (% of GDP)
Source: SSI statistics (05.01.2020), TÜİK

Graph 1 above indicates the budget transfers to the SSI. According to this, the ratio of "budget transfers to the SSI" to GDP has increased every year.

The criterion related to the financial survival of a social security system is the active/passive ratio. This ratio shows how many employees' premiums finance a retired person's pension payment. A low rate negatively affects the fiscal sustainability of the system. According to the generally accepted view, the active/passive insured ratio should be at least 4 to financially sustain the social security system. Today, in EU countries, 1 pensioner is financed by 4 insured people. In OECD countries, 1 pensioner is financed by 6 insured people. This rate is approximately 1 pensioner per 2 insured people in Turkey, as shown in Graph 2 below. This is because of the high number of retirees in our country; i.e. active employees who pay insurance premiums have to finance more pensioners than EU countries.

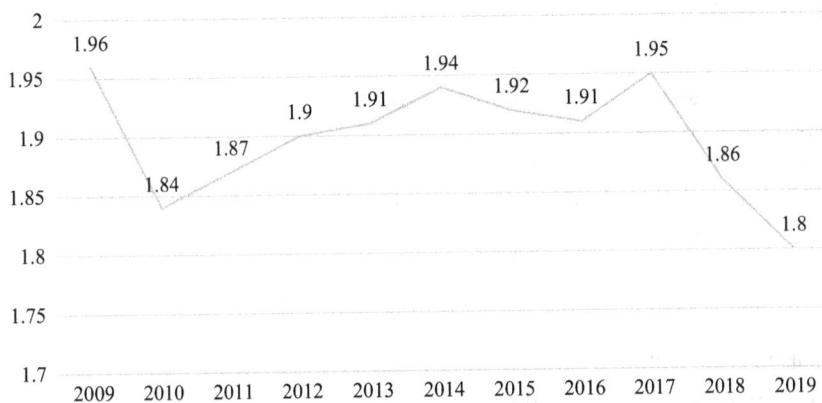

Graph 2: Active/Passive Ratio by Years in Turkey

Source: SSI (prepared by the authors by using the accountability reports of the SSI.)

The figures above show that the problem of premium revenue failing to cover social security payments continues to increase every year.

The income-expense imbalance of SSI, which provides the public financing of health expenditures, ultimately reflects negatively on the general government budget. This shows the importance of solving the financing problem of SSI for the development process of Turkey. This could be possible in two ways:

1. To reduce the health expenditures and pensions, which are the main expenditures of the SSI, or
2. To increase the premium revenues, which are the primary incomes of the SSI.

It does not seem possible both to reduce health expenditures, which are indispensable for human capital as one of the important production factors for development, and to ensure the right to health, which is the main duty of the state. Similarly, decreasing the income levels required to ensure people's right to life also causes social problems, so it should not be preferred in solving the SSI's financing problem. This shows that the only solution to increase the premium revenues.

The Ninth, Tenth, and Eleventh Development Plans of Turkey covering between 2007 and 2023 show that the main problems of the social security system include the inability of the SSI to meet its expenditures and the low premium collections. In this respect, a special emphasis is placed on increasing premium revenues among the policy priorities.

Conclusion

Having a healthy society should be a must for all countries, including Turkey. Therefore, having a healthy and educated society by increasing human capital investments is essential for Turkey to achieve sustainable economic growth and increase its socioeconomic development as a developing country. In this line, protecting public health is one of the fundamental duties of the state.

Indeed, Article 56 of the Turkish Constitution states that everyone should have the right to live in a healthy and balanced environment and that the state is in charge of planning and organizing the service-delivery of health institutions to ensure that people have physical and mental health. In addition, it states that the state will fulfil this task by utilizing and auditing the health and social institutions in the public and private sectors. This shows that the delivery and maintenance of healthcare services is one of the essential duties of the state.

A generation of healthy individuals is important for economic development. The health expenditure amounts of countries also differ according to their economic development levels. Moreover, per capita health expenditure in developed countries is higher than the one in developing countries. This can also be seen in the case of the budgets that countries allocate to health expenditures.

Although the per capita health expenditure in Turkey has increased over the years, the share of these expenditures in GDP decreased from 5.1 % in 2010 to 4.4 % in 2019. This rate is below OECD averages and the developed OECD countries in particular.

It can be said that health expenditures in Turkey are mainly financed by the social security system. Therefore, it is important to ensure its fiscal sustainability. The basic expenditures of the social security system are health expenditures and pensions, while its main income is the premium revenue paid by active employees. As of the end of 2020, 23.344.547 people in Turkey pay premiums as actively insured people, while 12.490.714 people paid pensions as passive. Because of the right to retirement at an early age in Turkey, every two employees must finance one pensioner. Since the active/passive ratio, which should be at least four for the fiscal sustainability of the social security system, is around two in Turkey, this places the system in an impasse.

Moreover, when we look at the ratio of premium revenue (except for state contribution) to total expenditures between 2008 and 2020, we see that it is between 62–80 %. Since social security deficits are financed from the state budget as duty losses, we see that the transfers to the SSI from the general state budget are increasing every year. Considering that the ratio of budget transfers to SSI to GDP was between 3.5–5 % between 2008 and 2020 in Turkey, the importance of increasing the premium revenue and ensuring the balance of income-expenditure becomes evident.

Governments set macroeconomic targets in line with long-term perspectives to maintain economic development, fight against poverty, prevent inequality in income distribution, create a healthy society, and ensure the fiscal sustainability of the social security system in all developed and developing countries. The Ninth, Tenth, and Eleventh Development Plans of Turkey covering between 2007 and 2023 show that the main problems of the SSI include the income-expense imbalance of the social security system and the low premium collections, but the proposed solutions for this problem cannot be fully implemented. For example, according to the said Development Plans, the main reason for the low premium collections is the frequent enactment of restructuring laws so the aim should be the enactment of restructuring laws only in exceptional cases. However, this measure cannot be implemented and a new restructuring law is implemented almost every year. The expectation that a new restructuring law will be enacted every year decreases the motivation of the insured to pay premiums and causes the premium revenue to be low and eventually the SSI cannot meet its expenses. Or similarly, while the aim is to increase the premium collections by closely monitoring the premium debts, there are problems in the premium tracking systems and the premium collections are not at a sufficient level.

Ensuring the right to health is among the fundamental duties of the state, and most of the public financing of health expenditures is covered by the SSI. However, as the SSI cannot provide the balance of income-expense adequately and as its financing deficits are covered by the state budget every year, it seems that the state poses a risk to the stable provision of the right to health. It is important to ensure the fiscal sustainability of the SSI to achieve the sustainable development goals, create a healthy society, and accelerate economic development. For this purpose, it is important to implement the policy goals and priorities planned in the development plans for increasing the premium revenues.

References

Ak, R. (2012). The Relationship between Health Expenditures and Economic Growth: Turkish Case. *International Journal of Business Management and Economic Research, 3(1)*, 404–409.

Akar, S. (2014). An Investigation of the Relationship among Health Expenditures, Relative Price of Health Expenditures and Economic Growth in Turkey (In Turkish). *Celal Bayar University, Journal of Management and Economics, 1(21)*, 311–322.

Akın, C. S. (2007). *Effect of the Health and Health Expenditure on Economy, Turkish Health Sector and Expenditures for Health* [Unpublished Master Thesis]. Adana: Çukurova University.

Akıncı, A., & Tuncer, G. (2016) The Relationship between Health Expenditures and Economic Growth in Turkey. *Journal of Turkish Court of Accounts, no. 102*, 47–61.

Blanco-Encomienda, F. J., & Ruiz-Garcia, A. (2017). Evaluating the Sustainability of Spanish Social Security System. *Economics and Sociology, 10(4)*, 11–20.

Demir, Ö., & Tanyıldızı, İ. (2017). Impact of Health Expenditures on Economic Growth. *Fırat University Journal of International Economic and Administrative Sciences, 1(1)*, 89–119.

Directorate of Presidential Strategy and Budget. (2018). *Sustainability of Social Security System*. Specialization Commission Report, Ankara.

Giray, F., & Çimen, G. (2018). Factors Determining the Level of Health Expenditures: Analysis of Turkey and OECD Countries. *Journal of Turkish Court of Accounts, no. 111*, 143–171.

International Social Security Association (ISSA). (2019). *10 Global Challenges for Social Security: Development and Innovation,* https://ww1.issa.int/sites/default/files/documents/publications/2-10-challenges-Global-2019-WEB-263629.pdf, Access date 20.04.2021.

Kekeç, H. M., Yıldırım, Z., & Polat, A. (2018). Analysis of Health Expenditures and Financial Periods in Turkey. *Gazi University Journal of Social Sciences, 5(14)*, 550–563.

Mazgit, İ. (1998). *Reconstruction of Turkey's Health Sector in the Process of Economic Development* (In Turkish) [Unpublished Doctoral Dissertation]. Dokuz Eylül University, İzmir.

Organization for Economic Cooperation and Development (OECD). (2020). *Health Statistics 2020*, Access date 19.04.2021.)

Republic of Turkey Social Security Institution, Statistical Bulletins. (2020). http://www.sgk.gov.tr/wps/portal/sgk/tr/kurumsal/istatistik/sgk_istatistik_yilliklari, Access date 15.04.2021.

Selim, S., Uysal, D., & Eryiğit, P. (2014). Econometric Analysis of the Effect on Economic Growth of the Health Expenditure in Turkey. *Niğde University Journal of Economics and Administrative Sciences, 7 (3)*, 13–24.

Turkish Statistical Institute (TÜİK). (2019). *Health Expenditure Statistics*. https://data.tuik.gov.tr/Bulten/Index?p=Saglik-Harcamalari-Istatistikleri-2019-33659.), Access date 20.04.2021.

World Health Organization (WHO). (2021). *Global Health Expenditure Database*. https://data.worldbank.org/indicator/SH.XPD.CHEX.GD.ZS?end=2018&start=2000&view=chart.), Access date 19.04.2021.

Mehmet Onur Yurdakul

Corruption and Money Laundering in the Health Sector

Introduction

Corruption is most commonly defined as "misuse of public office or public power for private gain" (Klitgaard, 1991:120; Bardhan, 1997:1321; World Bank, 1997:8; Transparency International, 2000:2; Treisman, 2000:399; OECD, 2008:22). Klitgaard (1988:75) also formulates corruption as, monopoly power + discretion – accountability of public officials. Rose-Ackerman (1999:75), Aktan (1999:20–21) and Mumcu (2005:1) associate corruption to political and social collusion. Moreover, Stapenhurst & Sedigh (1999:1) and Coase (1979:269) emphasizes that corruption may arise in private sector too.

The health sector is inherently vulnerable to corruption due to the global nature of the production chain, existence of various actors from public and private sectors, asymmetric information problem among the actors and the free-ridership phenomenon. Besides, for the purpose of freely benefiting the illegal proceeds acquired from corrupt acts, perpetrators of corruption or relevant third parties are needed to launder these revenues. Money laundering occurs in various ways. Nonetheless, laundering criminal proceeds acquired from corrupt acts in the health sector has not been subject to sufficient number of academic researches.

In this study, having provided the theoretical discussion and literature review on causes and effects of corruption in health sector in the first section, the concept of money laundering and the sector's vulnerability to this phenomenon is going to be discussed in the second section. The study concludes with policy proposals.

I. Corruption in the Health Sector

A. Classification of Corruption

As it is mentioned above, corruption definitions focus of misuse of power for private gain by public or private actors and lack of accountability. In order to better understand the definitions, some classifications exist on corruption types (Shah, 2007:235–236):

- Petty, Administrative or Bureaucratic Corruption: Public officials abuse their current authority to demand bribes, transfer public funds to their account or use them for personal gain (as embezzlement, fraud causing loss to public institutions). It frequently occurs.
- Grand Corruption: It is the abuse of public resources by public officials in senior positions defined as political or administrative elite for personal or interest group gain. It is a major corruption type in which decision makers involve.
- State Capture (and Regulatory Capture): Although it is a type of corruption that can be considered within grand corruption, it is a separate type as it is triggered by private sector agents. In cases the regulatory authority is exposed to pressures of interest groups, regulatory capture type major corruption cases occur (Le Grand, 1991:438–439).
- Patronage, paternalism, clientelism: Corruption occurs when officials use their official position to provide assistance to clients of the same geographic, ethnic, or cultural origin to get privileged services, including public sector employment.

Another classification of corruption is the distinction on legal and illegal corruption. Having developed by Kaufmann & Vicente (2005:1–4), this classification aims to draw attention to private sector linkage of corruption. Such private sector agents may exert undue influence on political and bureaucratic elite through lobbying activities assumed as "auction for favour". To illustrate, the legal corruption types are rent seeking, lobbying, vote trading and favouritism which are not criminalized in penal codes (TEPAV, 2006:29).

Apart from the above mentioned definitions, another distinction of corruption is the fact that whether it is prevalent in the society or not. In this regard, Klitgaard (1991:121) argues that systemic corruption will emerge as a result of the spread of corruption in a way that affects daily business life. An uncoordinated, "grabbing hand" type corruption type which causes more adverse results may happen as claimed by Shleifer & Vishny (1998:1–17).

On the other hand, Frye & Shleifer (1997:355) argues that state regulatory actions to correct market failures can lead to a politically organized "helping hand" type corruption, presumably with less negative effects. This approach is in line with "greese in the wheel" hypothesis developed by Leff (1964) and Huntington (1968) which claims that corruption might be beneficial to the economy in certain circumstances.

B. Reasons for State Intervention in the Economy and the Concept of Market and Government Failures

1. Market Failures

The failure of the market to produce the optimum amount of output is indicated as the main reason of state intervention in the economy. The state aims to overcome these failures through its economic functions to be summed up as allocation, redistribution and stabilizing as explained by Musgrave (1976:7–19). The argument that the market economy alone cannot achieve the optimum output is the main reason for state intervention to the economy. According to Stiglitz (2000:77–85), the failure of market to achieve Pareto efficient resource allocation is called "market failure", and its types are classified under six headings:

   i. Failure of Competition,
   ii. Public Goods,
   iii. Externalities,
   iv. Incomplete Markets,
   v. Information Failures,
   vi. Unemployment, Inflation and Disequilibrium.

In order to eliminate these failures, government can use regulation, financing, public production tools which have direct impacts on the market mechanism and income transfer tool which have indirect effects (Barr,1993:79). Musgrave (1976:10–12) is of the view that production of semi-public goods, the supply of which is inelastic, should be either ensured or subsidized by state. Education, healthcare and public housing can be illustrated in this regard. However, state intervention to prevent market failures is likely to cause government failure through expanding bureaucracy, generating rent for bureaucrats, distorting fair resource allocation and possibly causing corruption (Schultze, 1977:10–14, Acemoğlu & Verdier, 2000:209). How and to what extent to intervene in the economy is shaped as a political decision, and the differentiation of non-market supply and demand conditions leads to the emergence of "non-market failures" (Wolf, 1978:10–14).

2. Government Failures and Implications for the Health Sector

As stated above, healthcare services being considered as semi-public goods are deemed a cause of market failure per se. Thus, it is argued that these services should be offered by state. The health sector is subject to all kinds of market failures pointed out by Stiglitz (2000) due to positive externalities of services, information asymmetry in the sector, differentiation of the development level of the markets for its financing, imperfect market conditions and employment problems.

The positive externalities of services produced in the health sector constitute the main rationale for state intervention. There may be health services that have the characteristics of competitiveness in consumption and exclusion from using it as well as health services the benefit of which cannot be divided and consumers cannot be deemed rival in consumption as they are not excluded from using it. Health services produced by the state are mostly stated under this second group. For example, no one will be deprived of obtaining this benefit if the government vaccinates its citizens in relation to a pandemic and provides sanitation services. On the other hand, this situation will spread the "free rider" behaviour in the sector, increase health expenditures, and prepare the ground for corrupt relationships involving patients, doctors, pharmaceutical companies and hospitals (Tosun, 2002:56).

If health services are produced through a non-market resource allocation mechanism, the question on how much and in what quality they will be produced arises. Healthcare demand is not a static and predictable demand (Arrow, 1963:948). Moreover, governments lack performance indicators such as price and profitability in terms of deciding the quantity and quality of these goods and this may result in creating "internal" performance criteria (number of personnel, office, use of technology etc.) that undermine cost control of these goods. Thus Pareto efficient resource allocation would not be achieved[1] and such internalities would cause failure of government (Wolf, 1978:18–26).

In addition, the information asymmetry between the service providers (i.e. doctors, their institutions) and the consumers (i.e. patients) results in supplier-induced demand which may shift the patient's demand curve according to supplier's self-interest. This might happen by misleading a patient into accepting an inappropriate or less appropriate treatment (Ensor & Moreno, 2002:111). Although insurance practices are used to solve this uncertainty, "moral hazard" problem, to be explained as (i) the service demand exceeds the service requirement, (ii) reduced sensitivity of the individual to adopt a healthier lifestyle (iii) insurance also has an effect on the doctor's behaviour, is likely to arise (Yıldırım, 1999:6). In this context, state intervention in the market in the form of public

---

1   Pareto efficiency demonstrates a situation that no individual can be better without making at least one individual worse off.

production or regulation is unavoidable; but herein we encounter excessive consumption problem.

Moreover, health sector service providers such as hospitals, insurance companies and pharmaceutical companies operate within imperfect competition markets. In case of patent rights on certain drugs or devices, it is possible for those who produce them to form a monopolistic structure. Notwithstanding this, it appears that oligopoly market conditions prevail in the sector. Increasing concentration in the market allows rent seeking behaviour and "regulatory capture" type corruption (Kang, 2002:15).

Finally, although the unemployment problem of health sector workers requiring qualified workforce appears to be lower than other sectors, labour shortage is faced in this sector. Nonetheless, because of the economic downturn during the Covid-19 pandemic and the fact that routine healthcare services have been delayed or cancelled, unemployment has risen in the sector. In the USA, employment in the health sector was estimated to have fallen by 7.8 % in April 2020 compared to the previous year's same month (Health System Tracker, 2020).

C. Actors and Volume of Corruption in the Health Sector and Vulnerable Areas

As it is mentioned above, a wide variety of actors involve in the health sector and this may cause free-ridership, asymmetric information and moral hazard problems which increases sector's vulnerability to corruption. Furthermore, high amount of money is spent in the sector.

It is estimated that high income countries spend approximately 7 % of their GDP to health while low income ones spend on average 4.2 % (U4 Anti-Corruption Resource Centre, 2008:4). According to forecasts made by WHO (2020:2), cumulative global healthcare expenditures has reached $8.3 trillion in 2018 which is about 10 % of global GDP. The share of public sources was about $4.9 trillion, while private health spending was at $3.4 trillion level. Moreover, an average of 6.19 % of annual health spending is estimated to be lost to fraud (Button & Gee, 2015:6) which corresponds to almost $514 billion. Taking into account that these figures are pre-COVID-19 pandemic values, it is apparent that current expenditures would have exceeded such amounts.

Investigation based measurement techniques and perception based surveys are used to estimate the volume of fraud in the sector. Investigation-based measurement techniques take into account administrative or criminal investigations, audits, data-mining and price comparisons (Couffinhal & Frankowski, 2017:269). In the National Money Laundering Risk Assessment of the USA,

Mehmet Onur Yurdakul

annual healthcare fraud based on investigative techniques was estimated as $100 billion (US Treasury, 2018: 8) and it was supposed to be the most essential money laundering threat as well as drugs trafficking. In an assessment made for Colombia in 2017, it was estimated that their healthcare system had lost $160 million through fraudulent activities (Begue, 2018., Kussmann, 2020: 14–15). Estimation for Russia revealed that informal payments had posed 56 % of the health expenditures (WHO, 2006: 84).

Perception of corruption in the health sector has also been subject to surveys (Fig. 1). According to Transparency International's study on Global Corruption Barometer (2013:5) which includes views of citizens from 107 countries, average perception of health sector corruption was rated as 3.3 over 5 where the high score represents extreme corruption. In Albania, Armenia, Azerbaijan, Ethiopia, Morocco and Serbia, health sector was reported as the most corrupt sector. By the way, the highest corruption perception is gathered in Albania, Serbia, Tanzania and Kyrgyzstan while lowest perception was obtained in Denmark (Transparency International, 2013: 35–38).

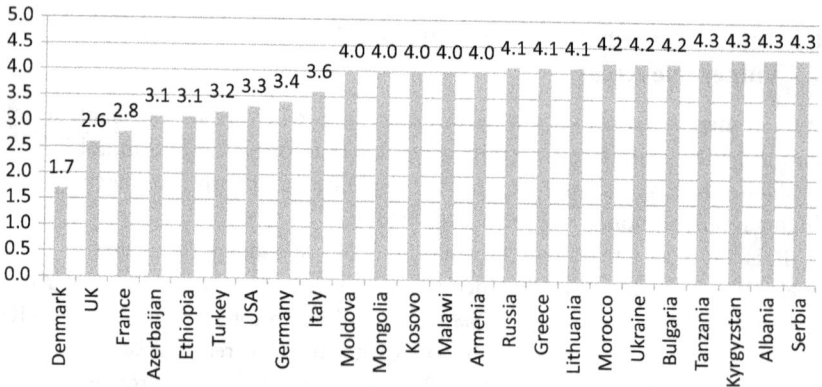

Fig. 1: Perception of Health Sector Corruption: Results of Several Countries
Source: Transparency International (2013)

In regard to the European Commission's Updated Study on Corruption in the Healthcare Sector report, corruption perception in healthcare services is estimated as 33 % in European Union. However, there are several outliers such as Greece with 81 %, Lithuania 74 %, Romania 67 % (European Commission, 2017:103). In another survey made for Africa, it is found out that 69 % of Liberian citizens believe that corruption was widespread in their health services (Mackey et al, 2018:635). In another study, bribery rate varied between 1 % and 51 % among countries (Kusmann, 2020:2).

The relationship between the actors in the health sector can be denoted by principal-agent-client models initially developed by Rose - Ackerman (1978) to reflect conflicts of interest. Here, the "principal" is the state which regulates healthcare services, the "agent" can be formulated as the healthcare bureaucrats and personnel providing healthcare service; the "client" represents patients who demand healthcare services. Advanced versions of this model also exist. In case the clients demand privileged treatment from their agents and the auditors interact with service units, the relations can be subject to principal, agent, organization, client network model developed by Jain (1998:15–17).

If we adapt this model to the health sector, the client would be patients who get service either from "proceeds generating organizations", such as insurance companies and pharmaceutical companies, or from "service organizations" working on healthcare such as hospitals, private clinics. In this model, companies operating on procurement (i.e. construction, medical equipment) services can also be deemed a proceeds generating organization, although they do not have direct contact with the clients. The model limits the role of principal to assign and delegate authority. The role of agent is to regulate the organizations within the scope of healthcare legislation and it controls the auditors who supervise healthcare service providers.

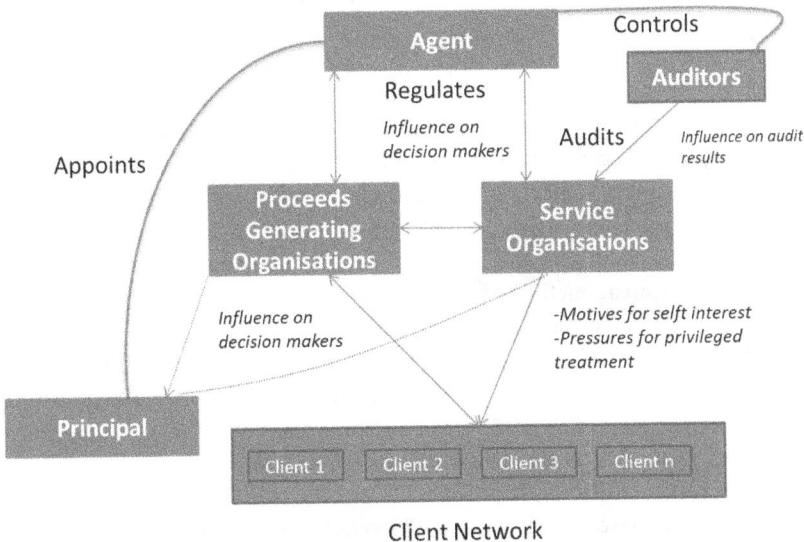

Fig. 2: Principal, Agent, Organization, Client Network Model
Source: Adapted from Jain (1998:15)

According to Fig. 2, an organization aiming to maximize profit can increase its share in the sector and service prices by penetrating government policy (through lobbying activities) as a result of rent-seeking activities. An organization that aims to be provided with undue privilege does not always pay bribes to the agent; instead it may seek lobbying activities (i.e. receiving a license, granting permission on marketing a product, etc.). Organizations may put pressure on the agent to adopt a regulation that will address their own interest at the expense of clients. Accordingly, pressure may be put on the agent for:

i. producing a medicine or equipment with appropriate quality and reliability,
ii. performing a tender service in accordance with the specification,
iii. completing the final acceptance procedures for the service received.

Moreover, the organizations may negotiate with the principal directly and the principal may act biased in the appointments to the health bureaucracy. The model described so far reveals state or regulatory capture styled, grand corruption cases (Savedoff & Hussmann, 2006:5–7, UNDP, 2011:12).

In the right part of the Fig. 2, the second circumstance regarding the model appears. In this case, the agent controls the supervisors who audit service providers and therefore their financial transactions with the proceeds generating organizations. In this example, the information asymmetry problem arises again and the auditors may have incentive to use the irregularities to their own interest rather than directly reporting to agent (Jain, 1998:17–19).

In addition, similar problems can be observed in the relationship between clients and organizations due to information asymmetry. Clients can incline toward paying bribery in the names of gifts, kickbacks, surgery money etc. in order to get privileged treatment from healthcare institutions. Moreover, they may further seek to benefit from social insurance opportunities by declaring their incomes underestimated.

Healthcare institutions and doctors can decide to implement unnecessary expensive treatment methods too. Furthermore, considering the size of the expenditures made in the health sector, it appears that the sector is also prone to embezzlement, bid rigging, fraud type corruption threats. Next, if sufficient number of personnel does not work in healthcare institutions, the client would not get healthcare services effectively. If requests for favouritism in appointment process of healthcare personnel are taken into account, absenteeism-styled corruption might occur (Vian, 2008:84).

Apart from these circumstances, the relationship between insurance and pharmaceutical delivery companies may cause adverse selection problem due to information asymmetry. In some cases, a payment can be requested with misleading documents for a service, medicine or equipment that is not actually got by the clients. In this regard, when recipients of services interact with public officials, petty corruption may arise (UNDP, 2011:11).

D. Consequences of Health Sector Corruption

As explained above, both grand and petty corruption types can be encountered in the health sector. In case of a state or regulatory capture type corruption, costs of healthcare programs increase and this adversely affects the allocation of resources at the expense of disadvantageous groups and regions. It also results in inappropriate usage of technology, (outdated or unnecessary), procurement of inappropriate standard of medicines, healthcare equipment and hospital facilities. In many cases, the quality of treatments and competence of healthcare professionals can be questioned or absenteeism of them in unfavourable regions may reduce the efficiency in distribution of services. Demands for informal payments deteriorate public trust, social justice and faith to government. As a result, unfair distribution of income is likely to rise and it prevents health reforms due to corrupt nature of healthcare services (Lewis, 2000:5–26, Kirigia & Diarra Nama, 2008:891; U4 Anti-Corruption Resource Centre, 2008:10; Vian, 2008:84–85; Vian, 2020:6; WHO, 2020:8–21).

Furthermore, permission of marketing of counterfeit (both branded and generic) or sub-therapeutic drugs poses important health risks to the communities and it increases corruption risk as well. Accordingly, a shortage of genuine drugs may be encountered. Developing countries are affected by this problem more than developed ones; but its negative externalities affect all over the world (Chika et al, 2011:260). Besides, drug promotions between pharmaceutical companies and doctors can influence doctors to engage in corruption. Such financial subsidies may distract research activities into profitable ones (Kassirer, 2006:86–89).

In addition to aforementioned implications, effects of corruption in the health sector has been analysed in several empirical studies. For example, Gupta et al. (2001:15–26), found evidence that corruption had significant negative impacts on indicators of healthcare such as mortality of infants and children by employing cross-sectional regressions on 128 developing and developed countries for the period of 1985–1987. Using cross-sectional data of World Value and WHO surveys on more than 120 countries, Holmberg & Rothstein (2011:537–541) found that quality of government corresponds to lower level of mortality rates for children and their mothers and increases life expectancies. Similarly, Sommer (2020:690–717) used a two way fixed effects panel data model for a sample of 90 countries and found that health expenditures decrease infant and child mortality more when perceived public sector corruption is lower.

Aside from above, Akçay (2006:40–46) employed a cross-sectional analysis of 63 countries in regressions which aim to explain human development index (1998) and concluded that corruption decreases the pace of growth, reduces healthcare spending and GDP per capita and both life expectancy and human capital accumulation decreases accordingly. Factor and Kang (2015:637–638) reached to similar results as they employed a structural equation model regression for 133 countries in 2003 and 2009 and suggested that corruption rises as GDP p.c. falls as the regime becomes more autocratic and higher corruption is associated with lower health expenditures. Azfar & Gurgur (2008:241–242) analysed the results of a survey made in Philippines in 2000 and concluded that corruption had adverse impacts on immunization and vaccination rates, public services in rural areas and increased unfair distribution of income.

Taking into consideration the relevant studies illustrated above, Vian (2005:45–46) summed up sector's vulnerabilities to corruption as it is shown in Tab. 1.

Tab. 1: Types of Corruption and Vulnerabilities in Health Sector and Their Possible Consequences

Field and Process	Corruption Types & Vulnerabilities	Possible Consequences
Construction and Maintenance of Health Facilities	- Bribery, kickbacks and political influence - Lack of accountability	- Deterioration in cost-benefit balance of services - Deterioration in distribution of services which do not focus on disadvantages groups and regions - Investment on unnecessary technology
Procurement of equipment and drugs	- Bribery, kickbacks and political influence - Bid rigging in tenders - Lack of incentives to ensure efficiency - Unethical drug promotions - Lack of accountability	- Deterioration in cost-benefit balance and appropriateness of drugs and equipment - Procuring Inappropriate standard of drugs and equipment
Distribution and usage of drugs	- Theft and stockpiling of drugs -Sale of drugs being supposed to be free	- Deterioration in quality of health services and effectiveness of drugs - Incentives for informal payments for patients - Incomplete treatments leading to anti-microbial resistance
Regulation of products, services, facilities and healthcare professionals	- Bribery, kickbacks and political influence - Biased application of sanitary regulations and procedures on certification, accreditation and licensing	- Sub-therapeutic or fake drugs are allowed on market - Poor quality facilities and incompetent professionals are allowed to operate - Rise in food poisoning - Emergence of infections and pandemics
Training of healthcare professionals	- Bribery, kickbacks and exposing political influence for being selected to medical schools, training and certificate programs	- Lack of quality in healthcare trainings and lack of competence in professionals - Loss of trust to healthcare mechanism
Medical research	- Clinical trials for marketing purposes - Trials without ensuring full consent of subject persons because of information asymmetry	- Biases and unfairness in research activities - Breaches of human rights

(continued on next page)

Tab. 1:   Continued

Field and Process	Corruption Types & Vulnerabilities	Possible Consequences
Services by healthcare professionals	- Use of public facilities and equipment to see private patients - Unnecessary referrals privately owned ancillary services - Absenteeism - Theft and embezzlement of budget allocation - Demanding informal payments	- Loss of trust and faith to healthcare mechanism and government - Unmet demand of healthcare services - Reduced availability to utilize from governmental healthcare programs - Increasing poverty

Source: Adapted from Vian (2008: 85)

Aside from the findings summed up in the Tab. 1, a natural consequence of health sector corruption is the money laundering phenomenon as explained in the next section.

II. Money Laundering Through Health Sector

A. The Concept of Money Laundering

Money laundering is defined as an autonomous criminal economic activity whose essential function lies in the transformation of liquidity of illicit origin, or potential purchasing power, into actual purchasing power usable for consumption, saving, investment or reinvestment (Masciandaro, 2007:2). Robinson (1998:3), described money laundering as a cycle of transactions to illegal or dirty money in order to attain legal or clean money. These transactions or actions are explained in the recommendations of Financial Action Task Force (FATF) and several international conventions in detail.

The FATF's recommendation 3 stipulates that countries should criminalize money laundering on the basis of the Vienna and Palermo Conventions, and that the predicate offenses of money laundering should include all serious offences. Apart from this, this offence has been defined in the UN Convention against Corruption (Merida Convention) and the Council of Europe's Strasbourg and Warsaw Conventions. In the relevant articles of the aforementioned conventions, it is seen that the acts associated with the money laundering offense are classified under three groups, and fourthly, participation and attempts to offence are regulated.

In this regard, when committed intentionally:

- The conversion or transfer of property, knowing that such property is the proceeds of crime, for the purpose of concealing or disguising the illicit origin of the property or of helping any person who is involved in the commission of the predicate offence to evade the legal consequences of his or her action [Vienne Convention art. 3(1)(b)(i), Palermo Convention art. 6(1)(a) (i), Merida Convention art. 23(1)(a)(i), Strasbourg Convention art. 6(1)(a), Warsaw Convention art. 9(1)(a)],
- The concealment or disguise of the true nature, source, location, disposition, movement or ownership of or rights with respect to property, knowing that such property is the proceeds of crime; [Vienne Convention art. 3(1)(b()ii), Palermo Convention art. 6(1)(a)(ii), Merida Convention art. 23(1)(a)(ii), Strasbourg Convention art. 6(1)(b), Warsaw Convention art. 9(1)(b)],
- The acquisition, possession or use of property, knowing, at the time of receipt, that such property is the proceeds of crime [Vienne Convention art. 3(1)(c() i), Palermo Convention art. 6(1)(b)(i), Merida Convention art. 23(1)(b)(i), Strasbourg Convention art. 6(1)(c), Warsaw Convention art. 9(1)(c)],
- Participation in, association with or conspiracy to commit, attempts to commit and aiding, abetting, facilitating and counselling the commission of any of the offences established in accordance with this article [Vienne Convention art. 3(1)(c()iv), Palermo Convention art. 6(1)(b)(ii), Merida Convention art. 23(1)(b)(ii), Strasbourg Convention art. 6(1)(d), Warsaw Convention art. 9(1)(d)].

These arrangements are also set forth in article 1(13) of the EU's Anti-Money Laundering Directive no 2015/849 and articles 3, 8, 10 of the EU Directive on Money Laundering by Criminal Law no 2018/1673. Therefore, mental and material elements of money laundering offense are constituted when the proceeds obtained from a predicate offense is subjected to the above-mentioned actions. However, in order to initiate a prosecution on money laundering, there is no need for predicate offence conviction. Particularly in offences committed via false or misleading documents, the predicate offence and acts of concealing or disguising the proceeds can be committed by the same act and this may lead to money laundering offence as well. Whether two penalties can be imposed cumulatively is another matter of discussion due to "non bis in idem" principle.[2]

---

2 Non bis in idem is an legal term transpose from Latin languange which means "not twice in the same thing". It effects that no legal action can be imposed twice for the same act.

B. Methods and Stages of Money Laundering

In terms of laundering methods, FATF (2006:1) makes a triple classification as laundering methods based on the financial system, cash couriers, trade - physical transportation of goods. In essence, money laundering is mostly committed within the financial system through "smurfing" and "restructuring" methods. In smurfing method, it is aimed to integrate the illegal proceeds into the financial system through a number of customers having transactions under the threshold of customer identification obligation. In restructuring method, number of transactions below customer identification threshold increases rather than customers.

Money laundering occurs in three successive stages within the financial system. In the first, "placement" stage, the proceeds of crime are entered into the financial system. The preventive measures, such as customer identification, mostly focus on this stage as the possibility of being noticed in this step is higher than other stages. The second stage is called, "the layering stage" and the illegal proceeds placed in the financial system must be moved away from its source. The main purpose of this stage is to make it difficult to trace the money. The final stage is called "integration stage" in which the money is now returned to the criminals as if it was legitimately acquired (Yurdakul, 2015:42–43).

It is observed that laundering activities committed outside the financial system are mostly carried out by purchasing various assets (real estate, etc.) or misusing corporate vehicles in order to conceal or disguise the proceeds of crime. It is also a common method to establish shell companies inside or outside the country and carry out cash movements through these companies (Yurdakul, 2013:23). The use of cash couriers is another laundering method (FATF, 2010:3).

Within these methods, Baker (2005:172), emphasized that trade based illicit financial flows and money laundering have gone up. Trade base money laundering mostly occurs via (I) Invoicing goods and services with higher or lower prices, (ii) Duplicate invoicing, (iii) Different description of the quantity and type of goods, (iv) Delivering more or less goods in comparison to the invoices, (v) Fictitious exports (FATF, 2006:3–7; 2008:3).

C. Vulnerabilities of Health Sector with Respect to Money Laundering

The health sector poses significant risks for obtaining illegal proceeds. Theoretically, perpetrators of corrupt acts being criminalized in penal codes or any third parties need to launder the revenues obtained from corruption in order to freely use them. Thus, perpetrators of corruption should feel to have required laundering the illegal proceeds in order to keep these proceeds away from being confiscated.

Especially, the conversion of large amounts of corruption revenues to give impression that they are obtained from a legitimate source is a significant laundering risk. These large amounts may be obtained either through grand corruption cases or unorganized minor corruption acts, the cumulative values of which may correspond to high amounts too. As stated by Schleifer and Vishny (1993:20–21), such type of corruption may have more negative effects on efficient resource allocation. In this context, proceeds obtained through corruption and money laundering actions in the health sector should be taken into consideration (Fig. 3).

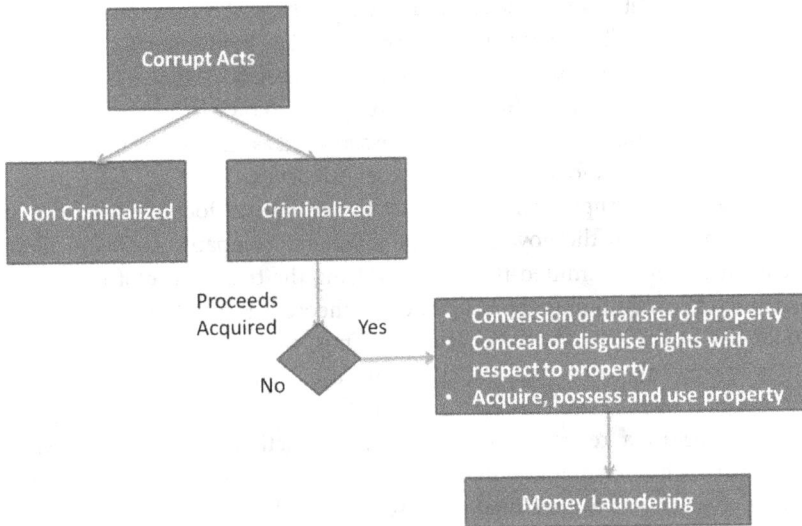

Fig. 3: Corruption and Money Laundering

In the regulatory capture or state capture styled grand corruption cases, the most prevalent laundering method has been the misuse of corporate vehicles as mentioned in "The Puppet Masters" book, in which 150 grand corruption cases were examined through UN's Stolen Asset Recovery Initiative (Willebois et al., 2011:20). Irrespective of the sector that the grand corruption occurred, the common features of these cases in terms of money laundering were summed up below (Willebois et al, 2011:171–217):

- A corporate vehicle (either a company or non-profit organization) was misused in order to conceal or disguise monetary transactions;
- Proceeds or instruments of corruption is partly deposited in bank accounts that banking system was abused. In some cases real estate is purchased.
- The corporate vehicle was either established or managed by a professional intermediary (including lawyers, accountants, company and trusts service providers) and complex shareholdership structure existed.

When it comes to petty corruption types, proceeds acquired through health sector can be laundered via a number of methods including banking and insurance transactions, purchasing real estate or securities etc. In regard to insurance, life insurance policies might pose higher money laundering risks than the remaining insurance products as new beneficiaries can be assigned by the insurer so as to ensure that payments are made to them and it might be used as collateral to purchase other financial instruments (IAIS, 2004:4). In addition, health insurance policies might be misused via unjust reimbursement claims. Purchase of a policy that does not meet the customer's needs, unrelated to his/her health or age (in example policy sold to disabled or elderly persons or for doing extreme sports exercises) can be supposed as an indicator for misuse of health insurance policy for laundering purposes (Moneyval, 2010:61).

In cases the corrupt act is committed by fraudulent documents to receive unjust benefit from the government or insurance company, as the predicate offence has been committed through disguising the true nature of the case, it is also worth mentioning about laundering theoretically as the unjust benefit would also be laundered with the same act. Thus, banking transactions, fraudulent invoicing and reimbursement claims, misuse of shell companies are among the common ways of laundering.

According to a review made on suspicious activity reports received by FinCEN, which is the financial intelligence unit of the USA attached to Treasury, insurance payments for personal purposes or quickly moving (layering) insurance payments through accounts of the same or other financial institutions, withdrawal or depositing of these funds were deemed suspicious. In regard to accounts, it was noted that the account might be held in the name of a licensed medical professional or healthcare institution, or it may be held in the name of a shell company (US Treasury, 2018:8–9). Shell companies might be used in trade based money laundering schemes as well (Citibank, 2016:8).

D. Case Studies

The case studies below reveal the practices for misuse of health sector for corruption and money laundering.

Case 1. Federal Level Healthcare Fraud: The Largest Ever Law Enforcement Action against 601 Individuals in the USA

On 28 June 2018, a law enforcement operation was conducted against 601 individuals in 58 federal districts. Among the persons in charge, 165 doctors, nurses and other licensed medical professions exist. They are accused for participating in commission of health sector fraud through false invoicing with a cumulative amount of $2 billion, approximately by billing to health insurance programs Medicare,[3] Medicaid,[4] Tricare[5] and private insurance companies for medically unnecessary medicines and equipment that were not even purchased and/or distributed to beneficiaries. Because of fraudulent insurance billings, many of these persons were also accused for money laundering (US Department of Justice, 2021a).

Case 2. Three persons charged in $180 Million Healthcare Fraud (via Overbilling Medications) and Money Laundering Scheme

Similar to case 1, on 27 May 2020, an indictment was presented before a court in the Southern District of Mississippi regarding 3 individuals for fraudulent billing actions to health insurance programs in the USA. Using several pharmacies, the defendants were alleged to overbill the medications to the insurance companies. Further, they are charged to involve in a laundering scheme through monetary transactions and purchase of numerous assets including real estates, luxury cars, diamonds etc. (US Department of Justice, 2021b).

Case 3. Health and Injury Insurance Fraud and Money Laundering[6]

In Moldova, an insurer in collusion with an insured person attempted to launder money through insurance transactions. The insurance company sold health insurance policies which also provide assurance against accidents to dummy persons. These persons paid a low premium rates and then, when claims were received with false documents to substantiate the losses, the insurer paid the claims promptly. The reality is understood when the company took legal actions against businesses where the alleged accidents took place, as no such accidents occurred (Moneyval, 2010:45–46).

Case 4. Trade Based Money Laundering Example[7]

---

3   Medicare is the federal health insurance program for people at the age of 65 or older.
4   Medicaid provides health coverage to disadvantaged groups in USA such as low income adults, children, people with disabilities and pregnant women.
5   Health insurance program for members and veterans of the armed forces and their families.
6   Date of the case was not provided in the source document.
7   Date and locale of the case was not provided in the source document.

A transferable letter of credit for a million dollars trade relationship was issued by one of Bank A's correspondent banks (issuing bank) at the request of that country's Bureau of Health. The first beneficiary which is an intermediary institution in this trade network, was to supply medical goods; but this beneficiary was a small scale company without any experience in hospital/equipment contracts at millions dollar scale. Bank A (the advising bank) was asked to confirm the credit (Citibank, 2016:8).

Subsequently, the ultimate beneficiary presented invoices for a certain amount, and the first beneficiary substituted its invoices with a mark-up of more than 300 %. It also appeared to have a connection with the consulting firm acting as the agent for the Bureau of Health. As no satisfactory response was received from the issuing bank for price discrepancies, Bank A declined the letter of credit and then necessary actions were taken (Citibank, 2016:8).

Case 5. Fake Hospital Bills[8]

Payment requests were gathered via bills of a hospital which was closed previously and then re-opened in a different address, which was far away from the address provided by the claimant. The inquires confirmed that both bills and names on them were fake (CRI Group, 2020:11).

E. Impact of COVID 19 Pandemic to Health Sector Fraud and Money Laundering

The COVID-19 pandemic has led new opportunities for fraud and laundering activities. In this regard, Financial Action Task Force (2020) published a document on risks and policy responses for COVID-19 related money laundering. Within the report, increasing risks are attributed to FATF, (2020:5–6, 8):

- Using online systems (for governments and businesses) while prioritising resources towards responding to COVID-19 related needs,
- Significant increase of demand for medical supplies,
- The fact that financial institutions operate via few personnel, prefer to offer services online,
- Adverse impact of lockdown measures on employment, trade and growth.

The most common fraud types deemed as threats for money laundering are (FATF, 2020:6–7):

---

8   Date and locale of the case was not provided in the source document.

- Impersonation of public officials to demand additional payments (i.e. for treatment),
- Counterfeiting of medical supplies and medicines,
- Fundraising for fake charities,
- Fraudulent investment scams (claiming to prevent, detect and cure COVID-19).

F. Implications for Turkey

As depicted in the Chart 1, according to a survey made by Transparency International, perception of corruption in health sector in Turkey was estimated less than global average (Transparency International, 2013:35–38). In advance of this study, a domestic survey was carried out by Şahin et al. (2009) in order to estimate the perception of corruption among health sector professionals.

In this regard, a questionnaire was prepared and responses of 4.075 Ministry of Health personnel was gathered. Accordingly, it was found out that acceptability of presumptive corruption aside from favouritism is very low while frequency of petty corruption types appears rather high in Turkey.

The most severe corruption type was perceived as political favouritism (such as nepotism, patronage, clientelism) in appointments and personnel having executive titles such as directors, managers are perceived to be more prone to corruption (Şahin et al, 2009:123–128). Nonetheless, to our best knowledge, no other study exists which aim to estimate the volume of criminal proceeds acquired through health sector fraud through investigation based measurement techniques.

According to the statistical data in the Activity Report 2019 of the Department of Anti-Smuggling and Organized Crime (KOM) in Turkey, in 2019, number of suspects detained in planned operations on healthcare fraud was 236; which is higher than any other corruption types (KOM, 2019:21). Moreover, it should be noted that this data does not include the impact of COVID-19 pandemics which has emerged in 2020.

Thus, healthcare fraud seems to pose a nonignorable money laundering threat in Turkey as well. However, since the predicate offences of money laundering cases do not take place in Judicial Statistics published by Ministry of Justice (2019) or in any other publication, we do not have a concrete opinion about the majority of the threat in Turkey.

Conclusion

This study documented the concepts of market failure, rationale of government intervention and its failure in terms of ensuring efficient resource allocation in health sector as the sector is prone to corruption because of the asymmetric information and moral hazard problems among the various actors take role in decision making. Moreover, cultural perceptions also impact on the types and level of corruption. In this regard, both grand and petty types of corruption may be encountered. In this regard, this study provided a literature review about the effects of corruption and studies which aim to reveal the majority of threat. Furthermore, the concept of money laundering and money laundering risks and methods posed by health sector corruption has been discussed.

It is demonstrated that the health sector is prone to money laundering, particularly when the fraudulent documentation is used in order to disguise the proceeds gained through corrupt acts. Case studies reveal that health professionals, bureaucrats, pharmaceutical companies and even hospitals might involve in corruption and money laundering cycle. Moreover, since the COVID-19 pandemic resulted in an increase in demand to health services including medicines and vaccines and non-face to face financial transactions has risen, money laundering risks have scaled up globally.

In order to fight against these threats, ensuring collaboration among the relevant bodies (bodies responsible for inspection of health sector service providers, financial regulation and supervision authorities, financial intelligence units, law enforcement units etc.) at national and international levels is a must. In addition, in order to estimate the volume of corruption and money laundering in the sector, both surveys and investigation based measurement techniques should be employed, sector's inherent and residual risks should be estimated and mitigation measures should be considered.

In regard to the situation in Turkey, statistical information should be improved to come up with a judgement about the scale of the risk. Taking into account the globally increased money laundering threats during the COVID-19 pandemic, the situation in Turkey should be further evaluated by relevant authorities.

References

Acemoğlu, D., & Verdier, T. (2000). The Choice between Market Failures and Corruption. *The American Economic Review*, 90(1), 194–211.

Akçay, S. (2006). Corruption and Human Development, *CATO Journal*, 26(1), 29–48.

Aktan, C. C. (1999). *Kirli Devletten Temiz Devlete*. Yeni Türkiye.

Arrow, K. J. (1963). Uncertainty and the Welfare Economics of Medical Care. *The American Economic Review*, 53(5), 941–973.

Azfar, O., & Gurgur, T. (2008). Does Corruption Affect Health Outcomes in the Philippines? *Economics of Governance*, 9, 197–244.

Baker, R. W. (2005). *Capitalism's Achille's Heel, Dirty Money and How to Renew the Free Market System*. Chichester: John Wiley and Son.

Bardhan, P. (1997), Corruption and Development: A Review of Issues,.*Journal of Economic Literature*, 35(3) September, 1320–1346.

Barr, N. A. (1993). *The Economics of the Welfare State*, 2nd Edition. Stanford University Press.

Begue, M. (2018). Colombia Battles Corruption within Healthcare System, https://america.cgtn.com/2018/11/20/colombia-battles-corruption-within-healthcare-system, Access date 01.02.2021.

Button, M., & Gee, J. (2015). *The Financial Cost of Healthcare Fraud 2015: What Data from around the World Shows*. University of Portsmouth Centre for Counter Fraud Studies.

Chika, A., Bello, S. O., Jimoh, A. O., & Umar, M. T. (2011). The Menace of Fake Drugs: Consequences, Causes and Possible Solutions. *Research Journal of Medical Sciences*, 5(5), 257–261.

Citibank (2016). *Trade Based Money Laundering*. White Paper.

Coase, R. H. (1979). Payola in Radio and Television Broadcasting. *Journal of Law and Economics*, 22(2), 269–328.

Couffinhal, A., & Frankowski, A. (2017). Wasting with Intention: Fraud, Abuse, Corruption and Other Integrity Violations in the Health Sector, in OECD (Ed.), *Tackling Wasteful Spending on Health* (1st Edition, pp. 265–301). OECD Publishing.

CRI Group. (2020). *Pharma Case Studies Uncovered – Due Diligence Lessons Learned*. E book.

Ensor, T., & Moreno, A. D. (2002). Corruption as a Challenge to Effective Regulation in the Health Sector in Saltman, in Busse, R. & Mossialos (Eds), *Regulating Entrepreneurial Behaviour in European Health Care Systems*. European Observatory on Health Care Systems Series.

European Commission. (2017). *Updated Study on Corruption in the Healthcare Sector*. Ecorys Nederland B.V.

Factor, R., & Kang, M. (2015). Corruption and Population Health Outcomes: An Analysis of Data from 133 Countries Using Structural Equation Modeling. *International Journal of Public Health*, 60(6), 633–641.

FATF (2006). *Trade Based Money Laundering*. FATF Secretariat.

FATF (2008). *Best Practices on Trade Based Money Laundering*. FATF Secretariat.

FATF (2010). *International Best Practices on Detecting and Preventing the Illicit Cross-Border Transportation of Cash and Bearer Negotiable Instruments.* FATF Secretariat.

FATF (2020). *COVID-Related Money Laundering and Terrorist Financing Risks and Policy Responses.* FATF Secretariat.

Frye, T., & Shleifer, A.(1997). The Invisible Hand and the Grabbing Hand, *AEA Papers,* 87(2), May, 354–358.

Gupta, S., Davoodi, H. R., & Tiongson E. R. (2001). Corruption and the Provision of Health Care and Education Services, in Abed, G. T. & Gupta, S. (Ed.) (1st Edition), *Governance, Corruption, Economic Performance.* IMF.

Health System Tracker (2020). *What Impact Has the Coronavirus Pandemic Had on Healthcare Employment?* https://www.healthsystemtracker.org/chart-col lection/what-impact-has-the-coronavirus-pandemic-had-on-healthcare-employment/#item-start, Access date 05.01.2021.

Holmberg, S., & Rothstein, B. (2011). Dying of Corruption. *Health Economics, Policy and Law,* 6(4), 529–547.

Huntington, S. P. (1968). *Political Order in Changing Societies.* New Haven, CT: Yale University Press.

Hussman, K. (2020). *Health Sector Corruption: Practical Recommendations for Donors.* U4 Anti-Corruption Resource Centre, I4, issue no. 2020:10. CHR Michelsen Institute.

IAIS (2004). *Examples of Money Laundering and Suspicious Transactions Involving Insurance,* https://iaisweb.org/file/34375/examples-of-money-lau ndering-october-, Access date 12.02.2021.

Jain, A. K. (1998). Corruption: Quantitative Estimates, in Jain, A. K. (Ed.), *Economics of Corruption.* Kluwer Academic Publishers, 13–34.

Kang, D. C. (2002). *Crony Capitalis, Corruption and Development in South Korea and the Philippines.* Cambridge University Press.

Kassirer, J. P. (2006) The Corrupting Influence of Money in Medicine, in Transparency International (Ed.), *Global Corruption Report 2006,* 85–90.

Kaufmann, D., & Vicente, P. (2005). *Legal Corruption,* World Bank Institute Working Paper, http://siteresources.worldbank.org/INTWBIGOVANTCOR/Resources/Legal_Corruption.pdf, Access date 10.06.2015.

Kirigia, J. M., & Diarra-Nama, A. J. (2008). Can Countries of the WHO African Region Wean Themselves Off Donor Funding for Health? *Bulletin of the World Health Organization,* 86(11), 889–895.

Klitgaard, R. (1988). *Controlling Corruption.* University of California Press.

Klitgaard, R. (1991). *Adjusting to Reality, Beyond State versus Market in Economic Development.* ICS Press.

KOM (2019). *Anti-Smuggling and Organized Crimes 2019 Report,* https://www.egm.gov.tr/kurumlar/egm.gov.tr/IcSite/kom/YAYINLARIMIZ/%C4%B0NG%C4%B0L%C4%B0ZCE/2019-ENGLISH-REPORT.pdf, Access date 08.12.2020.

Le Grand, J. (1991). The Theory of Government Failure. *Britsh Journal of Political Sciences.* 21(4), 423–442.

Leff, N. (1964). Economic Development through Bureacratic Corruption. *American Behavioral Scientist,* 8(3), 8–14.

Lewis, M. (2000). *Who Is Paying for Health Care in Eastern Europe and Central Asia?* The World Bank.

Mackey, T. K., Vian, T., & Kohler, J. (2018). The Sustainable Development Goals as a Framework to Combat Health-Sector Corruption. *Bull World Health Organ,* 96, 634–643.

Masciandaro, D. (2007). Economics: The Demand Side, in Masciandaro, D., Takats, E., & Unger, B. (Eds) (1st Edition, pp. 1–26), *Black Finance, the Economics of Money Laundering.* Edward Elgar.

Ministry of Justice (2019). *Judicial Statistics 2019,* https://adlisicil.adalet.gov.tr/Resimler/SayfaDokuman/1092020162733adalet_ist-2019.pdf, Access date 08.12.2020.

Moneyval (2010). *Money Laundering Through Private Pension Funds and the Insurance Sector.* Typology Research.

Mumcu, A. (2005). *Osmanlı Devletinde Rüşvet (Özellikle Adli Rüşvet)* (3rd Edition). İnkılap Yayınları.

Musgrave, R. A., & Musgrave, P. B. (1976). *Public Finance in Theory and Practice* (2nd Edition). McGraw-Hill.

OECD (2008). *Corruption, a Glossary of International Standards in Criminal Law.* OECD Glossaries.

Robinson, J. (1998). *The Laundrymen: Inside Money Laundering, the World's Third Largest Business* (Rev. Ed.). Simon & Schuster Ltd.

Rose-Ackerman, S. (1978). *Corruption – A Study in Political Economy.* New York, Academic Press.

Rose-Ackerman, S. (1999). *Corruption and Government, Causes, Concequences and Reform.* Cambridge University Press.

Savedoff, W. D., & Hussmann, K. (2006) Why Are Health Systems Prone to Corruption? in Transparency International (Ed.), *Global Corruption Report 2006*, 4–16.

Schultze, C. L. (1977). The Public Use of Private Interest. *AEI Journal on Government and Society, Regulation*, 10, 10–15.

Shah, A. (2007). Tailoring the Fight against Corruption to Country Circumstances, in Shah, A. (Ed.), *Performance Accountability and Combating Corruption* (1st Edition, pp. 233–254). The World Bank.

Shleifer, A., & Vishny, R. W. (1993). Corruption, *The Quarterly Journal of Economics*, 108(3), 599–617.

Shleifer, A., & Vishny, R. W. (1998). *The Grabbing Hand, Government Pathologies and their Cures*. Harvard University Press.

Sommer, J. M. (2020). Corruption and Health expenditure: A Cross-National Analysis on Infant and Child Mortality. *The European Journal of Development Research*, 32, 690–717.

Stapenhurst, R., & Sedigh, S. (1999). *Curbing Corruption toward a Model for Building National Integrity*. The World Bank.

Stiglitz, J. (2000). *Economics of the Public Sector* (3rd Edition). W.W. Norton & Company.

Şahin, İ., Özbek, M. A., Güran, C., & Tosun, M. U. (2009). Sağlık Sektöründe Yolsuzluk: Sağlık Bakanlığı Çalışanlarının Yolsuzluk Algılamaları. *Amme İdaresi Dergisi*, 42(4), 101–136.

TEPAV (2006). *Yolsuzlukla Mücadele*, TBMM Raporu Bir Olgu Olarak Yolsuzluk: Nedenler, Etkileri, Çözüm Önerileri, TEPAV Yolsuzlukla Mücadele Kitapları 1.

Tosun, M. U. (2002), Bir Kamusal Başarısızlık Ürünü Olarak Yolsuzluk in Cingi, S., Tosun, M. U. & Güran, C.(Eds), *Yolsuzluk ve Etkin Devlet* (1st Edition, pp. 17–106). ATO Yayınları.

Transparency International (2000). *Source Book 2000: Confronting Corruption*. The Elements of a National Integrity System, Access date 11.02.2021

Transparency International (2013). *Global Corruption Barometer 2013*.

Treisman, D. (2000). The Causes of Corruption: A Cross National Study. *Journal of Public Economics*, 76, 399–457.

U4 Anti-Corruption Resource Centre (2008). *Corruption in the Health Sector*, I4, issue no 2008:10. CHR Michelsen Institute.

UNDP (2011). *Fighting Corruption in the Health Sector: Methods, Tools and Good Practices*. UNDP.

US Department of Justice (2021a). *National Health Care Fraud Takedown Results in Charges Against 601 Individuals Responsible for Over $2 Billion in Fraud Losses*, https://www.justice.gov/opa/pr/national-health-care-fraud-taked own-results-charges-against-601-individuals-responsible-over, Access date 05.01.2021.

US Department of Justice (2021b). *Three Charged in $180 Million Health Care Fraud and Money Laundering Scheme*, https://www.justice.gov/opa/pr/three-charged-180-million-health-care-fraud-and-money-laundering-scheme, Access date 05.01.2021.

US Treasury (2018). *National Money Laundering Risk Assessment*, https://home.treasury.gov/system/files/136/2018NMLRA_12-18.pdf, Access date 17.05.2019.

Vian, T. (2005). The Sectoral Dimensions of Corruption: Health Care. in Spector B.I. (Ed.), *Fighting Corruption in Developing Countries: Strategies and Analysis*, Bloomfield, CT: Kumarian Press Inc.

Vian, T. (2008). Review of Corruption in the Health Sector: Theory, Methods and Interventions. *Health Policy and Planning*, 23, 83–94.

Vian, T. (2020). Anti-corruption, Transparency and Accountability in Health: Concepts, Frameworks, and Approaches, *Global Health Action*, 13, 1–24.

WHO (2006). New Report on Corruption in Health. *Bulletin of the World Health Organization*. 84(2), 84–87.

WHO (2020). *Potential Corruption Risks in Health Financing Arrangements: Report of a Rapid Review of the Literature*, https://www.who.int/publications/i/item/potential-corruption-risks-in-health-financing-arrangements-report-of-a-rapid-review-of-the-literature, Access date 14.03.2021.

Willebois, E., Halter., E., Harrison, R., Park, J. W., & Scharman, J. C. (2011). *The Puppet Masters, How the Corrupt Use Legal Structures to Hide Stolen Assets and What to Do About It?* StAR Initiative.

Wolf, C. Jr. (1978). *A Theory of Non Market Failure Framework for Implementation Analysis*, The RAND Paper Series, P-6034, California.

World Bank (1997). *Helping Countries Combat Corruption: The Role of the World Bank*. Poverty Reduction and Economic Management Report, http://www1.worldbank.org/publicsector/anticorrupt/corrptn/corrptn.pdf, Access date 14.02.2019.

Yıldırım, H. H. (1999). Piyasa, Sağlık Bakımı ve Piyasa Başarısızlıkları. Amme İdaresi Dergisi, 32(1), 1–9.

Yurdakul, M. O. (2013). Uluslararası Sözleşmeler ve Avrupa Birliği Hukuku Çerçevesinde Suç Kaynaklı Malvarlıklarının Geri Alınması, Ülke Uygulamaları ve Türkiye İle Mukayese, MASAK Yayınları, No. 23.

Yurdakul, M. O. (2015). Aklanan Suç Gelirlerinin Ekonomik Boyutu ve Aklama ile Mücadelede Önleyici Tedbirlerin Finansal Gelişim Düzeyi Üzerindeki Etkileri Konulu Yatay Kesit Veri Analizi. *Bankacılar Dergisi*, 94, 40–64.

Ayşe Nur Songür Bozdağ

Funda Pınar Çakıroğlu

Diabetes in Turkey: A Review of Economic Burden and Medical Nutrition Therapy of the Disease

Introduction

Chronic diseases that affect people throughout their lives, that have various anthropic, financial, social negative effects and that require long term and costly care are defined as non-communicable diseases (NCD) (Wang et al., 2016). Due to changes in personal lifestyle, environmental factors, ageing, changes in eating habits, increased lifespan, non-communicable diseases such as cardiovascular diseases (CVD), cancer, chronic respiratory diseases and diabetes have become the primary causes of deaths around the world over the recent years (Health Institutes of Turkey, 2018). These four primary non-communicable diseases are responsible for approximately 82.0 % of deaths caused by NCDs (Republic of Turkey Ministry of Health and World Health Organization European Office, 2017). In 2012, approximately 65.5 % of deaths worldwide (Lozano et al., 2012) and approximately 87.5 % of deaths between the ages of 30 and 70 in Turkey (Turkish Statistical Institute, 2012) were caused by non-communicable diseases.

Diabetes, prevalence of which has increased in recent years, similar to other NCDs and which has become one of the biggest health problems of 21st century, is a serious chronic disease that occurs when pancreas fails to produce enough insulin or the body fails to utilize the produced insulin (WHO, 2016). According to the statistics in International Diabetes Federation (IDF) Diabetes Atlas, there are 451 million diabetes patients (18–99 years) living in the world as of 2017 and it is estimated that this number will reach 693 million in the year 2045 (Chou et al., 2018).

Diabetes, which was first classified by World Health Organization (WHO) in the year 1980, consists of four commonly used clinical types: Type 1 diabetes (T1D), Type 2 diabetes (T2D), other specific types of diabetes and gestational diabetes (ADA, 2020). Majority of diabetes patients consist of people with

T1D and T2D (Public Health Institution of Turkey, 2014). It is commonly seen in middle and advanced ages, however, in recent years, T2D cases have been observed in younger people. As obesity becomes more prevalent, a rapid increase in especially T2D is expected (Balkau & Eschwège, 2003).

Diabetes does not just affect the individual patient but also the family and the entire society. If the hyperglycaemia in diabetes is not controlled properly, besides acute complications, chronic complications that threaten health over the long term and that are life threatening such as retinopathy, nephropathy, neuropathy occur. Each year, the number of people who suffer from diabetes and complications caused by diabetes increase, quality of life of individuals significantly decrease and this situation creates economic burdens on both governments and individuals (Tuchman, 2009; IDF, 2015). Most of the economic burdens related to diabetes are caused by hospitalizations due to acute and chronic complications. World Health Organization foresees that the global diabetes spending will increase each passing year (WHO, 2016). According to IDF, 12.0 % (727 billion dollars) of global health spending in 2017 was spent for diabetes (IDF, 2017). When Turkey is considered, according to the year of 2012 data of Republic of Turkey Social Security Institution, the total cost of diabetes patients were 9,992.88 million TL and approximately 22.6 % of total health spending were allocated for diabetes (Republic of Turkey Ministry of Health, 2016).

Researches show that diabetes complications can be reduced with proper diabetes control. Each 1 mmol/L decrease in fasting blood glucose corresponds to 23.0 % reduced risk of CVD (Lawes, 2004) while each 1 % increase in HbA1c can cause 20–30 % increase in mortality and CVD risk (Khaw et al., 2004). 5–10 % decrease in body weight in moderately overweight and overweight individuals provides increased glycemic control and decreases the risk of CVD (ADA, 2017).

One of the most important components of diabetes control is Medical Nutrition Therapy (MNT). The purpose of MNT is to maintain metabolic equilibrium and the intake of necessary nutrients by control blood glucose levels and lipid profiles and to reduce risks of acute and chronic complications. With an effective MNT, patients see weight loss and improvements in blood glucose levels, blood pressure and blood lipids, thus, HbA1c is lowered and accordingly, complications related to diabetes are reduced (ADA, 2014).

In this research, in light of information in literature, the current status and economic burden of diabetes and medical nutrition therapy used in the treatment of diabetes will be evaluated.

I. What Is Diabetes? What Are Its Diagnosis and Screening Criteria, Types and Risk Factors?

A. *Definition and Epidemiology*

Diabetes is a metabolic disease that causes acute metabolic and chronic degenerative complications that is the result of total or partial deficiency of insulin hormone, which is secreted by the pancreas and which regulates the use of blood glucose in body and it is characterized by hyperglycaemia and progresses with dysfunctions in carbohydrate, lipid, protein metabolisms (Public Health Institution of Turkey, 2014; Turkish Diabetes Foundation, 2019).

Diabetes is accepted as an important public health problem as its prevalence rapidly increases, both in Turkey and in the world and as it frequently affects the adult age group. It is foreseen that the number of individuals with diabetes will reach 578 million in 2030 and in 2045, it will increase by 50 % to 700 million individuals. The regions with highest diabetes prevalence are Middle East, America and South East Asia (Public Health Institution of Turkey, 2014). It is estimated that 59 million people had diabetes in 2019 in Europe and this number will reach 68 million while the 6.6 million people with diabetes in Turkey will rise to 10.4 million in 2045. Age-standardized diabetes prevalence in Turkey is 11.1 % while it is 6.3 % in IDF Europe region and 8.3 % worldwide. Among European countries, Turkey was the country with the highest prevalence of diabetes in the 20–79 age group in 2019 and was followed by Germany (10.4 %) and Portugal (9.8 %). Germany ranked first with 9.5 million diabetes patients and was followed by Russian Federation (8.3 million) and Turkey (6.6 million). When mortalities related to diabetes is analysed, mortality rate in individuals under 60 years of age was 29.3 % in Turkey, 31.2 % in IDF Europe region and 46.2 % in the world (IDF, 2019).

The first study conducted in Turkey to determine the prevalence of diabetes between the years of 1997 and 1998 was Turkish Diabetes Epidemiology Study I (TURDEP-I) and the second study was TURDEP-II conducted in 2012 (International Diabetes Leadership Forum, 2013). According to the TURDEP-I study, the diabetes prevalence in Turkey was 7.2 % (2.6 million), the prevalence of impaired glucose tolerance (IGT) was 6.7 %. According to TURDEP-II study, it was determined that the prevalence of diabetes increased by 90 % to 13.7 % (6.5 million adults). In TURDEP-II the regional diabetes prevalence was the lowest in Northern Anatolia with 14.5 % and the highest in Eastern Anatolia with 18.2 %. When the diabetes prevalence was evaluated according to age groups, it was determined that at least 10 % of the population from the age group 40–44 and upwards had diabetes (Public Health Institution of Turkey, 2014).

According to the data of Heart Diseases and Risk Factors in Turkish Adults study (TEKHARF) published in 2009, diabetes prevalence in the population over the age of 35 was estimated to be 11.3 % (3.3 million) (Onat, 2009). According to the PURE-Turkey (The Prospective Urban Rural Epidemiology – Turkey) study published in 2018, diabetes prevalence in Turkey rose to 21 % (Oğuz et al., 2018).

B. Diagnosis and Screening Criteria

There are various indicators and symptoms in diagnosing diabetes. The primary indicators and symptoms are dry mouth, polyphagia (increased appetite) or lack of appetite, polydipsia (increased thirst), polyuria (increased urination), nocturia (waking up at night once or multiple times with a need to urinate), weight loss, blurred vision, numbness, tingling, burning in feet, urinary tract infections, vulvovaginitis (inflammation or irritation of vagina or vulva), fungal infections, itchiness, dryness of skin and fatigue (TEMS, 2019). Various diagnosis methods are used along with these clinical indicators and symptoms. Those methods are presented in the Tab. 1:

Tab. 1. Diagnostic criteria of diabetes mellitus and other disorders of glucose metabolism [*] (TEMS, 2019)

	Overt DM	Isolated IFG	Isolated IGT	IFG + IGT	High Risk Group for DM
FPG (≥8 hr fasting)	≥126 mg/dl	100–125 mg/dl	<100 mg/dl	100–125 mg/dl	-
OGTT 2 hr PG (75 g glucose)	≥200 mg/dl	<140 mg/dl	140–199 mg/dl	140–199 mg/dl	-
Random PG	≥200 mg/dl + Diabetes symptoms	-	-	-	-
A1c[**]	≥6.5 % (≥48 mmol/mol)	-	-	-	5.7–6.4 % (39–47 mmol/mol)

Notes: [*]Glycaemia measured in venous plasma using glucose oxidase method, and quantified as "mg/dL." Either one of four diagnostic criteria is sufficient for "Overt DM" diagnosis, whereas, both criteria are required for "Isolated IFG", "Isolated IGT", and "IFG+IGT". [**] Must be measured with a standardized method.
DM: Diabetes mellitus, FPG: Fasting plasma glucose, 2 hr PG: 2 hour plasma glucose, OGTT: Oral glucose tolerance test, A1c: Glycated haemoglobin A1c, IFT: Impaired fasting glucose, IGT: Impaired glucose tolerance

Measurement of fasting plasma glucose (FPG): It is the measurement of plasma glucose following a fasting of at least 8 hours through the night. If FPG level is 126 mg/dL or above, diabetes is diagnosed. It is an inexpensive and easy method to apply. American Diabetes Association defined the situation in which fasting blood glucose is between 100–126 mg/dL as "Impaired Fasting Glucose (IFG)" (Ovayolu & Ovayolu, 2016).

Oral glucose tolerance test (OGTT): The test with the highest sensitivity that is used for diabetes diagnosis. If the blood glucose level is 200 mg/dL after 2 hours of consuming a liquid with 75 grams of glucose, diabetes diagnosis becomes definite (Ovayolu & Ovayolu, 2016).

Random blood glucose measurement: Diabetes is diagnosed if the plasma glucose level is 200 mg/dL or above when measured at a random time with the existence of diabetes symptoms. (Public Health Institution of Turkey, 2014).

Glycated haemoglobin (A1c): A1c denotes the glucose that is attached to haemoglobin. HbA1c value of $\geq$6.5 % (48 mmol/mol) is accepted as a threshold value for diabetes diagnosis. The advantages of HbA1c are the facts that it does not require fasting and it does not vary during situations such as acute diseases or stress. Its disadvantages are the facts that it is expensive, it is not as common as plasma glucose measurement, it is affected by hemolysis and anaemia (Public Health Institution of Turkey, 2017).

C. Types of Diabetes (Classification) and Risk Factors

Diabetes is etiologically classified into 4 types as Type 1 diabetes, Type 2 diabetes, other specific types and gestational diabetes (Tab. 2).

Tab. 2. American Diabetes Association (ADA) Classification of Diabetes (2020)

Type 1 Diabetes	Beta cell destruction that commonly leads to total insulin deficiency - Autoimmune - Idiopathic
Type 2 Diabetes	Insulin resistance, relative insulin deficiency, insulin secretory defect with insulin resistance
Other Specific Types	- Genetic defects of Beta cell functions - Genetic defects in insulin action - Diseases of exocrine pancreas - Endocrinopathies - Drug or chemical induced diabetes - Infections - Uncommon forms of immune-mediated diabetes - Other genetic syndromes sometimes associated with diabetes
Gestational Diabetes	- Carbohydrate intolerance defined during pregnancy

1. Type 1 Diabetes

Type 1 diabetes is the type of diabetes that causes insulin deficiency as a result of autoimmune destruction of beta cells in pancreas and presents with hyperglycaemia and ketoacidosis. The incidence of T1D is continuing to increase worldwide. Approximately 5–10 % of all diabetes cases are T1D cases (ADA, 2014). 90 % of the patients have autoimmune causes while 10 % have idiopathic causes. T1D is one of the most common chronic diseases observed in children and the age group with the most prevalence is ages 10–15 (Boztepe, 2012; Eroğlu, 2017). Number of newly diagnosed T1D patients in the ages 0–19 group in Turkey is 2.8 thousand, in IDF Europe region is 31.1 thousand and in the world is 1.110.100 thousand (IDF, 2019).

The most common symptoms of T1D are extreme thirst, blurry vision, frequent urination, fatigue, extreme hunger and rapid weight loss (IDF, 2019). Patients are usually underweight or normal weight and are prone to diabetic ketoacidosis (DKA) (TEMS, 2019). Even though the exact cause is unknown, the risk factors are:

Genetics: T1D is seen in genetically susceptible individuals. There is a multifactorial inheritance rather than a mendelian inheritance (Haller et al., 2005). It is stated that if the mother has T1D, her children has a 2 % risk of diabetes while if the father has T1D, his children has a 7 % risk of diabetes (Hämäläinen & Knip, 2002). Multiple genes related to T1D were determined. It is stated that genes in the gene region of human leukocyte antigens (HLA) on the 6. chromosome that causes genetic susceptibility to T1D are related to genetic susceptibility or prevention (Demirbilek, 2018).

Autoimmunity: T1D occurs due to the destruction of Beta cells which are responsible for insulin synthesis and secretion, via autoimmune mechanisms. Environmental and genetic factors play parts for the start of this autoimmune destruction (Haller et al., 2005; Hämäläinen & Knip, 2002). Antibodies that affect diabetes development are antibodies such as islet cell antibodies (ICAs), glutamic acid decarboxylase (GAD65A) and transmembrane protein tyrosine phosphatase (Abacı et al., 2007).

Environmental factors: It is thought that T1D not occurring in everyone with genetic risk shows that environmental factors that start autoimmune events have effects. One or more environmental factors may cause the disease to occur in individuals with genetic susceptibility (Köksal and Özel, 2019). Primary environmental factors responsible for the occurrence of the illness are diet, past infections, hygiene and toxins and it is stated that the exposure time to these factors and diabetes occurrence have a relation (Haller et al., 2005). Moreover, it is also stated that psychological stress is a risk factor for T1D (Sharif et al., 2018).

2. Type 2 Diabetes

Type 2 diabetes (T2D) is the most common type of diabetes and is characterized with hyperglycaemia, insulin resistance and relative insulin deficiency. Approximately 90 % of all diabetes cases are T2D (Maitra and Abbas, 2005; Turkish Diabetes Foundation, 2017). T2D has high morbidity and mortality due to complications such as cardiovascular risk and kidney failure and is becoming a more important health problem due to increased prevalence (Feero and Guttmacher, 2010). T2D more often occurs after the age of 30, however, as obesity has increased and daily activities have changed over the last 10–15 years, T2D showed and increase in children and adolescent individuals (TEMS, 2015; WHO, 2016).

T2D presents sneakily and the patients continue their lives for a long time without diagnosis. The complaints of individuals are similar to T1D but milder. Therefore, the disease is detected years after its original beginning and sometimes it is diagnosed after its complications occur (Durna, 2013). It is stated that 1/3-1/2 of T2D cases aren't diagnosed and therefore aren't treated (Engelgau et al., 2000).

The development of T2D is multifactorial: Socio-demographic risk factors (age, ethnicity etc.), genetic risk factors, body weight, intrauterine and early childhood periods, risk factors associated with nutrition, risk factors associated with lifestyle (exercise, smoking etc.)

Age: Risk of T2D increase significantly with age. The reasons for this are the facts that people exercise less as they age, people lose muscle mass as they age and they tend to gain weight. However, over the recent years the occurrence age of T2D has dropped to younger adults and even adolescents (Alberti et al., 2007).

Ethnicity: It is determined that Asians, Hispanics and African Americans have higher risks of diabetes compared to Caucasians (Shai et al., 2006).

Socio-economic status: It is stated that the T2D risk is increased in individuals of lower socioeconomic status including lower levels of education, employment and income (Agardh et al., 2011). Even though the causes of the relationship between T2D and socioeconomic status are not completely known, it is thought that socioeconomic status may cause problems in accessing healthcare, healthy foods, places to exercise etc., and cause an unhealthy lifestyle, thus contributing to T2D development (Brown et al., 2004).

Genetics: Increased T2D risk is associated with family history of diabetes. When compared to individuals without family history of T2D, it is stated that individuals with a history of diabetes in a first degree relative have 2–3 times the risk of developing diabetes (The InterAct Consortium, 2013).

Body weight: Increased body weight and body fat are among the biggest risk factors of type 2 diabetes (Menke et al., 2015). It is found that weight gain during young adulthood between the ages 25 and 40 has a stronger relationship to diabetes risk than weight gain during late adulthood between the ages 40 and 55. Correction of obesity, which is among the redeemable risk factors, reduces the risk of T2D (Schienkiewitz et al., 2006).

Intrauterine and early childhood period: Children who are exposed to maternal diabetes during intrauterine period have a higher possibility of becoming overweight in childhood and having impaired glucose tolerance (IGT) during young adulthood (Baz et al., 2016; Lawlor et al., 2011).

A significant relationship between birth weight and T2D risk is determined. Compared to normal birth weight (2500–4000 g), lower birth weight (<2500 g) is determined to be related to high T2D risk. Additionally, it is also presented that when the birth weight is above 4000 g, the risk of diabetes also increases (Harder et al., 2007). Mean childhood period body mass index is also determined as a risk factor independent of birth weight (Bjerregaard et al., 2018). It is stated that during infancy, short term severe malnutrition may increase T2D risk in adulthood (van Abeelen et al., 2012).

Risk factors associated with nutrition: Factors increasing diabetes risk associated with nutrition are Western diet, red meat, processed meats, high energy density foods, refined grains or sugar sweetened drinks. Factors reducing diabetes risk associated with nutrition are Mediterranean diet, plant-based foods, fermented milk products, milk-yoghurt consumption, hazelnuts, whole grains, diet rich in olive oil, consumption of green leafy vegetables, fruits, foods rich in anthocyanin and coffee. On the other hand, grain fibres are shown to have a preventative effect against T2D development (Al-Goblan et al., 2014; Carter et al., 2010; Ding et al., 2014; Koning et al., 2011; Tong et al., 2011; Wedick et al., 2012; Wu et al., 2014).

Smoking: Even though the underlying mechanism is not completely explained, it is determined that smokers have a higher risk of developing T2D than non-smokers (Willi et al., 2007). Additionally, it is stated that being exposed to second hand smoke at work or home is also associated with increased risk of developing diabetes (Zhang et al., 2011).

Exercise: It is stated that physical inactivity is responsible for 7 % of T2D cases worldwide (Lee et al., 2012; WHO, 2010). Sedentary lifestyle of continuous, long duration TV watching is associated with obesity and diabetes development (Grøntved & Hu, 2011). It is known that medium and high intensity exercise has beneficial effects on preventing T2D (Meisinger et al., 2005).

Sleep: Researches show that common sleep disorders are associated with risk of T2D development. People with especially short (shorter than 5–6 hours) and long (longer than 8–9 hours) sleep durations have a higher risk of developing T2D (Cappuccio et al., 2010).

3. Other Specific Types

These are types of diabetes that are not related to type 1 and type 2 diabetes and their aetiologies are known (Tab. 2). In this group, the causes of diabetes development are situations that disrupt the beta cell function and insulin secretion of pancreas (pancreas diseases, hormonal disorders, medications, chemical agents, insulin receptor anomalies, genetic syndromes) (ADA, 2020).

4. Gestational Diabetes

Gestational diabetes mellitus (GDM) is the glucose tolerance disorder that first occurs during pregnancy. GDM usually develops after the 24th week of pregnancy due to the increase of insulin resistance caused by placenta hormones (Public Health Institution of Turkey, 2017). It is seen in 2–5 % of all pregnancies (Ovayolu & Ovayolu, 2016). Today, the prevalence of GDM is increasing and correspondingly, development of maternal and perinatal complications are also increasing (Özkaya and Köse, 2014). Even though GDM gets better after birth, those women need to be followed after birth as they have increased risk of T2D development (Public Health Institution of Turkey, 2017).

II. Complications of Diabetes

Many biochemical, morphological and functional changes occur in the tissues and organs of individuals with diabetes. If diabetes is not managed properly, health threatening complications develop. These complications are classified into two as acute and chronic (ADA, 2015) (Figure 1).

```
┌─────────────────────────────┐        ┌─────────────────────────────┐
│                             │        │                             │
│     Acute Complications     │        │    Chronic Complications    │
│                             │        │                             │
└─────────────────────────────┘        └─────────────────────────────┘
```

┌─────────────────────────────┐   ┌─────────────────────────────────┐
│   *Hypoglycemia   │   │ Macrovascular Complications   │
│   *Diabetic Ketoacidosis   │   │   *Cardiovascular Diseases   │
│ *Hyperosmolar Hyperglycemic │   │   *Cerebrovascular Diseases   │
│   Nonketotic Coma   │   │ *Peripheral Vascular Diseases │
└─────────────────────────────┘   └─────────────────────────────────┘

                                       ┌─────────────────────────────────┐
                                       │ Microvascular Complications   │
                                       │   *Retinopathy   │
                                       │   *Nephropathy   │
                                       │   *Neuropathy   │
                                       │   *Diabetic Foot   │
                                       └─────────────────────────────────┘

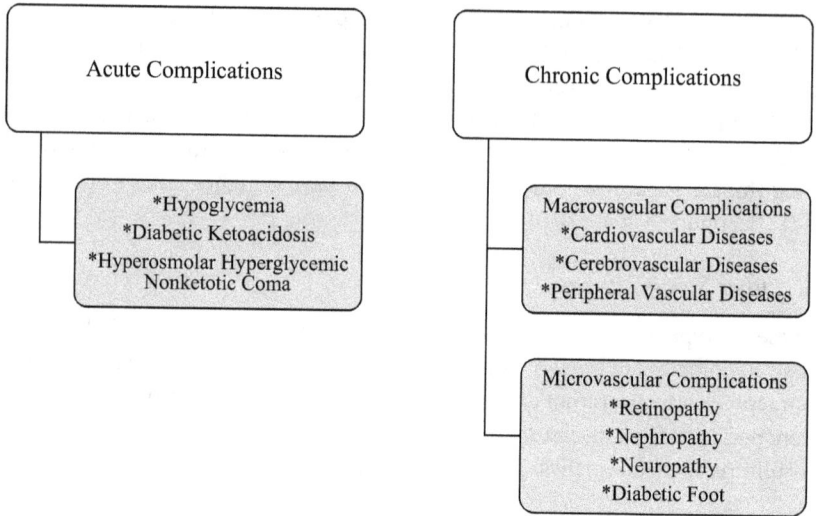

Fig. 1. Complications of Diabetes (ADA, 2015)

A. Acute Complications

1. Hypoglycaemia

It is one of the acute complications that is seen especially in patients that use insulin and is the biggest obstacle of tight glycemic control and one of the most feared complications. It is accepted as the blood glucose level below 70 mg/dL (TEMS, 2019). Among the causes of hypoglycaemia are overdosing insulin, timing errors in insulin application, inappropriate insulin choice, use of high doses of oral antidiabetics, adrenal failure, over exercising, insufficient energy intake due to diarrhoea and vomiting, skipping meals, insufficient carbohydrate intake and increase in insulin sensitivity (Turkish Diabetes Foundation, 2017). Hypoglycaemia causes symptoms such as shivering, cold sweating, anxiety, tachycardia, numbness and hunger, vertigo, headache, clammy skin, paleness, mental changes, lack of concentration, difficulty speaking and fatigue (TEMS, 2019). If no precautions are taken, these symptoms may be followed by blurry vision, loss of concentration, clouding of consciousness or even loss of consciousness (Ovayolu & Ovayolu, 2016). For treatment of hypoglycaemia, if the patient in conscious, 15–20 g of glucose should be administered orally. In an unconscious patient with impaired chewing-swallowing functions, parenteral treatment must be used. Patient who receive insulin treatment must be educated for hypoglycaemia (Turkish Diabetes Foundation, 2019).

2. Diabetic Ketoacidosis (DKA)

DKA is a complication that is resulted by significant decrease in insulin or complete lack of insulin and is characterized by hyperglycaemia, dehydration, loss of electrolytes, high ketone levels in urine and acidosis. Infections, errors in infection technique, expired insulin, quitting insulin treatment, use of medication that disrupts carbohydrate tolerance, alcohol and cerebrovascular events play roles in its development (Eroğlu, 2017). DKA starts with nausea, vomiting, stomach ache, excessive hydration, excessive urination complaints and may develop to cloudiness of consciousness and coma and it may require emergency intervention (Akdemir & Birol, 2011). DKA is managed by fluid and electrolyte treatment, insulin treatment and treatment of the underlying causes (Farsani et al., 2017).

3. Hyperosmolar Hyperglycemic Nonketotic Coma

Hyperosmolar hyperglycemic syndrome (HHS) is a complication characterized by dehydration, loss of consciousness caused by lack of hydration due to diuresis. In contrast with DKA, there are no ketones in the urine or the plasma and plasma glucose levels and osmolarity are high (Yılmaz et al., 2003). Reasons such as chronic diseases, infections, cerebrovascular diseases, alcohol and trauma are among the reasons of HHS occurrence (Pasquel & Umpierrez, 2014). The treatment of HHS is similar to that of DKA and consists of fluid replacement, correcting electrolyte imbalance and administering insulin. Moreover, patients may require airway support, nasogastric aspiration (Ul Abideen et al., 2017).

B. Chronic Complications

1. Macrovascular Complications

a. Cardiovascular Diseases

Cardiovascular diseases (CVD) are the most important reasons of morbidity and mortality in diabetes patients. Primary cardiovascular diseases seen in diabetes are hypertension, myocardial infarction, coronary artery disease (CAD), heart failure and cardiomyopathy. It is though that in development of cardiovascular complications, endothelial dysfunction and accelerated atherosclerosis occurring in diabetes patients have a large effect (Bernstein, 2008). The incidence of cardiovascular diseases in diabetes patients are 2–4 times more frequent (Turkish

Diabetes Foundation, 2019). CVD screening in diabetic patients must be done using resting electrocardiography. Stress test must be applied for individuals with symptoms or other accompanying diseases (Shaw & Iskandrian, 2004).

b. Cerebrovascular Diseases

Incidence rates of cerebrovascular diseases in addition to coronary artery disease is also increased in diabetes patients and it is seen more frequently in people with diabetes compared to the normal population. 25 % of diabetes patients die from cerebrovascular diseases. Advanced age, atherosclerosis, hyperlipidaemia and the existence of cardiac diseases may increase the risk of cerebrovascular diseases (Biberoğlu, 2003).

c. Peripheral Vascular Complications

Metabolic status change in diabetes causes pro-atherogenic changes that affect the structure and functions of veins. Peripheral vascular diseases (PVD) that are characterized by atherosclerotic clogging disease of lower extremities are frequently seen in diabetes (Huysman & Mathieu, 2009). Peripheral vascular diseases (PVD) start at a much earlier age in people with diabetes compared to nondiabetics and it progresses worse. 20 % of symptomatic patients with PVD have diabetes (Hiatt, 2001). Medical treatment has no role in the treatment of PVD, stent and graft applications are preferred (İlicin et al., 2003).

2. Microvascular Complications

a. Retinopathy

Retinopathy is a complication that causes functional and structural changes in retina and it is the most important preventable and/or treatable reason for blindness that is seen in the age group of 20–65 years worldwide. It is developed due to micro-occlusions and vascular permeability disruptions (Önmez, 2017). Factors that accelerate the development of retinopathy are bad glycemic control, especially with diabetes age, puberty, pregnancy, hypertension, hypothyroidism, dyslipidaemia, inflammation, anaemia, pregnancy and alcohol use (ADA, 2019). As retinopathy may progress slowly, symptoms such as blurry vision or loss of vision may not be seen in patients until it develops into macular edema and/ or proliferative diabetic retinopathy. Therefore, after the individual is diagnosed with diabetes, follow up exams (at least once a year) are important for early diagnosis (Durna & Akın, 2012). For protection against retinopathy, optimal glycemic control, blood pressure control and lipid control are extremely important. Medical treatment is limited to blood glucose control. If there is hypertension, it must be treated aggressively. Retinal photocoagulation is the most common treatment method (Satman, 2007).

b. Nephropathy

Diabetic nephropathy is the most important cause of morbidity and mortality and is seen in 20–40 % of patients with diabetes (Tuttle et al., 2014). Diabetic nephropathy, which has been determined as the most common cause of kidney disease recently, primarily occurs due to damage of intraglomerular arterioles (Ivanac-Janković et al., 2019). Diabetic nephropathy is clinically characterized with hypertension, edema, proteinuria and kidney failure. Early sign of diabetic nephropathy is increased urine albumin discharge. In prevention and treatment of diabetic nephropathy, glycemic control and optimal blood pressure control are very important. In individuals with diabetes, lifestyle changes such as salt and protein restriction, blood pressure and blood glucose level control, regular exercise, quitting smoking and alcohol should be ensured (ADVANCE Collaborative Group, 2008).

c. Neuropathy

Neuropathy, which is the most common chronic complication of diabetes, is an important complication that shows symptoms related to peripheral or autonomous nervous system by affecting the nervous system, lowers the quality of life of patients and progresses with high morbidity and mortality (Turkish Diabetes Foundation, 2019). It is thought that lipotoxicity or high blood sugar toxicity cause the development of neuropathy (Kasper et al., 2015). Neuropathy especially affects lower extremities and is the most important cause of foot amputations along with infection and ischemia (TEMS, 2019). Diabetic neuropathy can be classified into two groups as peripheral and autonomous neuropathy. Peripheral neuropathy is very common and affects peripheral nerves. Autonomous neuropathy affects cardiovascular, genitourinary and gastrointestinal nerves (Katsarou et al., 2017).

There is no specific treatment for neuropathy occurring in diabetes however, it is shown a good glycemic control slows the start of neuropathy by 70 % and progression of early neuropathy by 57 %. Additionally, blood pressure control, lipid profile control, lifestyle changes and proper foot care are very important in treatment (Tesfaye et al., 2010).

d. Diabetic Foot

It is defined as the impairment of foot health due to neuropathy, micro and macrovascular complications caused by diabetes. The most important cause is not noticing repeated trauma due to the numbness caused by diabetic neuropathy (Eldor et al., 2004). The purposes of diabetic foot treatment are protecting tissue integrity, preventing complications that may develop in other organs and systems, preventing the development of new ulcers and infections and ensuring the fastest recovery of the scar with a good scar care. Regular following after diagnosis and education of the individual with diabetes in preventive behaviours are important (Ovayolu & Ovayolu, 2016).

III. Treatment of Diabetes

Patients with diabetes require lifelong care and specialist treatment. A successful diabetes treatment and control is only possible with medicine treatment, medical nutrition therapy (MNT), regular exercise schedule, diabetes education and proper coordination of individual blood sugar monitoring (Eroğlu, 2017).

A. Medical Treatment

1. Antihyperglycemic (Oral Antidiabetic and Insulinmimetic) Drugs other than Insulin

As blood glucose of individuals with T2D cannot be controlled with diet and exercise, oral antidiabetics (OAD) are used for these patients. With appropriate oral antidiabetic choice, the aim is to keep the fasting blood sugar and HbA1c of the individual within target limits (Çubuk & İnce, 2015). OADs usually work by increasing insulin secretion from pancreas, increasing insulin sensitivity or reducing carbohydrate absorption in intestines (Atmaca & Ecemiş, 2012). If the desired glycemic target cannot be reached with the use of a single drug, combination drug treatment is applied. If the desired glycemic target cannot be reached even with combination treatment, insulin therapy must be started. It is not recommended to use OADs in T1D or during pregnancy (Kasper et al., 2015).

2. Insulin Therapy

Insulin is a protein secreted by pancreas cells. It facilitates the entry of glucose into cells, increases glycogen storage, prevents hepatic glucose output, increases peripheral and hepatic insulin sensitivity and prevents the destruction of fats and proteins (TEMS, 2019). Insulin therapy is applied when diet and OAD combinations fail to provide desired glycemic control, when glycemic control is disrupted due to various stress sources, when acute and chronic complications develop, in situations such as pregnancy, surgery and severe hyperglycaemia and also in all T1D patients (Tüfekçi Alphan, 2013).

When insulin doses for individuals are determined, the age of the individual, their body weight, the socioeconomic and psychological situation of the family must be taken into consideration. Insulin is generally used subcutaneously (Public Health Institution of Turkey, 2014). Insulin intake are done through multiple daily injections to simulate endogenous insulin physiology or through an insulin pump (Biester et al., 2018).

Insulins are classified according to the onset of action, peak effect and duration of action (TEMS, 2019). Short acting insulins have onsets of action after 30–60 minutes of injection, their peak effect occurs after 2–4 hours and their duration of action is 5–8 hours. Short acting insulin must be applied 30 minutes before eating. Rapid acting insulins have onsets of action after 15 minutes of injection, they reach peak effect in 30–90 minutes and their duration of action is 3–5 hours. Rapid acting insulins are usually applied before meals (Swinnen et al., 2009). Intermediate acting insulins have onsets between 1–3 hours, they peak in 8 hours and their duration of action is 12–16 hours (TEMS, 2019). There is a high risk of nocturnal hypoglycaemia. Long-acting insulins provide 24 hours of basal insulin level. Their use have low risk of hypoglycaemia. Long-acting insulins are applied at the same time everyday regardless of meals. As the regular insulin in those mixed insulins have late onsets, they are required to be injected half an hour before meals (usually breakfast and dinner) (Swinnen et al., 2009).

The most important and most common side effect in insulin therapy is hypoglycaemia and other side effects are weight gain, massive hepatomegaly, edema, immunogenicity, lipohypertrophy-atrophy, bleeding, leakage, pain, hyperinsulinemia, atherosclerosis and risk of cancer (TEMS, 2019). During diabetes treatment, patients who start insulin therapy should be educated on recognizing, preventing and treating hypoglycaemia. Patient should be educated on dose titration. After beginning insulin therapy, glucose monitoring should continue after reaching ideal blood glucose (TEMS, 2019).

B. Medical Nutrition Therapy

Medical nutrition therapy (MNT) is the sufficient and balanced nutrition program designed towards the needs of the individual and it is an inseparable part of diabetes treatment. MNT creates healthy dietary habits in diabetes patients, it provides improvements in blood glucose levels, body weight and blood pressure, prevents complications or reduces the risk of developing complications (TEMS, 2019).

Medical nutrition therapy consists of four stages: General assessment, education, determining a goal and evaluating the therapy (Eroğlu, 2017). In a patient who is diagnosed with diabetes and referred to a dietitian, MNT application consists of 3–4 visits with 45–90 minute durations and is completed over 3–6 months. To support lifestyle changes and to evaluate the therapy, it should continue with at least one visit each year. In required circumstances, dietitian can change the number of visits and their durations (Evert et al., 2014).

When MNTs of individuals with diabetes are constructed, a personal program should be created appropriate to dietary habits of individuals, their lifestyles, metabolic goals, preferences and socioeconomic statuses (Smart et al., 2014). During MNT, monitoring all metabolic parameters is required for both quality of life and for assessing the needs for the changes in treatment, thus providing successful results. Nutrition program should be usable for individuals with diabetes (Franz et al., 2010).

Dietary habits of individuals should be assessed and arrangements should be made as 2–3 main meals and 2–4 snacks each day. 45–60 % of energy requirements may be fulfilled by carbohydrates, 10–20 % by proteins and 20–35 % by fats. It is important in terms of cardiovascular disease prevention that <30 % of energy must come from fats, <7 % from saturated fats and trans-fat intake must be <1 %. In the therapy, low carbohydrate diets which provide less than 130 g of daily carbohydrates are not recommended (TEMS, 2019). Healthy carbohydrate sources such as whole grain bread, grains, legumes, fruits and vegetables, low fat dairy products lower glycemic variation during postprandial period and increase the quality of the diet (Sacks et al., 2017). Saturated fat intake must be limited to 7–8 % of daily energy. Trans fat intake should be reduced as it increases LDL-cholesterol levels and reduces HDL-cholesterol levels. Cholesterol intake should be less than 300 mg daily (TEMS, 2019). Consuming 1.6–3 g/day of plant stanols or sterols may prove effective in reducing total and LDL-cholesterol levels of individuals with dyslipidaemia. Two or more servings of fish per week provide omega-3 polyunsaturated fatty acids and this amount must be recommended for consumption (Diabetes Dietitian Association, 2019). In individuals with diabetes (if renal functions are normal), it is recommended that 15–20 % of daily energy (0.8–1 g/kg/day) comes from proteins, similar to general population (TEMS, 2019). Similar to the general population, arrangements should be made to provide dietary fibres from various sources as 14 g/1000kcal (Diabetes Dietitian Association, 2019). All foods, primarily vegetables and fruits, contain various vitamins and minerals. Healthy eating diabetes patients do not require additional vitamin and mineral supplements. Less than 5 g of table salt consumption is suitable for individuals with diabetes. Sufficient water consumption is very important for the body. On average, 8–10 cups of water must be consumed daily (Public Health Institution of Turkey, 2017).

The first step of MNT for gestational diabetes is to reach glycemic goals. Medical nutrition therapy is constructed specifically for the individual by calculating nutritional need during pregnancy. Additionally, MNT aims to prevent ketosis and provide appropriate weight gain for the mother (ADA, 2015).

In medical nutrition therapy, eating in the recommended time is as important as the amount and type of food. To eat sufficiently and healthy and to keep blood sugar in balance, meal schedule should be followed and meals must not be skipped. Irregular eating causes hypoglycaemia and hyperglycaemia. With foods spread through the day, endogenous insulin production is better and insulin requirement is lower. Number of meals vary depending on the type of diabetes, the received medical treatment, level of physical activity, the blood sugar level at that time and life conditions. Diabetes patients who use short acting insulin might eat in three meals and three snacks, a total of 6 meals. Type 2 diabetes patients who do not receive insulin therapy should eat in 4–6 meals including main meals and snacks. It is recommended for them to eat in the same hours (Bozkurt & Yıldız, 2011; Public Health Institution of Turkey, 2017)

1. Carbohydrate Counting

Carbohydrate counting (CC) is a meal preparation method that helps to adjust the amount of carbohydrate to be consumed in a meal, to adjust the dosage of insulin according to the amount of carbohydrate to be consumed or to adjust the dosage of insulin according to the blood glucose level before the meal (TEMS, 2019). It is considered a fundamental part of dietary care for children and adolescents with T1D to apply carbohydrate counting in MNT. Carbohydrate counting method for those age groups aims to provide sufficient and appropriate energy as well as macro and micronutrients for optimal growth, development and glycemic control (Bayrak, 2013; Yalçınkaya, 2007). CC has positive effects on metabolic control and HbA1c concentrations. Additionally with this method, the frequency of hypoglycaemia may decrease and food choice may become more various and flexible to help children and adolescents manage their lifestyles more effectively (Gökdoğan and Akıncı, 2001; Gökmen Özel, 2010). CC consists of 3 consecutive steps:

1st step (beginner level/basic level): Is the level in which carbohydrate counting skill is taught (foods that contain 15g of carbohydrates and calculations). In this step, dietitian determines the amount of carbohydrates the patient needs to consume according to the patient's eating records.

2nd step (intermediate level): Portion sizes and weights of foods are practiced (this step is very important for people with diabetes who do not receive insulin therapy)

3rd step (advanced level): The blood sugar control must be ensured and the basal insulin dosage of the patient must be adjusted properly. Determining, calculating and using the carbohydrate/insulin ratio and the insulin sensitivity factor are taught to the patient by the dietitian (diabetes dietitian). It is applied to the patients who receive multiple insulin therapy or who use insulin pumps (Tüfekçi Alphan, 2013).

C. Exercise

Insufficient physical activity and exercise cause diabetes, complications related to diabetes and increases in morbidity and mortality. Exercise has positive effects on lowering blood glucose level, increasing the number of insulin receptors, increasing insulin sensitivity in peripheral tissues, reducing the need for insulin, controlling blood pressure, reaching and maintaining ideal weight and lowering cholesterol level. Therefore, a scheduled exercise program is an important step of the treatment plan of a patient with diabetes (Tura Bahadır and Atmaca, 2012).

In order to prepare a safe exercise program for individuals with diabetes; physical limitations, heart diseases, possible leg pains from walking, rheumatic diseases, heart rate, blood pressure, hypoglycaemia/hyperglycaemia episodes and other situations of the individual that may affect physical activity must be taken into consideration. Turkey Endocrinology and Metabolism Society (TEMS) exercise recommendations are as follows (TEMS, 2019):

1. It must be ensured that adult individuals with diabetes must exercise at least 3 times per week for a total of 150 minutes without taking a break longer than 48 hours.
2. Exercise must start with low intensity and slowly increase to intermediate intensity.
3. Exercise must be stopped if there are indicators such as vertigo, sweating, shortness of breath, nausea, pain.
4. Individuals with diabetes must not remain still longer than 30 minutes, they must stand up for a short time or take a walk
5. Ideal blood glucose level before exercise must be between 90–250 mg/dL.

D. Education

Diabetes education is important as it is the fundamental approach that increases the quality of diabetes care and provides the success of the self-management of the individual. The purpose of this education is to make the adaptation of the patient to the disease and the treatment easier, to prevent possible complications, to keep blood pressure and blood glucose levels within normal limits and to provide ideal body weight and optimal blood pressure control (Bayrak & Çolak, 2012). Diabetes education may be conducted by authorized health personnel towards the patients or their relatives individually or in groups (Hashempour, 2018). Education must start as soon as diabetes is diagnosed and it must be planned specifically according to the personal characteristics and level of education of the patient and the progression of the disease. During the education, the educator and the individuals with diabetes must have mutual interaction and cooperative relationships. Sustainability of the educations must be ensured with regular attendance (Bayrak & Çolak, 2012). It is stated that individuals with diabetes who were included in an education program presented 80 % less damage to other organs caused by the disease, 50 % less leg and foot amputations caused by diabetic foot and 70 % less diabetes complications which require emergency treatment (Karadeniz, 2008).

E. Individual Blood Sugar Monitoring

Individual blood sugar monitoring, which is an irreplaceable part of treatment in patients that receive insulin therapy makes individuals with diabetes achieve responsibility over their own health. Additionally, it prevents fluctuations in blood glucose levels and helps reduce micro and macro complications (Knapp et al., 2016).

IV. Economic Burden of Diabetes

The number of people who live with diabetes and complications related to diabetes is increasing every year. This situation causes a large economic burden due to increase in healthcare use, loss of manpower and occurrence of long-term complications such as kidney failure, blindness and cardiac problems (IDF, 2015).

Diabetes causes a serious financial burden on individuals and their families because of the cost of insulin and other important medications. Moreover, it also has a considerable effect on countries and their national health systems (IDF, 2015). Cost calculation has 2 components as direct (diabetes monitoring, treatment and medication) and indirect (absence from work, working despite the disease, disability caused by the disease) (ADA, 2013). In the study by NCD Risk Factor Collaboration (NCD-RisC) published in 2016, annual direct cost of diabetes was determined as 825 billion dollars. When direct costs were analysed by country, top ranking countries were China with 170 billion dollars, USA with 105 billion dollars, India with 73 billion dollars and Japan with 37 billion dollars. Moreover, approximately 60 % of the global cost of diabetes originated from low- and middle-income countries (NCD Risk Factor Collaboration, 2016). According to the 2015 data by IDF, 75.4 % of people with diabetes lived in low- and middle-income countries but only 19 % of global health spending towards diabetes was from those countries. It is seen that mean per capita expenditure for people with diabetes varied between 401 and 688 dollars in low- and middle-income countries while this value was between 5374 and 9641 dollars in high income countries (IDF, 2015). Data from 2017 show that total health spending for diabetes reached 727,000 million US dollars (between the ages 20 and 79). This equates to an 8 % increase from 2015 calculations (IDF, 2017).

Gordois et al. (2003) researched the healthcare costs of peripheral neuropathy, one of diabetes complication, in USA and determined the total cost as $10.9 billion. In another study in which economic burden related to diabetes in the United States of America, annual per capita expenditures for undiagnosed patients were $2864, it was $9975 for diagnosed patients and $443 for prediabetes (Dall et al., 2010). According to 2012 predictions of American Diabetes Association (ADA), it is estimated that the 174 billion dollars of total cost of diabetes in 2007 is estimated to have increased to 245 billion dollars with a 41 % increase. The direct cost was 176 billion dollars and it constituted 72 % of total cost. Total health expenditure in the USA was 1.3 trillion dollars and 306 billion dollars of this were spent for the population with diabetes, which corresponds to the 23 % of total expenditure. Indirect cost was 28 % of the total cost with 69 billion dollars (ADA, 2013).

In a study in Pakistan, cost of diabetes care outside the clinic were analysed and it was estimated that each individual with diabetes has an annual direct cost of $197 (Khowaja et al., 2007).

In a study in which early-stage nephropathy in diabetes patients and the resource use and cost caused by it and the effect of these costs on the economy of Germany are analysed, it was determined that as the disease progressed, the costs increased significantly, main cost parameters were dialysis and hospitalizations and total estimated cost of nephropathy was €1332 in terms of health insurance and €2019 in terms of society (Happich et al., 2008).

Van Der Linden et al. (2009) calculated the direct costs of diabetes in Netherlands as €1283 and determined that 65 % of the calculated cost was due to hospitalizations.

Hall et al. (2011) calculated the total cost of diabetes in Sub-Saharan Africa as 67.03 billion dollars and the cost per capita as $8836. In a study estimating the economic burden related to diabetes in WHO Africa Region countries, it is stated that in the year 2000, 7.02 million diabetes cases caused 25.51 billion dollars of economic loss in Africa Region countries and it was determined that diabetes was an important economic burden in the countries of the region (Kirigia et al., 2009).

When the situation in Italy is considered, mean annual cost of diabetes is €2450 and of the total cost, 71.2 % was for insulin therapy and blood glucose monitoring for the patients, 18 % was for hospitalizations, 4 % for visits, 3.9 % was for tests conducted and 2.9 % was for medicines and microvascular and macrovascular complications doubled the cost of treatment (Franciosi et al., 2013).

Lee et al. (2013), in the study in which cost of adult diabetes patients were analysed in Australia, stated that annual direct cost of diabetes per capita was $4390, annual total cost related to diabetes was 4.5 billion dollars and the cost of diabetes for individuals and the government was high.

In a study conducted to determine the health inequalities caused by economic burden of diabetes in Mexico, it is determined that health expenditures caused by the economic burden of diabetes are one of the primary reasons of health inequalities in middle income countries. In the study, total cost of diabetes was calculated as 7.7 billion dollars (3.4 billion dollars of which were direct costs and 4.3 billion of which were indirect costs) (Arredondo and Reyes, 2013).

In a study evaluating the direct and indirect costs of T1D and T2D in Poland, it was determined that the direct costs of medical services for both of those types doubled between the years 2005 and 2009 and the fact that diabetes caused absence from work and disability to work was one of the most important reasons of the decreasing productivity in Poland. It was determined that the total cost of diabetes and its complications to Polish health budget was €654 million and this number corresponded to 2.8 % of total cost of healthcare services of Poland and in 2009 in Poland, total cost of diabetes was €1.5 billion (Lesniowska et al., 2014).

In their study, Chevreul et al. (2014) states that diabetes was the most common chronic disease among those that are 100 % covered by the official health insurance of France and the number of patients who were covered by the insurance had doubled over the past 10 years. It is stated that in 2007, mean annual cost was €6930 for T1D patients and €4890 for T2D patients and the large increase in costs were due to complications.

Png et al. (2016) determined the total economic burden of T2D in Singapore in 2010 as $5646 (42 % of which is direct and 52 % of which is indirect) and concluded that diabetes was a growing economic burden in Singapore.

It is stated that the direct cost of insulin induced hypoglycaemia in individuals with T1D and T2D in Denmark was 96.2 million DKK which equated to 1.9 million euros (Hoskins et al., 2016).

In a recent study conducted as part of the WHO global action plan for the prevention and control of non-communicable diseases, the global burden of diabetes was calculated as 1.3 trillion dollars and was foreseen that global costs were going to increase significantly until the year 2030 (Bommer et al., 2018).

When the studies on the economic burden of diabetes in Turkey are evaluated, it is seen that the data on the subject are insufficient.

In Turkey, the number of individuals with diabetes and the burden of the disease is rapidly increasing. Number of individuals with diabetes increases 8 % each year and the cost of treatment increases 18 % each year. According to a report of Republic of Turkey Social Security Institution (SSI) on diabetes, it was determined that the total cost of T1D and T2D to Turkish health system was approximately 10 billion TL in 2012 and this constituted approximately 23 % of the total health expenditure of SSI (Republic of Turkey Social Security Institution, 2014). However, those cost approximations do not take indirect costs such as the loss of productivity of the individual with diabetes, their caregiver, and the family into consideration and does not reflect the effect of low quality of life.

As the prevalence of T2D increase worldwide, the disease and accompanying complications cause a significant increasing burden on both the health system and the society. When the economic burden of T2D in Turkey is analysed, according to the patient records of a tertiary hospital in Turkey, it was calculated that the cost burden of T2D as of 2010 was between 11.4 billion and 12.9 billion TL. It was seen that approximately 12 % of the cost was for diabetes medications, 15 % was for medications not for diabetes and 73 % was for complication screening and treatment (Malhan et al., 2014).

When the distribution of total cost of diabetes in Turkey is analysed, it is stated that 26 % of the costs were direct and 74 % of the costs were for complications caused by diabetes and cardiovascular disease had the highest share (28 %) among those complications (Public Health Institution of Turkey, 2014).

Total cost of NCD treatment of outpatients in both hospitals and family health centres (FHC) in 2016 was 2.1 billion TL, 7.1 % of which were caused by diabetes. When the hospitalizations related to NCDs in the same year are analysed, total cost was 420,649,702 TL, 45,076,864 TL of which were for diabetes (World Health Organization European Office, 2018).

In a recent study analysing the cost of T1D in terms of annual specific costs, treatment costs to reimbursement institution was estimated as 204 TL and the cost of medicine was estimated as 1602.65 TL. The cost to reimbursement institution of patients who do not use insulin pumps was calculated as 3129.15 TL and of patients who use insulin pumps was calculated as 5990.92 TL and of patients who use sensors was calculated as 17,945.25 TL. Total costs were 6807.25 TL for patients who do not use insulin pumps, 11,753.4 TL for patients who use insulin pumps and 23,711.42 TL for patients who use continuous blood sugar measuring systems (Sarı, 2020).

Conclusion and Suggestions

NCDs are global threats that cause high mortality rates, decrease in productivity, increase in health and health system sustainability spending. With effective management of NCDs, decreases in emergency room visits, symptoms and complications of diseases, rates of hospitalizations and increases in quality of live are possible. The burden of diabetes, prevalence of which is constantly increasing, is a topic that has been emphasized by public stakeholders for a long time. Effective management of the disease is very important to reduce burden brought by the disease.

Until now, initiatives such as awareness campaigns for the prevention of T2D and early diagnosis, understanding the current T2D burden on the country and diagnosis for effective diabetes management, developing and applying policies on treatment and monitoring standards, providing effective treatments for diabetes and its complications by improving diabetes education, supporting the access of individuals with diabetes to healthy foods and physical exercise facilities, improving the treatment and care of diabetes and taking steps towards preventing the disease in children, including childhood obesity which is an important T2D risk in adults have been attempted in Turkey. Recently, the government revealed the 5-year Turkey Diabetes Program (2015–2020). The aims of this program were determined as "developing and applying policies for effective diabetes management, preventing diabetes and facilitating early diagnosis, providing effective treatments of diabetes and its complications, developing diabetes care and treatment in children, preventing T2D and obesity, effective monitoring and evaluation of diabetes and the diabetes program". In order to reduce the burden of diabetes on the individual and the society, earliest possible diagnosis is needed. In order for the individuals with diabetes, number of which is increasing each day, to maintain their lives healthy and problem free, they need to have sufficient information and skill (IDF, 2019). Therefore, it is important for individuals with diabetes to be educated in diabetes and to ensure that those individuals receive the education. Thus, the success rate in the management of the disease increases and the individual can take responsibility of their own health.

It is important to provide healthy eating conditions and to ensure access to those by everyone in order to prevent diabetes, its complications and obesity. Medical nutrition therapy must be applied during the treatment of the disease. MNT has a complementary role in the management of diabetes and it contributes to metabolic control in individuals who follow appropriate nutrition therapy after diagnosis. Physical activity is also very effective in preventing possible complications and providing metabolic control. Individuals can be made to help reduce the burden on themselves and the society caused by diabetes by creating accessible physical activity opportunities. Moreover, it is important for policy makers to continue disease prevention and health improvement efforts with a multi-disciplinary approach in order to improve the quality of life of sick individuals and to reduce the economic burden on the health system.

References

Abacı, A., Böber, E., & Büyükgebiz, A. (2007). Tip 1 diyabet. *Güncel Pediatri*, 5(1), 1–10.

ADVANCE Collaborative Group, Patel, A., MacMahon, S., Chalmers, J., Neal, B., Billot, L., Woodward, M., Marre, M., Cooper, M., Glasziou, P., Grobbee, D., Hamet, P., Harrap, S., Heller, S., Liu, L., Mancia, G., Mogensen, C. E., Pan, C., Poulter, N., Rodgers, A., … Travert, F. (2008). Intensive blood glucose control and vascular outcomes in patients with type 2 diabetes. *The New England Journal of Medicine*, 358(24), 2560–2572.

Agardh, E., Allebeck, P., Hallqvist, J., Moradi, T., & Sidorchuk, A. (2011). Type 2 diabetes incidence and socio-economic position: A systematic review and meta-analysis. *International Journal of Epidemiology*, 40(3), 804–818.

Akdemir, N., & Birol, L. (2011). *İç hastalıkları ve hemşirelik bakımı*. Sistem Ofset.

Alberti, K. G., Zimmet, P., & Shaw, J. (2007). International Diabetes Federation: A consensus on type 2 diabetes prevention. *Diabetic Medicine: A Journal of the British Diabetic Association*, 24(5), 451–463.

Al-Goblan, A. S., Al-Alfi, M. A., & Khan, M. Z. (2014). Mechanism linking diabetes mellitus and obesity. *Diabetes, Metabolic Syndrome and Obesity: Targets and Therapy*, 7, 587–591.

American Diabetes Association (ADA). (2013). Economic costs of diabetes in the U.S. in 2012. *Diabetes Care*, 36(4), 1033–1046.

American Diabetes Association (ADA). (2014). Standards of medical care in diabetes. *Diabetes Care*, 37(Supplement 1), S14–S80.

American Diabetes Association (ADA). (2015). Standards of medical care in diabetes. *Diabetes Care*, 29 (Supplement 1), 43–48.

American Diabetes Association (2017). 7. Obesity management for the treatment of type 2 diabetes. *Diabetes Care*, *40*(Suppl 1), S57–S63.

American Diabetes Association (ADA). (2019). 11. Microvascular complications and foot care: Standards of medical care in diabetes-2019. *Diabetes Care*, *42*(Suppl. 1), S124–S138.

American Diabetes Association (ADA). (2020). 2. Classification and Diagnosis of Diabetes: Standards of Medical Care in Diabetes – 2020. *Diabetes Care*, *43*(Suppl. 1), S14–S31.

Arredondo, A., & Reyes, G. (2013). Health disparities from economic burden of diabetes in middle-income countries: Evidence from México. *Plos One*, *8*(7), e68443.

Atmaca, M. H., & Ecemiş, G. C. (2012). Oral antidiyabetik ajanlar. *Journal of Experimental and Clinical Medicine*, *29*(1s), 23–29.

Balkau, B., & Eschwège, E. (2003). The Diagnosis and Classification of Diabetes and Impaired Glucose Regulation. In: Pickup, J. C., & Williams, G. (Eds), *Textbook of Diabetes* (3rd ed., ch. 2.1–2.13). Wiley-Blackwell.

Bayrak, G., & Çolak, R. (2012). Diyabet tedavisinde hasta eğitimi. *Journal of Experimental and Clinical Medicine*, *29* (1s), 7–11.

Bayrak Özarslan, B. (2013). *Diyabetik koroner arter hastalarında sağlıklı yaşam biçimi davranışları ve yaşam kalitesinin belirlenmesi* [Unpublished master thesis], University of Hacettepe.

Baz, B., Riveline, J. P., & Gautier, J. F. (2016). Gestational diabetes mellitus: Definition, aetiological and clinical aspects. *European Journal of Endocrinology*, *174*(2), R43–R51.

Bernstein, R. K. (2008). *2008 American diabetes association clinical guidelines comments.* http://www.diabetes-book.com/2008-american-diabetes-association-clinical-guidelines/, Access date 14.02.2021.

Biberoğlu, İ., & Süleyman, Ü. (2003). Diyabetin Komplikasyonları. In: İliçin, G. (Ed.), *Temel İç Hastalıkları* (pp. 2311–2331). Güneş Kitapevi.

Biester, T., Kordonouri, O., & Danne, T. (2018). Pharmacotherapy of type1 diabetes in children and adolescents: More than insulin?. *Therapeutic Advances in Endocrinology and Metabolism*, *9*(5), 157–166.

Bjerregaard, L. G., Jensen, B. W., Ängquist, L., Osler, M., Sørensen, T. I., & Baker, J. L. (2018). Change in overweight from childhood to early adulthood and risk of type 2 diabetes. *New England Journal of Medicine*, *378*(14):1302– 12.

Bommer, C., Sagalova, V., Heesemann, E., Manne-Goehler, J., Atun, R., Bärnighausen, T., Davies, J., & Vollmer, S. (2018). Global economic burden of diabetes in adults: Projections from 2015 to 2030. *Diabetes Care*, *41*(5), 963–970.

Bozkurt, N., & Yıldız, E. (2011). Diabetes Mellistus ve Beslenme Tedavisi. In: Baysal, A., Aksoy, M., Besler, H. T., Bozkurt, N., Keçecioğlu, S., et al. *Diyet El Kitabı* (6th Press, pp. 257–297). Hatipoğlu Yayınları.

Boztepe, H. (2012). Tip 1 diyabetin yönetiminde riskli bir dönem: Ergenlik. *Hacettepe Üniversitesi Hemşirelik Fakültesi Dergisi, 19*(1), 82–89.

Brown, A. F., Ettner, S. L., Piette, J., Weinberger, M., Gregg, E., Shapiro, M. F., Karter, A. J., Safford, M., Waitzfelder, B., Prata, P. A., & Beckles, G. L. (2004). Socioeconomic position and health among persons with diabetes mellitus: A conceptual framework and review of the literature. *Epidemiologic Reviews, 26*, 63–77.

Cappuccio, F. P., D'Elia, L., Strazzullo, P., & Miller, M. A. (2010). Quantity and quality of sleep and incidence of type 2 diabetes: A systematic review and meta-analysis. *Diabetes Care, 33*(2), 414–420.

Carter, P., Gray, L. J., Troughton, J., Khunti, K., & Davies, M. J. (2010). Fruit and vegetable intake and incidence of type 2 diabetes mellitus: Systematic review and meta-analysis. *BMJ, 341*, c4229.

Chevreul, K., Brigham, K. B., & Bouché, C. (2014). The burden and treatment of diabetes in France. *Globalization and Health, 10*(1), 1–9.

Cho, N. H., Shaw, J. E., Karuranga, S., Huang, Y., da Rocha Fernandes, J. D., Ohlrogge, A. W., & Malanda, B. (2018). IDF Diabetes Atlas: Global estimates of diabetes prevalence for 2017 and projections for 2045. *Diabetes Research and Clinical Practice, 138*, 271–281.

Çubuk, G., & İnce, S. (2015). Oral antidiyabetik ilaçlar. *Kocatepe Veterinary Journal, 8*(1), 95–102.

Dall, T. M., Zhang, Y., Chen, Y. J., Quick, W. W., Yang, W. G., & Fogli, J. (2010). The economic burden of diabetes. *Health Affairs, 29*(2), 297–303.

Demirbilek, H. (2018). Tip 1 Diyabet: Patofizyoloji ve Klinik. Aycan, Z. (Ed.). *Çocukluk Çağı Diyabeti: Tanı ve Tedavi Rehberi.* Buluş Matbaa.

Ding, M., Bhupathiraju, S. N., Chen, M., van Dam, R. M., & Hu, F. B. (2014). Caffeinated and decaffeinated coffee consumption and risk of type 2 diabetes: A systematic review and a dose-response meta-analysis. *Diabetes Care, 37*(2), 569–586.

Diabetes Dietitian Association. (2019). *Diyabetin önlenmesi ve tedavisinde kanıta dayalı beslenme tedavisi rehberi.* https://f3e89f52-6f04-4783-b858-156511f9e8f9.filesusr.com/ugd/d8e695_1202327d321b4867aa2cdbd7f48d5222.pdf, Access date 14.02.2021.

Durna, Z. (2013). *İç hastalıkları hemşireliği.* Akademi Basın ve Yayın.

Durna, Z., & Akın, S. (2012). *Kronik hastalıklar ve bakım.* Nobel Tıp Kitapevleri.

Eldor, R., Raz, I., Ben Yehuda, A., & Boulton, A. J. M. (2004). New and experimental approaches to treatment of diabetic foot ulcers: A comprehensive review of emerging treatment strategies. *Diabetic Medicine, 21*(11), 1161–1173.

Engelgau, M. M., Narayan, K. M., & Herman, W. H. (2000). Screening for type 2 diabetes. *Diabetes Care, 23*(10), 1563–1580.

Eroğlu, N. (2017). *Tip 2 diyabetli hastalarda eğitimin diyabet öz yönetim ve öz etkililiklerine etkisi* [Unpublished doctoral thesis]. University of Halic.

Evert, A. B., Boucher, J. L., Cypress, M., Dunbar, S. A., Franz, M. J., Mayer-Davis, E. J., Neumiller, J. J., Nwankwo, R., Verdi, C. L., Urbanski, P., & Yancy, W. S., Jr. (2014). Nutrition therapy recommendations for the management of adults with diabetes. *Diabetes Care, 37*(Suppl. 1), S120–S143.

Farsani, S. F., Brodovicz, K., Soleymanlou, N., Marquard, J., Wissinger, E., & Maiese, B. A. (2017). Incidence and prevalence of diabetic ketoacidosis (DKA) among adults with type 1 diabetes mellitus (T1D): A systematic literature review. *BMJ Open, 7*(7), e016587.

Feero, W. G., & Guttmacher, A. E. (2010). Genomics, type 2 diabetes and obesity. *New England Journal of Medicine, 363*, 2339–2350.

Franciosi, M., Lucisano, G., Amoretti, R., Capani, F., Bruttomesso, D., Di Bartolo, P., Girelli, A., Leonetti, F., Morviducci, L., Vitacolonna, E., & Nicolucci, A. (2013). Costs of treatment and complications of adult type 1 diabetes. *Nutrition, Metabolism, and Cardiovascular Diseases: NMCD, 23*(7), 606–611.

Franz, M. J., Powers, M. A., Leontos, C., Holzmeister, L. A., Kulkarni, K., Monk, A., Wedel, N., & Gradwell, E. (2010). The evidence for medical nutrition therapy for type 1 and type 2 diabetes in adults. *Journal of the American Dietetic Association, 110*(12), 1852–1889.

Gökdoğan F., & Akıncı F. (2001). Bolu'da yaşayan diyabetlilerin sağlık ve hastalıklarını algılamaları ile uygulamaları. *Cumhuriyet Üniversitesi Hemşirelik Yüksekokulu Dergisi, 5*(1). 10–17.

Gökmen Özel, H. (2010). Tip 1 diabetes mellitus ve beslenme. *Diyabet ve Obezite, 23*, 20–26.

Gordois, A., Scuffham, P., Shearer, A., Oglesby, A., & Tobian, J. A. (2003). The health care costs of diabetic peripheral neuropathy in the US. *Diabetes Care, 26*(6), 1790–1795.

Grøntved, A., & Hu, F. B. (2011). Television viewing and risk of type 2 diabetes, cardiovascular disease, and all-cause mortality: A meta-analysis. *JAMA, 305*(23), 2448–2455.

Hall, V., Thomsen, R. W., Henriksen, O., & Lohse, N. (2011). Diabetes in Sub Saharan Africa 1999–2011: Epidemiology and public health implications. A systematic review. *BMC Public Health, 11*(1), 1–12.

Haller, M. J., Atkinson, M. A., & Schatz, D. (2005). Type 1 diabetes mellitus: Etiology, presentation, and management. *Pediatric Clinics*, *52*(6), 1553–1578.

Hämäläinen, A. M., & Knip, M. (2002). Autoimmunity and familial risk of type 1 diabetes. *Current Diabetes Reports*, *2*(4), 347–353.

Happich, M., Landgraf, R., Piehlmeier, W., Falkenstein, P., & Stamenitis, S. (2008). The economic burden of nephropathy in diabetic patients in Germany in 2002. *Diabetes Research and Clinical Practice*, *80*(1), 34–39.

Harder, T., Rodekamp, E., Schellong, K., Dudenhausen, J. W., & Plagemann, A. (2007). Birth weight and subsequent risk of type 2 diabetes: A meta-analysis. *American Journal of Epidemiology*, *165*(8), 849–857.

Hashempour, L. (2018) *Sağlık ve diyabet okuryazarlığı: Hacettepe Üniversitesi Hastaneleri örneği* [Unpublished doctoral thesis]. University of Hacettepe.

Health Institutes of Turkey. (2018). *Bulaşıcı olmayan hastalıklar nelerdir?* https://www.tuseb.gov.tr/tuhke/makaleler/bulasici-olmayan-hastaliklar-nelerdir, Access date 12.02.2021.

Hiatt, W. R. (2001). Medical treatment of peripheral arterial disease and claudication. *New England Journal of Medicine*, *344*(21), 1608–1621.

Hoskins, N., Tikkanen, C. K., & Pedersen-Bjergaard, U. (2016). The economic impact of insulin-related hypoglycemia in Denmark: An analysis using the Local Impact of Hypoglycemia Tool. *Journal of Medical Economics*, *20*(4), 363–370.

Huysman, F., & Mathieu, C. (2009). Diabetes and peripheral vascular disease. *Acta Chirurgica Belgica*, *109*(5), 587–594.

İlicin, G., Biberoğlu, K., Süleymanlar, G., & Ünal. S. (2003). *İç hastalıkları*. Güneş Kitapevi.

International Diabetes Federation (IDF). (2015). *IDF Diabetes Atlas* (7th ed). https://www.idf.org/e-library/epidemiology-research/diabetes-atlas/13-diabetes-atlas-seventh-edition.html, Access date 15.02.2021.

International Diabetes Federation (IDF). (2017). *IDF Diabetes Atlas* (8th ed). https://diabetesatlas.org/upload/resources/previous/files/8/IDF_DA_8e-EN-final.pdf, Access date 15.02.2021.

International Diabetes Federation (IDF). (2019). *IDF Diabetes Atlas* (9th ed). https://www.diabetesatlas.org/en/resources/, Access date 15.02.2021.

International Diabetes Leadership Forum. (2013). *Türkiye'de ve bölge ülkelerinde diyabet sorunu.* http://www.diabetcemiyeti.org/c/turkiye-de-ve-bolge-ulkelerinde-diyabet-sorunu, Access date 13.02.2021.

Ivanac-Janković, R., Lovčić, V., Magaš, S., Šklebar, D., & Kes, P. (2019). The novella about diabetic nephropathy. *Acta Clinica Croatica*, *54*(1), 83–90.

Karadeniz, G. (2008). *İç hastalıkları hemşireliğinde teoriden uygulamaya temel yaklaşımlar*. Göktuğ Yayıncılık.

Kasper, D., Fauci, A., Hauser, S., Longo, D., Jameson, J., & Loscalzo, J. (2015). *Harrison's principles of internal medicine* (19th ed). McGraw Hill Education.

Katsarou, A., Gudbjörnsdottir, S., Rawshani, A., Dabelea, D., Bonifacio, E., Anderson, B. J., Jacobsen, L. M., Schatz, D. A., & Lernmark, Å. (2017). Type 1 diabetes mellitus. *Nature Reviews. Disease Primers, 3*, 17016.

Khaw, K. T., Wareham, N., Bingham, S., Luben, R., Welch, A., & Day, N. (2004). Association of hemoglobin A1c with cardiovascular disease and mortality in adults: The European prospective investigation into cancer in Norfolk. *Annals of Internal Medicine, 141*(6), 413–420.

Khowaja, L. A., Khuwaja, A. K., & Cosgrove, P. (2007). Cost of diabetes care in out-patient clinics of Karachi, Pakistan. *BMC Health Services Research, 7*, 189.

Kirigia, J. M., Sambo, H. B., Sambo, L. G., & Barry, S. P. (2009). Economic burden of diabetes mellitus in the WHO African region. *BMC International Health and Human Rights, 9*, 6.

Knapp, S., Manroa, P., & Doshi, K. (2016). Self-monitoring of blood glucose: Advice for providers and patients. *Cleveland Clinic Journal of Medicine, 83*(5), 355–360.

Köksal, G., & Gökmen Özel, H. (2019). *Çocuk hastalıklarında beslenme tedavisi* (2nd ed). Hatipoglu Yayınevi.

Koning, L., Chiuve, S. E., Fung, T. T., Willett, W. C., Rimm, E. B., & Hu, F. B. (2011). Diet-quality scores and the risk of type 2 diabetes in men. *Diabetes Care, 34*(5), 1150–1156.

Lawes, C. M., Parag, V., Bennett, D. A., Suh, I., Lam, T. H., Whitlock, G., Barzi, F., Woodward, M., & Asia Pacific Cohort Studies Collaboration. (2004). Blood glucose and risk of cardiovascular disease in the Asia Pacific region. *Diabetes Care, 27*(12), 2836–2842.

Lawlor, D. A., Lichtenstein, P., & Långström, N. (2011). Association of maternal diabetes mellitus in pregnancy with offspring adiposity into early adulthood: Sibling study in a prospective cohort of 280,866 men from 248,293 families. *Circulation, 123*(3), 258–265.

Lee, C. M., Colagiuri, R., Magliano, D. J., Cameron, A. J., Shaw, J., Zimmet, P., & Colagiuri, S. (2013). The cost of diabetes in adults in Australia. *Diabetes Research and Clinical Practice, 99*(3), 385–390.

Lee, I. M., Shiroma, E. J., Lobelo, F., Puska, P., Blair, S. N., Katzmarzyk, P. T., & Lancet Physical Activity Series Working Group. (2012). Effect of physical inactivity on major non-communicable diseases worldwide: An analysis of burden of disease and life expectancy. *Lancet, 380*(9838), 219–229.

Lesniowska, J., Schubert, A., Wojna, M., Baran, I. S., &ve Fedyna, M. (2014). Costs of diabetes and its complications in Poland, *The European Journal of Health Economics,* 15, 653–660.

Lozano, R., Naghavi, M., Foreman, K., Lim, S., Shibuya, K., Aboyans, V., Abraham, J., Adair, T., Aggarwal, R., Ahn, S. Y., Alvarado, M., Anderson, H. R., Anderson, L. M., Andrews, K. G., Atkinson, C., Baddour, L. M., Barker-Collo, S., Bartels, D. H., Bell, M. L., Benjamin, E. J., ..., & Memish, Z. A. (2012). Global and regional mortality from 235 causes of death for 20 age groups in 1990 and 2010: A systematic analysis for the Global Burden of Disease Study 2010. *Lancet, 380*(9859), 2095–2128.

Maitra, A., & Abbas, A. K. (2005). *Endocrine system. Robbins and Cotran Pathologic basis of disease* (7th ed). Saunders.

Malhan, S., Öksüz, E., Babineaux, S. M., Ertekin, A., & Palmer, J. P. (2014). Assessment of the direct medical costs of type 2 diabetes mellitus and its complications in Turkey. *Turkish Journal of Endocrinology & Metabolism, 18*(2), 39–43.

Meisinger, C., Löwel, H., Thorand, B., & Döring, A. (2005). Leisure time physical activity and the risk of type 2 diabetes in men and women from the general population. *Diabetologia, 48*(1), 27–34.

Menke, A., Casagrande, S., Geiss, L., & Cowie, C. C. (2015). Prevalence of and trends in diabetes among adults in the United States, 1988–2012. *JAMA, 314*(10), 1021–1029.

NCD Risk Factor Collaboration (NCD-RisC). (2016). Worldwide trends in diabetes since 1980: A pooled analysis of 751 population-based studies with 4.4 million participants. *Lancet, 387*(10027), 1513–1530.

Oğuz, A., Telci Çaklılı, Ö., Tümerdem Çalık, B., & PURE Investigators (2018). The Prospective Urban Rural Epidemiology (PURE) study: PURE Turkey. *Türk Kardiyoloji Derneği* Arsivi, *46*(7), 613–623.

Onat, A. (2009). *Türk erişkinlerinde diyabet ve prediyabet: Patogeneze önemli katkı. TEKHARF çalışması.* Figür Grafik ve Matbaacılık Tic. Ltd. Şti.

Önmez, A. (2017). Diabetes mellitus'ta mikrovasküler komplikasyonların yönetimi. *Düzce Üniversitesi Sağlık Bilimleri Enstitüsü Dergisi, 7*(2), 117–119.

Ovayolu, N., & Ovayolu, Ö. (Eds). (2016). *Temel İç Hastalıkları Hemşireliği ve Farklı Boyutlarıyla Kronik Hastalıklar.* Çukurova Nobel Tıp Kitabevi.

Özkaya, M. O., & Köse, S. A. (2014). Gestasyonel diyabet: Güncel durum. *Perinatoloji Dergisi, 22*(2), 105–109.

Pasquel, F. J., & Umpierrez, G. E. (2014). Hyperosmolar hyperglycemic state: A historic review of the clinical presentation, diagnosis, and treatment. *Diabetes Care, 37*(11), 3124–3131.

Png, M. E., Yoong, J., Phan, T. P., & Wee, H. L. (2016). Current and future economic burden of diabetes among working-age adults in Asia: Conservative estimates for Singapore from 2010–2050. *BMC Public Health, 16*(1), 1–9.

Public Health Institution of Turkey. (2014). *Türkiye diyabet programı 2015–2020.* https://extranet.who.int/ncdccs/Data/TUR_D1_T%C3%BCrkiye%20Diyabet%20Program%C4%B1%202015-2020.pdf, Access date 13.02.2021.

Public Health Institution of Turkey. (2017). *Birinci basamak sağlık kurumları için obezite ve diyabet klinik rehberi.* https://hsgm.saglik.gov.tr/depo/birimler/saglikli-beslenme-hareketli-hayat-db/Diyabet/diyabet-rehberleri/Obezite-ve-Diyabet-Klinik-Rehberi.pdf, Access date 16.02.2021.

Republic of Turkey Ministry of Health and World Health Organization European Office. (2017). *Türkiye bulaşıcı olmayan hastalıklar çok paydaşlı eylem planı 2017–2025.* https://sbu.saglik.gov.tr/Ekutuphane/kitaplar/%C3%A7ok%20payda%C5%9Fl%C4%B1%20eylem.pdf, Access date 16.02.2021.

Republic of Turkey Ministry of Health. (2016). *Diyabete göz yumma.* https://www.saglik.gov.tr/TR,2643/diyabete-goz-yumma.html, Access date 16.02.2021.

Republic of Turkey Social Security Institution (SSI). (2014). *Sosyal güvenlik kurumu bakış açısıyla Diyabet.* https://silo.tips/download/sosyal-gvenlk-kurumu-43, Access date 16.02.2021.

Sacks, F. M., Lichtenstein, A. H., Wu, J. H., Appel, L. J., Creager, M. A., Kris-Etherton, P. M., ... & Van Horn, L. V. (2017). Dietary fats and cardiovascular disease: A presidential advisory from the American Heart Association. *Circulation, 136*(3), e1–e23.

Sarı, M. (2020). *Tip 1 diyabet hastalığının maliyet analizi* [Unpublished master thesis], University of Düzce.

Satman, İ. (2007). Diabetes mellitus tanı ve izleminde yeni kriterler ve belirlenme gerekçeleri. *Türkiye Klinikleri Journal of internal Medical Sciences, 3*(3):1–15.

Schienkiewitz, A., Schulze, M. B., Hoffmann, K., Kroke, A., & Boeing, H. (2006). Body mass index history and risk of type 2 diabetes: Results from the European Prospective Investigation into Cancer and Nutrition (EPIC) – Potsdam Study. *The American Journal of Clinical Nutrition, 84*(2), 427–433.

Shai, I., Jiang, R., Manson, J. E., Stampfer, M. J., Willett, W. C., Colditz, G. A., & Hu, F. B. (2006). Ethnicity, obesity, and risk of type 2 diabetes in women: A 20-year follow-up study. *Diabetes Care, 29*(7), 1585–1590.

Sharif, K., Watad, A., Coplan, L., Amital, H., Shoenfeld, Y., & Afek, A. (2018). Psychological stress and type 1 diabetes mellitus: What is the link? *Expert Review of Clinical Immunology*, *14*(12), 1081–1088.

Shaw, L. J., & Iskandrian, A. E. (2004). Prognostic value of gated myocardial perfusion SPECT. *Journal of Nuclear Cardiology*, *11*(2), 171–185.

Smart, C. E., Annan, F., Bruno, L. P., Higgins, L. A., & Acerini, C. L. (2014). Nutritional management in children and adolescents with diabetes. *Pediatric Diabetes*, *15*(S20), 135–153.

Swinnen, S. G., Hoekstra, J. B., & DeVries, J. H. (2009). Insulin therapy for type 2 diabetes. *Diabetes Care*, *32*(Suppl. 2), S253–S259.

Tesfaye, S., Boulton, A. J., Dyck, P. J., Freeman, R., Horowitz, M., Kempler, P., Lauria, G., Malik, R. A., Spallone, V., Vinik, A., Bernardi, L., Valensi, P., & Toronto Diabetic Neuropathy Expert Group (2010). Diabetic neuropathies: Update on definitions, diagnostic criteria, estimation of severity, and treatments. *Diabetes Care*, *33*(10), 2285–2293.

The InterAct Consortium. (2013). The link between family history and risk of type 2 diabetes is not explained by anthropometric, lifestyle or genetic risk factors: The EPIC-InterAct study. *Diabetologia*, *56*, 60–69.

Tong, X., Dong, J. Y., Wu, Z. W., Li, W., & Qin, L. Q. (2011). Dairy consumption and risk of type 2 diabetes mellitus: A meta-analysis of cohort studies. *European Journal of Clinical Nutrition*, *65*(9), 1027–1031.

Tuchman, A. (2009). Diabetes and the public's health. *The Lancet*, *374*(9696), 1140–1141.

Tüfekçi Alphan, E. (2013). Hastalıklarda beslenme tedavisi. In Alphan, E. (Ed.), *Diabetes Mellitus ve Beslenme Tedavisi* (1st ed, pp. 415–502). Hatipoğlu YayıneviTürk Diyabet Vakfı.

Tura Bahadır, Ç., & Atmaca, M. (2012). Diyabet ve egzersiz. *Journal of Experimental and Clinical Medicine*, *29* (1s), 16–22.

Turkey Endocrinology and Metabolism Society (TEMS). (2015). *TEMD Diabetes Mellitus Çalışma ve Eğitim Grubu: Diabetes mellitus ve komplikasyonlarının tanı, tedavi ve izlem kılavuzu*. http://www.anadoluissagligi.com/img/file_1 539.pdf, Access date 17.02.2021.

Turkey Endocrinology and Metabolism Society (TEMS). (2019). *TEMD Diabetes Mellitus Çalışma ve Eğitim Grubu: Diabetes mellitus ve komplikasyonlarının tanı, tedavi ve izlem kılavuzu*. https://temd.org.tr/admin/uploads/tbl_kilavuz/ 20190819095854-2019tbl_kilavuzb48da47363.pdf, Access date 16.02.2021.

Turkish Diabetes Foundation. (2017) *Diyabet tanı ve tedavi rehberi* (7th ed). https://www.turkdiab.org/admin/PICS/webfiles/Diyabet_tani_ve_tedavi__ kitabi.pdf, Access date 17.02.2021.

Turkish Diabetes Foundation. (2019) *Diyabet tanı ve tedavi rehberi* (9th ed). https://turkdiab.org/admin/PICS/files/Diyabet_Tani_ve_Tedavi_Rehberi_2 019.pdf, Access date 17.02.2021.

Turkish Statistical Institute. (2012). *Ölüm nedeni istatistikleri.* https://tuikweb.tuik. gov.tr/PreHaberBultenleri.do;jsessionid=GB9kfF0RL2JTXJ4D82cglVnxn 8F7K2151ctmDyj0YTTqJYhbPqdd!857776220?id=15847#:~:text=2012%20 y%C4%B1l%C4%B1nda%20%C3%B61%C3%BCme%20sebep%20o lan,ve%20duyu%20organlar%C4%B1%20hastal%C4%B1klar%C4%B1%20 ve%20%25, Access date 15.02.2021.

Tuttle, K. R., Bakris, G. L., Bilous, R. W., Chiang, J. L., de Boer, I. H., Goldstein-Fuchs, J., Hirsch, I. B., Kalantar-Zadeh, K., Narva, A. S., Navaneethan, S. D., Neumiller, J. J., Patel, U. D., Ratner, R. E., Whaley-Connell, A. T., & Molitch, M. E. (2014). Diabetic kidney disease: A report from an ADA Consensus Conference. *Diabetes Care, 37*(10), 2864–2883.

Ul Abideen, Z., Mahmud, S. N., Rasheed, A., Farooq Qasim, Y., & Ali, F. (2017). Central diabetes insipidus and hyperglycemic hyperosmolar state following accidental carbon monoxide poisoning. *Cureus, 9*(6), e1305.

van Abeelen, A. F., Elias, S. G., Bossuyt, P. M., Grobbee, D. E., van der Schouw, Y. T., Roseboom, T. J., & Uiterwaal, C. S. (2012). Famine exposure in the young and the risk of type 2 diabetes in adulthood. *Diabetes, 61*(9), 2255–2260.

Van Der Linden, M. W., Plat, A. W., Erkens, J. A., Emneus, M., & Herings, R. M. (2009). Large impact of antidiabetic drug treatment and hospitalizations on economic burden of diabetes mellitus in The Netherlands during 2000 to 2004. *Value in Health, 12*(6), 909–914.

Wang, Q., Brenner, S., Kalmus, O., Banda, H. T., & De Allegri, M. (2016). The economic burden of chronic non-communicable diseases in rural Malawi: An observational study. *BMC Health Services Research, 16*(1), 1–9.

Wedick, N. M., Pan, A., Cassidy, A., Rimm, E. B., Sampson, L., Rosner, B., … & van Dam, R. M. (2012). Dietary flavonoid intakes and risk of type 2 diabetes in US men and women. *The American Journal of Clinical Nutrition, 95*(4), 925–933.

Willi, C., Bodenmann, P., Ghali, W. A., Faris, P. D., & Cornuz, J. (2007). Active smoking and the risk of type 2 diabetes: A systematic review and meta-analysis. *JAMA, 298*(22), 2654–2664.

World Health Organization (2010). *Global recommendations on physical activity for health.* Geneva, Switzerland. https://www.who.int/publications/i/item/ 9789241599979, Access date 13.02.2021.

World Health Organization (2016). *Global report on diabetes.* Geneva, Switzerland. https://www.who.int/publications/i/item/9789241565257, Access date 13.02.2021.

World Health Organization European Office. (2018). *Türkiye'de bulaşıcı olmayan (kronik) hastalıkların önlenmesi ve kontrolü içinyatırım gerekçeleri raporu.* https://hsgm.saglik.gov.tr/depo/birimler/kronik-hastaliklar-engelli-db/hast aliklar/kalpvedamar/raporlar/BizzCaseTrSS.pdf, Access date 14.02.2021.

Wu, Y., Ding, Y., Tanaka, Y., & Zhang, W. (2014). Risk factors contributing to type 2 diabetes and recent advances in the treatment and prevention. *International Journal of Medical Sciences, 11*(11), 1185.

Yalçınkaya, M., Özer, F. G., & Karamanoğlu, A. Y. (2007). Sağlık çalışanlarında sağlıklı yaşam biçimi davranışlarının değerlendirilmesi. *TSK Koruyucu Hekimlik Bülteni, 6*(6), 409–420.

Yılmaz, T. (2003). Diabetes Mellitus' un Tanı Kriterleri ve Sınıflaması. In Yılmaz T., Bahceci M., Buyukbeşe A. (Eds), *Diabetes Mellitusun Modern Tedavisi İstanbu* (1st ed, pp. 1–10).

Zhang, L., Curhan, G. C., Hu, F. B., Rimm, E. B., & Forman, J. P. (2011). Association between passive and active smoking and incident type 2 diabetes in women. *Diabetes Care, 34*(4), 892–897.

Part II The Impact of Europeanization in Health Law and Policy

Azer Sumbas

Re-thinking Health Law and Politics in Turkey: A Dynamic Perspective from the Implementation of the EU Acquis

Introduction

Turkey's long-term relation with the EU is particularly related to the implementation of the EU Acquis (*Acquis*) and it is inevitable not to consider the EU policy in line with the *Acquis* in order to frame health law and policy. Whilst national health policy is still at the heart of the discussions before politicians and health professionals, "European Healthcare Union" *(EHU)* has literally begun to be shaped as a new, divided and independent chapter in European integration. Even though a comprehensive legislation hasn't been set up, yet, the process is still being encouraged by the Court of Justice of the European Union (CJEU) and the European Commission (EC). One the other hand, this process of shaping resulted in a crucial discussion on the *Acquis* due to the fact that the creation of a single European market has always been the main aim.

   In this sense, first and foremost, this research lies in the realm of Europeanization in the context of applying the *Acquis* in the Member States and candidate states. For instance, the EU might have an indirect effect on amending health-related regulations and reinforcing institutional reforms. Therefore, the first question to be clarified is whether the implementation of the *Acquis* and the transformation of institutions affecting national health law and policy is a matter of Europeanization. This complex issue will be explained with the concept of supremacy in regard to the legal theory of the EU and supremacy because European integration has to be conceptualized as an intertwined process of deregulation, harmonization and subsidiarity. Later, the alignment to the *Acquis* will be underlined as how it penetrates into domestic law because health policy does not only refer to policies focusing on the legislation for healthcare, also focuses on the structure of institutions in a broader context.

   At the second chapter, the core elements of the *EHU* will be described before Turkish health's alignment with the *Acquis* will be explained via referring to recent adopted laws, Health Transformation Plan (HTP), National Action Plan of the Ministry of Health and country reports by the EC. As the *Acquis* is a large concept constantly evolving, and which is not solely comprised of EU law in a strict sense, principles and political objectives of the EU Treaties and case law of the CJEU will be mentioned when appropriate.

Consequently, two-sided conclusion will be reached: The Europeanization of health law and policy results from mostly indirect impacts and Turkey's obligations arising from the *Acquis* in order to achieve the ultimate goal of full EU membership show a massive normative and structural transformation.

I. Methodology

The field of legal research has been mostly dominated by normative analyses of the law as doctrinal legal research methodology, also called "black letter law" (Tyler, 2017). Due to the fact that legal rules in primary sources are analysed in a detailed and descriptive way, this method not only describes the law; but also enables to comment and interpret on the sources. However, a multi-method particularly composed of doctrinal legal research and empirical research methods has been increasingly using to address a variety of legal questions for the last decades. The main reason of pursuing such a multi-method is lying on the acceptation of law not solely as a text-based discipline. In this regard, this research will employ a multi-method considering the broad influence of the EU policy as benefiting from policy papers and reports shall reveal much more regarding this research subject.

My first method is collecting sources of law comprised drawing up a series of selected EU's legal texts, includes the Founding Treaties of the EU, regulations and directives and the decisions of the CJEU. Under this collection, a qualitative analysis of legal materials is intended to support my hypothesis by identifying specific principles. My second method to develop an alternative perspective is selecting HTP, European Council country reports (2019 and 2020), EU Health Strategy Paper (2020), Turkey's National Action Plan (2016) revealing whether and how the implementation of the *Acquis* is achieved in Turkey. Thus, consisting of legal texts and policy papers shall be analysed to fit all together in a coherent system.

II. Europeanization: A Core Phenomenon in Health Systems

This research adopts EU law and European studies. Doing so, some language and terminology of European studies and scholars shall be selected. As there isn't a widely recognized definition for the term of "Europeanization"[1] in the

---

1   See for more arguments: Ladrech, 1994; Olsen, 2002.

literature. Europeanization is defined as "a process by which domestic policy areas become increasingly subject to European policy-making" (Börzel, 1999) or Europeanization means "a process of change in national institutional and policy practices that can be attributed to European integration" (Goetz & Hitz, 2000). For the purpose of this research, Radaelli's (2000) definition shall be preferred, that Europeanization process is formal and informal rules, procedures, policy paradigms, styles, "ways of doing things" and shared beliefs and norms which are first defined and consolidated in the making of EU decisions and then incorporated in the logic of domestic discourse, identities, political structures and public policies.

While the impact of the EU is progressively heading towards a large extent of law and policy domains, doubtlessly, health is becoming Europeanized as well (Greer et al., 2013). As a fact, the EU is a supranational body whose policies effect a wide range of public and private services including health services. In this sense, this chapter seeks to describe the impacts of Europeanization while underlining how it goes far beyond the policies due to the involvement of the discussions in every aspects of state sovereignty and domestic law. Nevertheless, the real question is how and when the supremacy of EU law affects health policies and law or, how it contradicts with state sovereignty.

A. The Legal Theory of the EU Interrelating Supremacy

It's a matter of fact that establishing the economies of participating states in common as a first attempt of European Community, later on referred to European Integration,[2] has transformed to surrender national sovereignty in some policy areas (Bache et al., 2015). Given that the Community particularly evolved to the EU after the Maastricht Treaty, the legal theory became much more complex. The Community was used to refer to a way of cooperation, the EU is accepted as a supranational body, even in some cases a legal entity[3] (Wessel, 2003). On the one hand, the EU is now more ambitious than before by including social inclusion, human rights, scientific research, immigration and environment. Accordingly, economic development extends itself improving health, too. (Greer et al., 2013) and in relation with EU law and its supremacy, *inter alia* primacy, neither the traditional statist language of sovereignty nor the old language of international law is adequate fully to explain the complexity of the EU legal order

---

2   There are numerous scholars who theorized European Integration. For instance: Haas, 1958; Lindberg, 1963; Tiez & Wiener, 2009.

3   See: Curtin & Dekker, 2011.

(Walker, 2005). In fact, the EU "interests the 'High Contracting Parties' as well as the private persons and entities within the member states" (Wessel, 2003). By all means, although member states preserve their national identities and competences, it cannot be deemed that they are subject to a complete isolation from the legislation and policy of the EU (Wessel, 2003). Thus, the question of where supremacy of EU law and state sovereignty stand for in further.

From the beginning of European integration, member states were concerned about the principle of supremacy and how this is to be accommodated within domestic constitutional orders (Berry et al., 2017). However, the Treaty Establishing the European Community (1997) and subsequent treaties do not mention the supremacy of EU law (Berry et al., 2017). For instance;

> Member States shall take all appropriate measures, whether general or particular, to ensure fulfilment of the obligations arising out of this Treaty or resulting from action taken by the institutions of the Community. They shall facilitate the achievement of the Community's tasks. (Article 10, EC Treaty)
> …The Member States shall facilitate the achievement of the Union's tasks and refrain from any measure which could jeopardize the attainment of the Union's objectives. (Article 4(3), TEU)

Nevertheless, the supremacy was ruled by the CJEU in landmark case of *Van Gend en Loos* (*1963*). In this case, the principle of direct effect was established via acknowledging that EU law was intended to confer rights on individuals and thus these rights must be enforceable (Berry et al., 2017). The CJEU recognized the principle of direct effect and supremacy as forming part of the new legal order regulating the relationship between the Community and its member states, and the legal subjects within the states as well (Wessel, 2003).

On the other side, De Witte (2011) distinguishes that "direct effect can be provisionally defined as the capacity of a norm of Union law to be applied in domestic court proceedings; whereas primacy (or supremacy) denotes the capacity of that norm of Union law to overrule inconsistent norms of national law in domestic court proceedings". Relevantly, the principle of direct applicability is recognized in case of regulations and directives in the Treaty of the Functioning of the European Union (TFEU);

> A regulation shall have a general application. It shall be binding in its entirety and directly applicable in all Member States.
> A directive shall be binding, as to the result to be achieved, upon each Member State to which it is addressed, but shall leave to the national authorities the choice of form and methods. (Article 288, TFEU)

Also, the CJEU approved the direct applicability of regulations and directives in *Politie SAS v. Minsitero delle Finanze* (1971) and *Van Duyn v. Home Office* (1974) which resulted in EU law having at least an indirect effect since "all national authorities have the obligation to interpret national legislation and other measures as much as possible in the light of the wording and purpose of valid EU law" (Wessel, 2003).

The principle of supremacy has been evolved with the principle of subsidiarity accepted in the Maastricht Treaty and it resulted in the involvement of the EU not only in national legal order; but also in national policy and institutions.

B. Penetration of National and Subnational Authorities

Considering the transformation in nation states and sovereignty, supranational organizations directly and explicitly have a voice in national matters. They are able to interfere in unitary sovereign through economic and social policies which occasionally cause powers to become fragmented and diffused within the market and society. This poses an immense challenge to the traditional concepts and practices between sovereignty and society as well as between legitimacy and legality (Jayasuriya, 2002). In other words, state sovereign becomes fragmented and distributed across a range of institutions.

However this fragmentation did not instantly appear in history. The ideology of sovereignty with the culture of traditional nation state in France manifested itself in the legal literature of unitary sovereignty. For instance, after the establishment of the League of Nations, French representative Leon Bourgeois stressed the French approach (Borgeois, 2018) and stated that none of states' sovereignty is bypassed by becoming a member of the League of Nations (Larson & Jenks, 1967) as referring to the Westheplian sovereignty. Besides, the legal interpretation on the League of Nations supported the said statement:

> The League of Nations is neither a federal state nor a confederation nor a supranational organization. (Hoijer, 1926)

On the other side, this interpretation has been changed following the establishment of the European Coal and Steel Community. Robert Schumann defined the powers of the Community as a supranational power that "High Authority, as the representative of the European Steel and Coal Community, is not vested with the characteristic of a state as a supranational organization; however it has particular sovereign powers. In the presence of national governments it is independent solely within the frame of the Community Convention….High Authority is not responsible before the governements; yet, he is responsible to the Community institutions" (Vedel, 1954).

To-day, each member state has been facing challenges about how to give effect to EU Law in their domestic legal order (Berry et. al., 2017), *vice versa*, candidate states are concerned about the effects of the implementation of the *Acquis*. Prior to the evolvement to the EU, the CJEU interpreted the hierarchy between Community and national law in *Costa v. E.N.E.L*[4] by stating that member states have a legal obligation to ensure that the rights within the Treaty are equally available in all Member States and that no national rules can restrict Community law rights. As a fact, "Community law were in principle to be recognized as a valid and indeed superior source of law within the national legal systems" (Dougan, 2011). Besides, TFEU's objectives, in general, must be converted into detailed EU law and transposed and implemented into the national laws (Greer et al., 2013). Considering the principle of supremacy, direct effect, direct applicability and the CJEU's interpretation so far, there is no doubt that EU law has a decentralizing, and even de-regulating impact on national legal order.

Apart from the impact on national legal order, a significant change in subnational authorities have come to forward with the recognition of the principle of subsidiarity in the Maastricht Treaty:

> …In areas which do not fall within its exclusive competence, the Community shall take action, in accordance with the principle of subsidiarity, only if and in so far as the objectives of the proposed action cannot be sufficiently achieved by the Member States and can therefore, by reason of the scale or effects of the proposed action, be better achieved by the Community. (Article 5 TEU)

Allocation of competence between member states and the EU became a much more complex issue with the principle of subsidiarity due to the fact that "it goes to wider issues than legal effectiveness as member states' sense of self-government is at present" (Chalmers et al., 2014).

Tour court, while this research comes to the terms with a significant transformation on the theory of sovereignty, it is a fact that Western European states have already softened the barriers of state sovereignty through the European Union and EU law interpretation.

---

4   Case 6/64 *Costa* v. *E.N.E.L* [1964] ECR 585.

III. A European "Healthcare" Union: Normative or Structural Change?

As above-explained in detail, the conception of a new legal order resulted in the Member States transferring a part of their sovereignty powers to the EU and, now, EU law is a part of the legal systems of the Member States (Berry, 2017). However, healthcare didn't suddenly appear in the EU's policy agenda which caused a policy and law patchwork (Hervey, 2016) involving elements of the principle of free movement, single market and competition. On the other side, the CJEU's decisions, EU regulations, Health Strategy Reports cleared the fog and provided a replacement of a European Healthcare Union *(EHU)*. While the EC Treaty[5] essentially states that healthcare is the responsibility of the Member States, health systems interacts with people, goods and services which are clearly related to the core element of free movement (Mossialos et al., 2010). In accordance with Europeanization, the concept of a *EHU* consists of three components: European, health care which involves the organization and financing and union referring to healthcare systems as a distinct entity (Vollaard & Martinsen, 2017). In this sense, the common values and principles became a credible expression of the principles and themes of EU health law[6] (Hervey, 2016). On the one hand, the question of how far the *Acquis* pushing the Member States, even candidate states, for a *EHU* is raised as the supremacy of EU law is extendedly established.

A. EU Law v. EU Policy

Given that the EU principally recognizes the Member States' sovereign-powers on healthcare,[7] the EU has a complementary role in health policy:

> A high level of human health protection shall be ensured in the definition and implementation of all Union policies and activities. (TFEU, Article 168 (1))

In this sense, the EU issue recommendations, conclusions and reports as defining key measures including but not limited to patients' rights in cross-border health-care, medicines and medical devices, serious cross-border health threats, cancer,

---

5　Article 152(5) EC Treaty.
6　Hervey alleges that a distinct area of EU health law has been narrated into existence over the years and the legal regulation of healthcare in the EU is no longer a matter of EU law. However, within the purpose of this research paper, EU health policy and law shall be mentioned rather than solely the notion of "EU health law".
7　TFEU, Article 168 (7).

tobacco and promotion of good health and organs, blood, tissues and cells (EU Health Policy, 2020). In order to give a short explanation on the EU's (extending) health policy, Council Conclusions in 2006 and in 2011 will be referred to due to their direct relevance to health. Council's Conclusions[8] in 2006 put forward common values and principles in order to establish a *EHU*. Doing so, its statement cleared out the EU's policies and institutions' effect that removing healthcare from the Directive on Services in the Internal Market should result from political consensus, and not solely from case law (Council Conclusions, 2006). The values of universality, access to good quality care, equity, and solidarity and operating principles of quality, safety, patient involvement, redress, privacy and confidentiality and care based on evidence and ethics have been accepted relatedly. Later on, The Council Conclusion in 2011 particularly invited the Commission to promote an adequate role of the health sector in the implementation of the Europe2020 Strategy (Council Conclusion, 2011). Both the Council Conclusions indeed cleared the way for the EU Health Strategy Papers and EU4Health Programme.

Health Strategy Paper primarily recognized the achievement for the real improvements in health only in case of a work across government. In the meantime, it declared that "Good health benefits all sectors and the whole of society, making it a valuable resource. Health and well-being are essential for economic and social development and of vital concern to the lives of every person, family and community" (Health Strategy Paper, 2020).

Lately, EU4Health Programme for 2021–2027[9] aiming to support the national policies of the Member States and to promote coordination among them in order to improve human health throughout the EU, has been provisionally agreed by the Council and the European Parliament (Council of the EU, 2020). In a nutshell, it seems that integration of health aspects in all policies, as well as Europeanization of health systems are a fundamental part of Europe's social infrastructure. Thus, objectives, values and principles set up by various policy papers should not be underestimated in the discussion of European Healthcare Union and its impact on the Member States and candidate states.

---

8   Council's Conclusions do not have a legal impact on the Member States; however, they intend to express a political position on a topic related to the EU's areas of activity, i.e. health, education.

9   For updated news see: Council of the EU, Press Releases. https://www.consilium. europa.eu/en/press/press-releases/

1. Chapters of Acquis

The *Acquis*[10] comprises 31 chapters covering the entire of the EU policies. However, health in *acquis* are not covered by a single chapter but almost all have some references and implications on it. The chapters particularly relevant to health are Chapter 28, on health and consumer protection and, Chapter 19, on social policy and employment;

Chapter 19 includes minimum standards in the areas of labour law, equality, health and safety at work and anti-discrimination while Chapter 28 aims to protect consumers' economic interests in relation to product safety, dangerous imitations and liability for defective products. The EU also ensures high common standards for tobacco control, blood, tissues, cells and organs, patients' rights and communicable diseases (European Commission, 2019). Furthermore, the chapter on free movement of goods implies to the medical devices and health products and chapter on freedom to provide services and freedom of movement of workers involve health professions as the chapter on environment's relevance with health raises from, not limited to, water and air quality, industrial pollution control and risk.

B. The Alignment of Turkey

Turkey-EU relationship has commenced with the application for association to the European Economic Community in 1959 and the Association Agreement (Ankara Agreement) in 1963. Mid-1990s has been noted a milestone as Turkey entered the Final Period in 1995 by completing "Transition Period" which lasted 22 years and completed the process of Customs Union Period (Chronology of Turkey-European Union Relations, 2020). Turkey's candidate status after the decision in Helsinki Summit (1999) shouldn't be seen as an ordinary process in the EU relations due to the fact that this era overlaps neo-liberal policies and Europeanization as well. In this timeline Turkey's long-term and open-ended relations with the EU, eight chapters of *Acquis* have suspended due to the Turkey's failure to fulfil its obligations related to the Additional Protocol to the Ankara Agreement. Currently, 16 out of 35 chapters are opened (Current Status, 2021). In fact, some of them are directly, some are indirectly related to health.

The question of Turkish health law and policy's alignment with the *Acquis* and Europeanization does not only lie in with solely legislative dimensions; but

---

10 Acquis communautaire comprises EU law, including its objectives, policies, legislation and case law. It's simply shortened to the EU Acquis or the *Acquis*.

also historical and socio-legal. However, due to the its extent, this research will only deal with organization and legislation formulated by the EU. This formulation may be divided in *normative alignment* and *structural alignment* particularly considering that Turkey is the only country in the Customs Union without being a full member of the EU. Alignment in health law and policy in terms of *structural alignment* becomes distinct from *normative alignment* substantially in institutional transformation which is not to be restricted with national plans, progress reports, projects, research and education programmess, strength of NGOs, foreign investment and health tourism. *Structural alignment* mainly signifies adapting and amending a massive body of laws in accordance with principles, objectives and policies in harmony with the EU law. For instance, Turkish National Action Plan for EU Accession for the years of 2016–2019 resulted in adapting 25 health-related regulations covering five chapters (Ministry of Foreign Affairs, 2016).

1. Normative Transformation

Beginning from the 2000s, a massive adoption and amendment on legislation occurred in Turkey. Some were related to Europeanization and global change; others were lined with change in national policy. In the sense of the accession negotiations, Turkey substantiated its obligations to fully align to the *Acquis* and to enhance the adequate capacity to implement them via adopting health-related laws of which a selection can be seen in Tab. 1.

Tab. 1: Adopted Legislation and Change in Health Services

2003	Pilot scheme for wage system based on performance at the hospital.
2004	Publishing Memorandum (117) "Restructuring Ambulatory Care Services" to provide patients to select physicians at their own choice.
2005	Amending Law (5283) gathering all public hospitals under a single roof. Amending Law (3359) setting up a substructure for public-private partnership. Adopting By-Law to establish "Patient's Rights Branch", "Patient's Rights Provincial Coordinatorship", "Patient's Rights Committee" and "Patient's Rights Department in Hospital".
2006	Adopting Law (5510) to extend the scope of social security.
2007	Publishing Health Practices Statement. Abolishment of Compulsory referral chain.
2009	Launch of E-prescription.
2010	Establishment of Department of Health Tourism. Start of Health Services at home. Launch of Family physician services in all provinces. Amendment of Full-time employment law.
2011	Decree-Law (663) restructured central and provincial organization of the Health Ministry. Department of Health Tourism transformed within the body of General Directorate of Health Services. Central System for Physician Appointment carried in to effect.
2012	Establishment of Department of Accreditation and Quality in Health. Establishment of Public Hospital Associations at the provincial level.
2013	Practice of E-prescription in all provinces.
2015	Establishment of Council for Health Tourism Coordination.
2017	Launch of first "City Hospital".
2019	Amending Health Professions Act. Adoption of Personal Health Data By-Law.
2020	Amending Health Professions Act. Adopting Act of Project Support Program for Turkish Health Institutes. Amending Communiqué for Social Security Instution on Healthcare Practices. Amending Communiqué for the Ministry of Health's circulating capital enterprises.
2021	Publishing Statements regarding import control for the goods subjected to the supervision and permission of the Ministry of Health.

Notes: Some parts of this table were adopted from the research of Altındağ & Yıldız (2020). Some of those were acquired via the Official Gazette of the Republic of Turkey.

The normative transformation aiming at achieving a satisfied implementation of the *Acquis* also causes a significant transformation in socio-legal and economic aspects. Because neither the European Commission Reports show a significant progress nor the Turkish national plans provide a coherence.

2. European Commission Reports

Country reports which are one-sided documents, are prepared annually by the EC in order to evaluate the progress achieved by the candidate countries with respect to the Copenhagen criteria (Directorate of EU Affairs, 2020). So far, 22 reports were issued regarding the progress of Turkey in which health protection mainly mentioned under social policy and employment till the 2005 report. Europeanization and European integration deeming primarily as an economic integration progress was the reason. But then, as *EHU* was appeared, Commission reports started to focus on health and consumer protection. Thus, due to their recency, 2019 and 2020 reports shall be expressed here in below.

According to the both reports, Turkey is at a good level of preparation for legislative alignment and there has been some progress to implement the EU public health acquis; but recommendations for ensuring effective protection of consumers by better enforcement and better coordination of and cooperation with consumer groups and for increasing its institutional/administrative capacity, inter-sectoral cooperation, financial resources and appropriate diagnostic facilities to address public health issues at central and provincial level haven't been fully implemented in 2019 and 2020. (EC Report, 2020). Several reasons might lie behind the failure: Firstly, Covid-19 pandemic resulted in having a hitch in performing all public sectors. Secondly, social and financial burden cause Turkey to present a huge excuse while its administrative and institutional substructure do not facilitate, *per se* to improve its capacity.

3. National Action Plan and HTP

National Action Plan and HTP resulted in *structural alignment* and *normative alignment* at the same time. The finger-prints of the EU dynamics and policies can be traced not only in alignment with the *Acquis*; but also in policy impositions of the WHO and IMF via their financial and technical support including studies on Turkish healthcare reforms (Yıldırım et al., 2020). With the respect of those policy impositions, Turkey adopted a hybrid health model beginning from the 2000s and HTP (2003) which caused decentralization in healthcare system. This hybrid model is based on three main axes: compulsory premiums paid by every citizen, general taxation and complementary private insurance as transferring elements from the three main health care financing models of the social health insurance model, the Beveridge model and the liberal model (Demirci, 2012). HTP indeed embraced a free market perspective in line with the World Bank directives and Europeanization as of involving the principles of sustainability, human-centred, participatory, negotiating, embodying continuous quality improvement, voluntary, separation of powers, decentralization and competition (Ministry of Health, 2003).

Moreover, National Action Plan announced the adoption and amendment in primary and secondary legislation in addition to the restructuring the institutional capacity:

Tab. 2: Legislation and Institutional Capacity to be Changed-Adopted-Amended

Year	Legislation/Institution	Alignment with the Acquis	Responsible Turkish Authority
2016/1st half	Law on Product Safety and Technical Regulations	Regulation (EC) 764/ 2008 and 765/2008, Repealing Regulation 339/ 93, Decision 768/2008 of the European Parliament, Directive 2001/95/EC	Ministry of Economy
2016/1st half	Amending the By-Law on Organ and Tissue Transplantation Services	Directive 2010/53/EU	Ministry of Health
2016/1st half	Amending the By-Law on Principles and Procedures concerning the Production Type, Labelling and Inspection of Tobacco Products for the purpose of Protection from Harmful Effects of Tobacco Products	EU Directive 2014/40/EU	Tobacco and Alcohol Market Regulatory Authority
2017/1st half	By-Law on General Product Safety	Directive 2001/95/EC	Ministry of Economy, Ministry of Customs and Trade
2019/1st half	Appropriate legislation for serious cross-border threats to health	Decision 1082/2013/EU	Ministry of Health, Disaster and Emergency Management Presidency, Ministry of Food, Agriculture and Livestock
2016/2nd half	Work towards the safe blood supply	Instrument for Pre-Accession Assessment (IPA) programming project (2010)	Ministry of Health, Turkish Red Crescent Society, Ministry of National Education
2016/1st half	Improving the institutional capacity in the area of organ donation	IPA programming project on Organ Donation (2009)	Ministry of Health
2016/ 2nd half	Improving the institutional capacity in the area of cell and tissue	IPA programming project on Cell and Human Tissues (2009)	Ministry of Health

Note: National Action Plan for EU Accession: https://www.ab.gov.tr/files/5Ekim/eylem_plani_ing_ ic_sirali_internet_icin_tarandi.pdf

Conclusion

At the centre of removing barriers to trade and promoting competitive behaviour has always been with the aim to create the single market. However, it is arguable whether candidate countries, such as Turkey, are able to handle to be reinforced national authorities to transform their national regulations ensuring an appropriate area for its integration. As Europeanization of Turkish health law and policy became the ultimate goal of full EU membership, the problem occurs in the cases that socio-economic substructure aren't sufficient enough because while the real power in the EU lies in its law, and the law is sometimes deregulatory and disruptive rather than supportive (Greer et al., 2013). Harmonization, regulation and deregulation are gradually updated as a dynamic process of Europeanization. As Foreign Ministry of Turkey lately made a statement that Turkey is committed to immediately starting top-level dialogue serving common interests in all areas, including the economy, energy, not just regional and health-related issues (Berker & Cakmak, 2021). Yet, it seems that transmission and transformation of Turkish health law and policy is an ongoing process with its ups-and-downs.

Tout court, this research shows a two-sided picture: First, Europeanization in the health policy field results from mostly indirect impacts. Secondly, the obligations arising from the *Acquis* identifies a growing new, complex responsibilities to the national and subnational authorities while the applicability of some is not widely and easily transformed because the harmonization of national laws in the *Acquis* also requires a "harmonized" administrative and institutional capacity providing to implement them effectively. However, it seems that Turkey's progress on the harmonization in the sense of Europeanization does show a massive change in institutional capacity and legislation which is currently questionable considering its vertical and horizontal coherence in its socio-legal and economic situation.

References

Altındağ, Ö. & Yıldız, A. (2020). Türkiye'de Sağlık Politikalarının Dönüşümü (Transformation of Health Policy in Turkey). *Birey ve Toplum*, 10 (1), 157–184.

Bache, I., Bulmer, S., George, S., & Parker, O. (2015). *Politics in the European Union* (4th ed.). Oxford University Press.

Berker, M. & Cakmak B. N. (2021). *Turkey Welcomes Conclusion Adopted by European Council* (26.03.2021). Anadolu Agency. https://www.aa.com.tr/en/europe/turkey-welcomes-conclusion-adopted-by-european-council/2188 626#. Access date 12.06.2021.

Berry, E., Homewood, M. J. & Bogusz, B. (2017). *Complete EU Law: Text, Cases and Materials* (3rd ed.). Oxford University Press.

Bourgeois L. (2018) *L'œuvre de la Société des nations (1920–1923)* (ed. 1923). Hachette Livre, Paris.

Börzel, A. T. (1999). Towards Convergence in Europe? Institutional Adaptation to Europeanization in Germany and Spain. *Journal of Common Market Studies*, 37 (4), 573–596.

Chalmers, D., Davies, G. & Monti, G. (2014). *European Union Law* (3rd ed.). Cambridge University Press.

Council Conclusions on Common Values and Principles in European Union Health Systems (2006). OJ C146/1. https://eur-lex.europa.eu/legal-cont ent/EN/TXT/PDF/?uri=CELEX:52006XG0622(01)&rid=1. Access date 09.05.2021.

Council Conclusions: Towards Modern, Responsive and Sustainable Health Systems. (2011). OJ C202/10. https://eur-lex.europa.eu/LexUriServ/LexUriS erv.do?uri=OJ:C:2011:202:0010:0012:EN:PDF. Access date 09.05.2021.

Council of the EU, Press Release. (15 December 2020). *EU4Health Programme for 2021–2027.* https://www.consilium.europa.eu/en/press/press-releases/ 2020/12/15/protecting-people-s-health-the-council-and-the-european-par liament-agree-provisionally-on-the-eu4health-programme-for-2021-2027/. Access date 09.05.2021.

Current Status. (2021). *Delegation of the European Union to Turkey.* https://www. avrupa.info.tr/en/current-status-742. Access date 09.05.2021.

Demirci, B. (2012). *Transformation in the Organizational and Financial Set-up of the Health Care System in Turkey – Its Repercussions and Similarities with the English Model* (unpublished doctoral dissertation). Middle East Technical University, Ankara.

De Witte, B. (2011). Direct Effect, Primacy, and the Nature of the Legal Order. In Craig, P. & De Burca, G. (eds.), *The Evolution of EU Law* (2nd ed., pp. 323–363). Oxford University Press.

Directorate for EU Affairs of the Ministry of Foreign Affairs of the Republic of Turkey. (2020). *Chronology of Turkey-EU Relations (1959–2019).* https://www. ab.gov.tr/siteimages/birimler/kpb/chronology-_en-_1959-_ocak2020.pdf. Access date 10.06.2021.

Dixon, A. & Poteliathoff, E. (2012). Back to the future: 10 years of European health reforms. *Health Economics, Policy and Law*, 7, 1–10.

Dougan, M. (2011). The Vicissitudes of life at the Coalface: Remedies and Procedures for Enforcing Union Law before the National Courts. In Craig,

P. & De Burca, G. (eds.), *The Evolution of EU Law* (2nd ed, pp. 407–439). Oxford University Press.

European Commission. (2019). *Chapters of EU Acquis.* European Neighbourhood Policy and Enlargement Negotiations. https://ec.europa.eu/neighbourhood-enlargement/policy/conditions-membership/chapters-of-the-acquis_en. Access date 11.05.2021.

European Commission. (2020). *Commission Staff Working Paper: Turkey 2020 Report (10.06.2020),* SWD (2020) 355 Final https://www.ab.gov.tr/siteima ges/trkiye_raporustrateji_belgesi_2020/turkey_report_2020.pdf. Access date 10.05.2021.

European Council (2020). *European Health Policy.* https://www.consilium.eur opa.eu/en/policies/eu-health-policy/. Access date 04.05.2021.

Flaminio Costa v E.N.E.L. (Case 6/64), [1964] ECR 585. https://eur-lex.eur opa.eu/legal-content/EN/TXT/?uri=CELEX%3A61964CJ0006. Access date 10.05.2021.

Greer Scott, L., Hervey, T. K., Mackenbach, J. P. & McKee, M. (2013). Health law and policy in the European Union. *The Lance,* 381 (9872), t1135–1144.

Goetz, K. & Hix, S. (eds.) (2000). *Europeanised Politics? European Integration and National Political Systems,* London: Frank Cass.

Hervey T., K. (2016). Telling stories about European Union Health Law: The emergence of a new field of law. *Comparative European Politics,* 15(3), 352–369.

Hoijer, O. (1926). *Le Pacte de la Société des Nations: Commentaire Théorique et Pratique: Préface de M. André.* Paris: Editions Spes.

Jayasuriya K. (2002). Globalization, Sovereignty, and the Rule of Law: From Political to Economic Constitutionalism? *Constellations,* 8(4), 442–460.

Ladrech R. (1994). Europeanization of Domestic Politics and Institutions: The Case of France. *Journal of Common Market Studies,* 32-(1), 69–88.)

Larson A. & Jenks C. W. (1967. *Sovereignty Within the Law.* London: Oceana Publications.

Ministry of Health. (2003). *Turkey Health Transformation Plan: Assessment Report (2003–2011).* https://sbu.saglik.gov.tr/Ekutuphane/kitaplar/SDPturk. pdf. Access date 05.05.2021.

Mossialos E., Permanand, G., Baeten, R. & Hervey (2010). The Role of European Union Law and Policy. In Mossialos, E., Permanand, G., Baeten, R. & Hervey, T. (eds.). *Health Systems Governance in Europe: The Role of EU Law and Policy* (1st ed., pp. 1–84). Cambridge University Press.

Politie SAS v. Ministero delle Finanze, (Case 43/71), [1971] ECR 1039. https:// eur-lex.europa.eu/legal-content/EN/ALL/?uri=CELEX%3A61971CJ0043.

Radaelli, C. M. (2000). Wither Europeanization: Concept Stretching and Substantive Change. *European Integration Online Papers*, 4 (8), 1–25. Access date 08.05.2021.

The Ministry of Foreign Affairs. (2016) *Turkey's National Action Plan for the EU Accession*. https://www.ab.gov.tr/turkeys-national-action-plan-for-the-eu-acc ession_50083_en.html. Access date 05.05.2021.

Tyler, T. R. (2017). Methodology in legal research. *Utrecht Law Review*, 13 (3), 130–41.

Van Gend en Loos v. Netherlandse Administratie de Belastingen, (Case 26/ 62) [1963] E.C.R. 1. https://eur-lex.europa.eu/legal-content/EN/TXT/?uri= CELEX%3A61962CJ0026. Access date 11.05.2021.

Vedel G. (1954) Reuter (Paul) – La Communauté européenne du charbon et de l'acier. Préface de Robert Schuman, *Revue française de science politique, 4ᵉ année*, n°4, 899–901.

Vollaard, H. & Martinsen D. S. (2017). The Rise of a European Healthcare Union. *Comparative European Politics*, 15 (3), 337–351.

Walker, N. (2005). Legal Theory and the European Union: A 25th Anniversary Essay. *Oxford Journal of Legal Studies*, 25 (4), 581–601, doi: 10. 1093/ojls/ gqi031.

Wessel Ramses, A. (2003). The Constitutional Relationship between the European Union and the European Community: Consequences for the Relationship with the Member States. Max Planck Institute for Comparative Public Law and International Law. *Jean Monnet Working Paper*, 9/0 Heidelberg, 24–27 February 2003. https://jeanmonnetprogram.org/archive/papers/03/030901- 09.pdf. Access date 29.04.2021.

World Health Organization. (2013). *Health 2020. A European policy framework and strategy for the 21st century*. https://www.euro.who.int/en/publications/ abstracts/health-2020.-a-european-policy-framework-and-strategy-for-the- 21st-century-2013. Access date 08.05.2021.

Yıldırım, H., Yıldırım, T., Bilir, M. K., Arı, H. O., Özkan, O. & Giray, H. (2020). Europeanization of the Turkish Health Policy: A Historical Exploration. *Journal of Health Systems and Policies*, 2 (1), 87–136.

Yvonne van Duyn v Home Office, (Case 41/74), [1974] ECR 1337. https://eur- lex.europa.eu/legal-content/EN/TXT/?uri=CELEX%3A61974CJ0041. Access date 03.05.2021.

Sezgin Mercan

Europeanization of Health Policies after Covid-19: Politicization, Governance and Coordination

Introduction

In a speech made at the end of 2020, the President of France, Emmanuel Macron questioned the possibility of global access to the Covid-19 vaccine. His another question was about the possibility of creating a two-speed world in which only the richest would be protected from the virus. The first signs in this respect do not give hope. Covid-19 has shown that European integration is not rooted geopolitically and industrially. A geopolitical and industrial competition has begun in terms of vaccine development among China, the USA, Germany, England, Israel. and Russia. The European Union (EU) fell behind in this competition (Pierru, Stambach & Vernaudon, 2021).

President of the European Commission von der Leyen underlined the importance of EU preparation for pandemics in a speech. She said this preparation of the EU and other international actors should include increasing reaction to health crises. Difficulties in reaction to health threats and diffusion of Covid-19 vaccine triggered this type of response (Fleming, 2021). According to von der Leyen,

> It's an era of pandemics we are entering. If you look at what has been happening over the past few years, I mean from HIV to Ebola to MERS to SARS, these were all epidemics which could be contained, but we should not think it is all over when we've overcome Covid-19. The risk is still there. (Fleming, 2021)

In addition, she emphasized EU's failure in vaccination initiative and campaign in comparison with the US and the UK (Fleming, 2021).

The EU was highly criticized by some member states which pointed out its inability to display a strong profile against Covid-19. It took time to clarify what kind of reaction to develop in terms of economic costs. In the context of the EU, this was not surprising. Because the health sector or health-related issues have been recognized as an area of responsibility for national governments. EU institutions such as the European Commission have been accepted as coordination and suggestion promoter to combat with Covid-19. However, member states have luxury of accepting or rejecting suggestions. Article 168 of the Treaty on the

Functioning of the European Union clearly defined this situation. This treaty has made the EU a complementary to the national health policies of the member states. But Covid-19 required the EU to do more. This requirement addresses the Europeanization of health policies. Europeanization includes cooperation, coordination, and common policies, interests, values from the European level in classical sense. It requires to follow European level social interests sometimes substituting for national preferences. Besides, Europeanization includes a form of governance based on some rules and procedures. Europeanization based convergence in policy areas of the EU has begun to reflect a modest domestic change of health policies with Covid-19.

This chapter is planned to be based on parts including new Europeanization effect on health policies of the EU members, sustainability of convergence in decision-making on health policies, and governance and politicization issues at the EU level under Covid-19. In this framework, some specific arguments that address public health, intergovernmentalism vs. supranationalism, decision-making, security-health relations, and Turkey-EU relations based on health are concerned. The main argument of this chapter is high politicization of health thanks to Covid-19 pandemic has increased EU level cooperation and Europeanization of it. The first section of this chapter introduces literature review and theoretical background of Europeanization concept. The second section presents decision-making forms with reference to the discussion based on intergovernmentalism, supranationalism, and complexity. The following section contains basic findings and discussions on Europeanization effect in health issues. Then a brief evaluation on Turkey-EU relations is included. The method of the article is to apply the concept of Europeanization to the case of EU's health policy. For this purpose, various secondary sources were used for conceptual and empirical analysis, as well as official EU documents that constitute the primary sources.

I. The Conceptual Framework: Europeanization

Since 1980s, Europeanization has become a significant reference for European studies. This concept is related with identity and legitimacy issues, social and cultural matters, economic and political subjects. It is also related with domestic and international changes. EU membership is basic motivator for domestic or national changes. Reflections of some domestic or national preferences to EU level are another dimension of Europeanization. Because this chapter addresses the Europeanization of health policies, it requires to concentrate on changing domestic or national preferences on this subject.

Europeanization has different meanings. It means regional integration and convergence based on political, social, economic, institutional, and ideal changes. It also means export of norms, beliefs, values, behaviour, and practices. Europeanization includes transnationalism which reflects spread of norms, values, ideas, and practices on European scale. Transnational spread can be accepted for different sectors from sport to education (Featherstone, 2003). As a comprehensive definition,

> Europeanization consists of processes of construction, diffusion, and institutionalisation of formal and informal rules, procedures, policy paradigms, styles, ways of doing things, and shared beliefs and norms which are first defined and consolidated in the EU policy process and then incorporated in the logic of domestic (national and subnational) discourse, political structures and public policies. (Radaelli, 2004)

Europeanization has a quality beyond transnational effects, meanings, and practices. It is also a result of market dynamics. Establishment of a single market, competition standards, standards for social security, and regulations for welfare state have become basic pillars of this dynamics. There are three properties of Europeanization (Bulmer & Radaelli, 2004): Firstly, Europeanization derives from some stages and forms as construction in the sense of policy formulation; institutionalization in the sense of putting policy into practice; and diffusion in the sense of EU's limited role forming an attitude. Secondly, Europeanization is related with policy rules, norms, values, and beliefs. Thirdly, this concept includes effects of the EU policies on member states. There are two steps for the effects as adoption at supranational EU level and integration at national level (Bulmer & Radaelli, 2004).

Common EU policies, laws, obligations, instruments, transnational pressures, different national inspirations in European area for learning construct the independent variable in European studies. The dependent variable can be found in Europeanized factor. Politics, polity, policy, and discourse are the factors that correspond to the Europeanization. Ideas, interests, strategies, governments, parliaments, institutions, norm, beliefs, agendas, practices, rhetoric, narratives, and legitimation constitute the content of these four factors. In addition to this, the extent of Europeanization is also significant as another dimension of the dependent variable. Effects, transformation, absorption, accommodation, and strategies are different factors of the Europeanization. Depth, degree of change, the situation of affected and unaffected features, and preferences of member states accepting Europeanization constitute the content of these five factors (Featherstone & Papadimitriou, 2008).

Europeanization requires to consider two types for integration called positive and negative integration. Positive integration necessitates supranational policies. In other words, the EU decides whatever is negotiated and member states apply the negotiated output. Market rules, common policies, regional decisions are components of positive integration. Under the conditions of negative integration, neutralization of national limits become adequate to form a common EU policy. In order to realize a common EU policy, national legislation would not be an obligation. Border controls, tax regimes, telecommunication issues, transport services, and energy matters can be accepted as the subjects of negative integration. "In negative integration, it is the competition amongst rules or amongst socio-economic actors that accounts for Europeanization rather than the need for national policy to comply with EU policy templates, as under positive integration" (Bulmer & Radaelli, 2004). In short, positive integration has an analytical core of "market correcting rules" and "EU policy templates". Negative integration has analytical core of "market-making rules" and "absence of policy templates" (Bulmer & Radaelli, 2004).

In positive integration, coercive side of Europeanization can be followed. Some common policies like agricultural policy, monetary union, social policy, and environmental policy are accepted with supranational pressure for adaptation. In negative integration, regulatory pressure is not so much compared to positive integration. But, competition is a propellant for member states to take position in common policies. Intergovernmental processes correspond coordination in common policies like foreign and security policy, employment policy, research and development (Bulmer & Radaelli, 2004).

Europeanization is about compatibility between national and supranational dynamics. "The lower the compatibility between European and domestic processes, policies, and institutions, the higher the adaptational pressure" (Börzel & Risse, 2000). Adaptational pressure becomes effective when EU policies may challenge national preferences and policies. In addition, it becomes effective when EU policies and rules challenge position of national institutions. The EU can give some national or domestic actors privileged positions in decision-making mechanism against other actors (Börzel & Risse, 2000).

Policy uploading and downloading processes are two-ways for Europeanization. It creates some benefits and costs for member states of the EU. In order to increase benefits and reduce adaptation costs of EU policies, uploading national policies to the EU level is accepted as a significant method. This method may ensure national governments to create a way solving domestic problems effectively. Organized crime, pollution, immigration, and also health problems may be stood up in this way. Conflictual nature of different preferences, regulations, and policies of member states may trigger rise of liberalization or protection and social or industrial principles, etc. (Börzel, 2002).

Member states pursue their own preferences inherently. They follow three strategies to protect their preferences in the EU level. Firstly, member states try to change EU policies considering their interests. In this way, domestic preferences can be accepted by other EU members. This is the strategy of "pace-setting" (Börzel, 2002). On the opposite side, "foot-dragging" includes stopping or restricting other EU members to upload their national policies to the EU level. Foot-dragging prevents full compliance with the EU law (Börzel, 2002). There is "fence-sitting" between these two strategies. Fence-sitting may reflect an impartial attitude or changing position considering different conditions and issues. Thus, EU policies do not have to face obstacles (Börzel, 2002). Economically developed states tend to be pace-setters, less developed states are foot-dragging. So, economic development is a main determinant in the approach to Europeanization. Those with economically similar levels of development form a preference group. Different similarities may construct coalitions of common interests. These coalitions may become actors of disagreements on common EU policies like environment, transport, and health (Börzel, 2002).

II. Decision-making Forms: Intergovernmentalism, Supranationalism, and Complexity

Theorizing European integration reflects a division between intergovernmentalism and supranationalism. Intergovernmentalism sees the EU members as the main actors in controlling European integration. In this integration, national governments are able to protect the interests of their own people. Intergovernmentalism necessitates considering the meetings of the European Council, Council of Ministers, and EU Summits in the pandemic. These organizations accept governments of the EU members as basic actors in decision-making process. On the opposite side, national governments are not authoritative bodies in supranationalism. The basic institutions of European integration are acceptable as long as they increase the control of national governments on internal matters. As seen in European integration, supranational institutions can also increase the power and effectiveness of governments (Schmidt, 2020).

From the perspective of intergovernmentalism, the EU's health policy is not shaped by the European Summits, EU level negotiations, etc. The EU members' collective interests and consent are driving forces in the way of constructing and funding common health policy. Generally, this perspective accepts that member states prefer behaviour or policies that match their interests (Schmidt, 2020).

From the perspective of supranationalism, the EU's health policy is shaped by the European Summits, EU institutions, EU level negotiations, etc. The Commission's and the Council's roles are considered with reference to proposals on health program, health policy, and funding of them. However, supranationalists accept the Commission's role in vaccine policies as a coordinator between the EU and its members (Schmidt, 2020).

Relationship between intergovernmentalism and supranationalism reflects politicization. Some crises of the EU like Eurozone and migration triggered disagreements between the EU institutions and member states. They criticized actions of eachother and increased politicization level. The pandemic conditions have also triggered politicization, but more cooperative attitude has been seen.

> For example, in a major break with what the traditional intergovernmentalists saw as the path-dependent pattern of the Council seeking to take back control from the Commission, in the current pandemic the Council instead gave the Commission more power and responsibility, by asking the Commission to provide new ideas for innovations across policy areas and then giving it greater responsibilities, such as with regard to the European recovery fund. (Schmidt, 2020)

In order to evaluate the decision-making process complexity perspective is beneficial. This perspective,

> combines two axes based on the degree of certainty and of agreement for a particular policy area. High levels of certainty indicate that the issue is well known and easily understood, while low levels of certainty imply that it is unknown/unknowable and that there are great differences in opinion over the issue, even among experts. Meanwhile, high levels of agreement denote substantial public agreement over the nature of, and solution to the issue, while low levels of certainty imply substantial public debate and disagreement. (Brooks & Geyer, 2020)

According to this perspective, there are five types of decision-making: Techno-rational decision-making, political decision-making, judgemental decision-making, mixed complex decision-making, and disorder intuition (Brooks & Geyer, 2020). Techno-rational zone reflects a high certainty, high agreement, and well understood subject. Political type reflects high certainty, low agreement on response, clear data, and well understood subject or problem. Because of low agreement, negotiations and bargaining processes become important between related actors. Judgemental decision-making includes low certainty, high agreement, but no simple response. There are different strategies to solve problems. Mixed complex decision-making includes complex certainty, complex agreement, and uncertain data. This type is the most common in decision-making considering flexibility. As last type, disorder intuition reflects low certainty, low agreement, high emotion, and high politicization (Brooks & Geyer, 2020). These decision-making types of complexity perspective can be accepted as facilitators in evaluating the EU's health policy. There are four aspects forming the EU's health policy. These are "the treaty base upon which health action is taken; Secondary EU law (regulations, directives and decisions adopted via the EU's legislative processes) that affect health; Soft law and policy initiatives (non-legislative action) relating to health; Institutional structures relating to health" (Brooks & Geyer, 2020).

In the Covid-19 period, treaty base does not include change to Article 168 of the Treaty on the Functioning of the EU. Considering techno-rational type, key secondary law includes rapid adoption of emergency legislation for medical device regulation and usage of EU structural funds for health problems in early months of pandemic. Key soft law and policy initiatives reflect short term agenda on testing, supply of medicines and devices, support to vulnerable groups, and agenda on strengthening health systems and preventing disease. EU action on these items may face with uncertainty and disagreement. Intergovernmental institutions may become more powerful on testing, contact tracing and public surveillance. The pharmaceutical strategy may confront powerful industries. At this point, other interventions from European structures may be activated beyond representatives of related industry. Building blocks of institutional structure includes strengthening and emerging roles of EU institutions like the Commission in the way of providing guidance (Brooks & Geyer, 2020).

> The impact of Covid-19 upon the EU's health policy agenda is likely to be an outward shift, deeper into the zone of mixed, complex decision-making. This trend had already started by 2020, as both the tractability and consensus of EU health policy had begun to decline and all four aspects of the agenda had moved into the political range. (Brooks & Geyer, 2020)

The EU has a potential to legislate in the techno-rational areas. Thus, it can promote development of vaccines and maintenance of supplies in health sector. Although there are different systems and approaches about health between the EU and its members, balancing between them demonstrates constructive complex system. Complexity perspective accepts that sustainable balancing and justification processes make the EU basic contributor for policymaking in health and Covid-19 agenda (Brooks & Geyer, 2020).

III. Europeanization in Health Issues

Towards the Europeanization of health issues, the basic treaty of preparing the EU as a legal contributor for health policies is Treaty establishing the European

Community, including Article 152, Article 129 of EC Treaty (Maastricht consolidated version). With this treaty, health policies were begun to be addressed at EU level. It reflects a reconciliation among member states about the EU's future in health. Article 152 includes that,

> a high level of human health protection shall be ensured in the definition and implementation of all Community policies and activities. Community action, which shall complement national policies, shall be directed towards improving public health, preventing human illness and diseases, and obviating sources of danger to human health. … The Community shall complement the Member States' action in reducing drugs-related health damage, including information and prevention. The Community shall encourage cooperation between the Member States in the areas referred to in this Article and, if necessary, lend support to their action. … The Community and the Member States shall foster cooperation with third countries and the competent international organisations in the sphere of public health. (Treaty establishing the European Community, 2002)

Maastricht Treaty and its Article 129 reflect the EU's necessity of disease prevention and health cooperation between the member states. It authorized the EU institutions on health issues. The European Commission prepared a proposal for public health policy after the Maastricht Treaty including eight priority areas to make the EU active in health sector. These areas were drug dependence; health promotion; cancer; AIDS and other communicable diseases; monitoring and surveillance of disease; injury prevention; pollution-related diseases; and rare diseases (Randall, 2000). After Maastricht Treaty, the European Council and European Parliament accepted the establishment of European Centre for Disease Prevention and Control in 2004. The establishment of the Health Security Committee was another decision to combat with pandemics in same year. In addition to Maastricht Treaty, Amsterdam and Lisbon Treaties enhanced the EU's potential of combating disease. Then, Article 168 of the Treaty on the Functioning of the European Union supported EU's initiatives on health sector (Cachia, 2021).

The health-related issues can be accepted as an area administered by national governments and health-related decisions are also initiatives of them. EU institutions such as the European Commission are coordinators of making recommendations for member states to combat with Covid-19. However, member states can afford to accept or reject them. Article 168 of the Treaty on the Functioning of the EU clearly defined this situation. With this Treaty, the EU has actually been kept in a complementary position to the national policies of the member states. The Treaty includes that,

... Union action, which shall complement national policies, shall be directed towards improving public health, preventing physical and mental illness and diseases, and obviating sources of danger to physical and mental health. ... The Union shall encourage cooperation between the Member States in the areas referred to in this Article and, if necessary, lend support to their action. ... The Union and the Member States shall foster cooperation with third countries and the competent international organisations in the sphere of public health. ...Union action shall respect the responsibilities of the Member States for the definition of their health policy and for the organisation and delivery of health services and medical care. (Treaty on the Functioning of the European Union, 2008)

Article 168 requires an intergovernmentalist analysis about health-related issues in the EU. Intergovernmentalism requires a demand of member states to create an EU level health policy. The keyword for intergovermentalist view is an agreement between member states on health policy (Greer, 2006). Besides, intergovernmentalism accepts member state's power on governance of the EU. But, European integration includes a hypothesis which assume sectoral cooperation spreads from one area to another. This type of extension shapes regional integration. Although the EU has limited capacity in health policies and member states have unique positions, institutions of the EU has become visible in health policies of the member states. As transnational institutions provide benefits, the interaction between member states and these institutions increases (Mnich, 2019). A rationale can be accepted suitable in the way of explaining Europeanization effect on health issues. So, health issues are related with political, economic, and social areas. Health has become a significant subject for international relations. Different areas, actors, and their interactions form a supranational authority which promotes cooperation and coordination in the EU inspiring integration in health policy (Mnich, 2019).

The interaction which promotes cooperation and coordination in health policy at the EU level makes the European Council responsible for lifting of restrictions on travel, cross-border tourism, common framework of antigen tests and mutual recognition of test results. Coordination in vaccination certificates, distribution of vaccines, and development of vaccination strategies are accepted as another subject which reflects the responsibility (European Council, 2020). Some reasons have caused negative opinions about vaccination. Fears about vaccine safety, accessibility and availability issues to health facilities and opportunities, lack of trust towards institutions, social norms, lack of encouragement and recommendation have been accepted as reasons to limit vaccination (Siciliani et al., 2020). Nevertheless, the EU is organizing an international reaction against

Covid-19 including the COVAX[1] facility for reaching to vaccines. As European Council meeting at the end of 2020 underlined, "to increase resilience in the area of health, including by taking forward the proposals for a Health Union and making full use of the potential of health data in Europe" became an aim to be achieved (European Council, 2020).

In order to form an international response to regional and global health problems, the EU's initiatives on health include some actions like joint procurement; clearing house to match supply and demand between manufacturers and member states; risk factors including data on trade flows and production capacity; enhanced monitoring to help anticipate drug shortages; strategic stockpiling including management of equipment for member states; manufacturing capacity to increase critical medicines; pharmaceutical ingredients and raw materials in Europe; trade policies to regulate exports and liberalize imports; anti-fraud measures including investigations of fake health products linked to COVID-19; simplifying standards to speed up market entry for essential medical items (OECD & European Union, 2020).

Although the EU had some difficulties in combating the Covid-19, its first attempts were remarkable. Beginning from March 2020 to July 2020, the EU introduced significant measures against Covid-19 (Cachia, 2021). These were European Central Bank's Pandemic Emergency Purchase Programme including €750 million support for member states; European Commission's decision of suspending Schengen practice, Coronavirus Response Investment Initiative including €37 billion support for member states, removal of custom duties on imports of medical production from third countries; European Parliament's approval of additional funds; European Council's acception on the new budget. European Central Bank was one of the EU's leading institutions to accept measures to combat Covid-19. European Commission failed to perform effectively on the issue of presenting a road map for member states to combat Covid-19 and protect their citizens from it. Although European Commission had an early warning opportunity to give member states information about Covid-19 pandemic, it could not do this duly. The resignation of Mauro Ferri on April 7th, 2020, who was the head of the European Research Council, became a symbolic action pointing out the EU's inefficiencies about plans and investments against

---

1   COVAX is co-led by Gavi, the Coalition for Epidemic Preparedness Innovations (CEPI) and WHO. Its aim is to accelerate the development and manufacture of COVID-19 vaccines, and to guarantee fair and equitable access for every country in the world. For details visit https://www.who.int/initiatives/act-accelerator/covax

Covid-19. European Commission's prominent contribution was Multiannual Financial Framework for 2021–2027 considering Covid-19, funds for the EU's health programs like €94 billion for Horizon Europe, and doctor support for Italy through the European Civil Protection Mechanism and the EU Medical Corps (Cachia, 2021).

The EU's increasing influence on health policies is a result of economic and financial actors of EU institutions like the Commission. These actors accept health policy at the EU-level as an indicator of a functional economy. Economic crisis consolidates interaction between health system and economy. Their efficiencies depend on each other. Thus, the EU becomes more visible in health system. Another reasons of this visibility are decreasing resources, difficulties in management of infectious disease cases, and transboundary health problems like Covid-19. Danger of non-action in the EU against these problems motivates the member states to cooperate on crisis-management. Besides, the EU influences to crisis-management processes emphasizing the role of the Commission with reference to the principle of supranationalism (Földes, 2016). In other word, health has been affected by the EU. Its common policies and spill-over transactions of them have made health systems and health care as cross-border subject of the EU market. Member states are subject to EU rules. These rules present a framework about the conditions of reaching health services. Although there is not an absolute harmonization, EU rules are becoming more effective in national-level on health issues. Population ageing, the growing burden of chronic diseases and multi-morbidity, increasing costs of health technology, and infectious diseases may accepted as the subjects of EU influence (Földes, 2016).

Europeanization of combating Covid-19 can be figured out with reference to top-down and bottom-up impact (see Fig. 1) (Cachia, 2021).

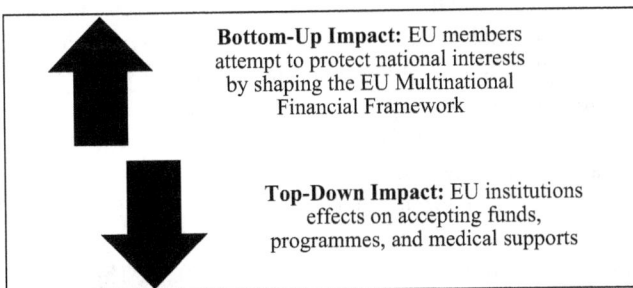

Bottom-Up Impact: EU members attempt to protect national interests by shaping the EU Multinational Financial Framework

Top-Down Impact: EU institutions effects on accepting funds, programmes, and medical supports

Fig. 1: Europeanization of combating Covid-19

Top-down impact faces with difficulties when member states can not agree with each other on common policies. The lack of agreement means lack of effects for the EU institutions on accepting funds, programmes, and medical supports to member states' combat Covid-19 (Cachia, 2021). Bottom-up impact underlines the importance of national interests over interests in the EU level. This situation puts the EU, which fails to cope with pop-up crisis, in an even worse position. Covid-19 pandemic has shown once again that the EU needs to deepen the integration project considering health sector to respond new type of international crises (Cachia, 2021).

The EU's influence on health policies or Europeanization of health policies considering Covid-19 can be analysed considering a classification based on three pillars (Wolff & Ladi, 2020). Firstly, "whether the existing tools for crisis management/preparedness have been used," secondly, "whether the EU was able to anticipate secondary/cascading effects of the early days of the crisis," and thirdly, "whether the EU has been 'projecting an image of competence' namely communicating well about the crisis and its management" should be defined (Wolff & Ladi, 2020; Rhinard, 2020).

First pillar about crisis management and preparedness were realized accepting some decisions on Protective Equipment which included buying equipment through EU funds like Solidarity Fund (Wolff & Ladi, 2020). Some decisions on vaccine research provided free movement of workers and patients in the EU, although Schengen practice was suspended because of rising pandemic. Integrated Political Crisis Response mechanism made information sharing possible in the EU against health crisis (Wolff & Ladi, 2020). Second pillar about cascading effect reflected that the EU could resist against the devastating side of the pandemic on economy (Wolff & Ladi, 2020). Some supports for businesses, workers, and unemployed reduced costs of it. €750 billion temporary recovery instrument to repair damages of pandemic was an example for the EU's position. €540 million for jobs, €200 million for companies, and €240 million for the EU members to remove public health expenses were basic steps of Europeanization in health policies. In addition to these resources, the EU's public health strategy adopted in July 2020 and its vaccines strategy adopted in June 2020 strengthened the EU's potential to combat pandemic. EU4Health is the EU's project on medical and healthcare staff, patients and health systems in Europe. In September 2020, the EU allocated €6.2 billion for the development of a Covid-19 vaccine (Wolff & Ladi, 2020; European Commission: Recovery Plan for Europe; European Commission: EU4Health 2021–2027). Third pillar included EU's struggle with disinformation (Wolff & Ladi, 2020; Loss & Puglierin, 2020). The European Council on Foreign Relations explained that "the media did not report that Poland sent medical personnel to Italy, the Czech Republic donated 200,000 respirators to Slovakia, and Lithuania supplied 35,000 protective gloves to the Croatian police. These transnational acts of support have sometimes been instrumentalized..." (Loss & Puglierin, 2020; Wolff & Ladi, 2020). This pillar created a crisis management deficit for the EU on health policies.

Health policies are not only a crisis management subject but also a politicization subject for the EU. Political, economic and social actors can be mobilized and polarized over health. Politicization can be at the top and the bottom of the EU (Wolff & Ladi, 2020). There are differences between politicization at the top and at the bottom (Wolff & Ladi, 2020). Politicization at the bottom reflects controversy on policies which create inequalities. This type of policies feeds distrust in national (member states level) and supranational (the EU level) governance. Politicization caused by Covid-19 was at the top level in first months and polarization between the Netherlands, Austria, Denmark and Sweden which were prudent about the usage of EU funds and France, Germany which were discussing a EU-level recovery plan. This politicization at the top promoted EU-level cooperation in many policy areas from disease prevention to health governance. Requiring cooperation between member states, Covid-19 made politicization positive in the EU. Before Covid-19, the EU did not experience such politicization. For example, there was a damaging competition in the EU to get vaccines at the time of swine flu (Wolff & Ladi, 2020).

Health subject can be accepted as creating job opportunities and growth for the EU market. Health services and goods have become mutual import instruments for the EU members. In order to decrease negative effects of different decision-making procedures which limit free trade and implementation of common market, the EU via the Commission tries to promote internal trade. Although the EU members are worried about their sovereignty, they follow welfare of their citizens considering health sector and EU level policies. In this way, their national resilience may also increase with reference to EU level cooperation. Besides, EU level cooperation makes the EU responsible for funding or unfunding treatment of some patients and decision on medical products. So, the EU members may charge responsibility of funding and usage decisions to the EU. Innovative treatments and new technologies in some EU members may be reached by other members' patients and doctors if not in their own states (Böhm & Landwehr, 2014). In short, "although there exist huge differences between national health care systems and member states are not willing to lose sovereignty in this health policy area, there are good reasons and strong interests that support further integration as well as further Europeanization" (Böhm & Landwehr, 2014). For example, Germany, Poland, Romania, Austria, and Slovakia were the states which provided first supports to other member states like Italy considering medical team supply and patient movement (Cachia, 2021).

The EU members have different economic conditions. So, member states' positions on health are affected by economic conditions. This situation does not completely undermine Europeanization effect on health. But it makes this effect more limited and softer (Böhm & Landwehr, 2014). Europeanization effect on health or agreement on health policy is related with the European social model and the EU's labour protection principle. In the context of labour standards, working hours for doctors became harmonization component in the EU. The EU requests all member states to harmonize their labour laws (Greer, 2006). The other request of the EU is mobility of medicine. It means mutual recognition of health professionals who are educated outside the EU and licensed in a member state. It is about

> the principle of non-discrimination thus means that it cannot be assumed that a national of, or a person educated in, a given country is better qualified or better than a person educated elsewhere in the EU who is licensed by the authorities of the state within EU standards. (Greer, 2006)

Although the EU has limited impact on member states about health services, administrative attempts are remarkable. These attempts lead to linkage between health and single market. The European Court of Justice can be accepted as a promoter of this linkage. The Court recognized health system activities as economic activities and associated them with internal market legislation. Health became an object of common market (Greer, 2006). Because common market is basic pillar of globalization, health is also a part of global interactions. Thus, health become a subject related with complexity. "The increasing interface between global public health and other sectors, such as trade, finance, communication and security, and the need to engage new discourses, has compounded this complexity" (Hill, 2011).

Although health issues are related with political, economic, and social areas primarily, it is also related with security area. Covid-19 has almost put security ahead of other areas. This relation has two dimensions. One is EU member states' unilateral actions to close national borders. The other is Covid-victim member states' rising need to the strengthened EU in health sector (Genschel & Jachtenfuchs, 2021). Covid-19 has made security as the main functional concern. Rebordering or renationalization in the EU single market and the Schengen area has limited the EU institutions dominance on common policy areas (Genschel & Jachtenfuchs, 2021). For example, at the beginning of the pandemic, the health ministers of the EU instructed the Commission to collect information about health equipment stocks. But, some member states did not accept to give information for security reasons (Genschel & Jachtenfuchs, 2021). "By the end of March, the Single Market and the Schengen area were rigidly rebordered. The distinction between internal and external frontiers lost meaning as governments refused entry to all non-nationals" (Genschel & Jachtenfuchs, 2021). Free movement of people was restricted to control pandemic. In the face of these developments, the Commission wanted to create a coordination on rebordering with the motto of "producing more, keeping it in the EU and sharing with each other" (Thompson, 2020).

IV. Unusual Aspect of Turkey-EU Relations: Covid-19

Covid-19 has promoted an international cooperation to combat pandemic in the world. It is also unavoidable for the EU-Turkey relations. Turkey followed a way in accordance with the EU until 2007, under the condition of the accession negotiations. However, the national concerns such as combatting terrorism had a priority due to the impact of regional and international security issues. The deadlock of negotiations with the EU disrupted accession process. An "a la carte" process started for Turkey in the way of constructing accession negotiations (Mercan, 2015).

The EU promotes norms and practices for the member states and candidates. They accept norm and practices as long as they provide benefits for national policies. This is also the case for Turkey. The accession process necessitates the adjustment of Turkey to the acquis communautaire and common EU policies. However, disagreements and estrangement increased at the beginning of the negotiation process between two parties. Then, the goal of membership was destructed and two parties concentrated on accession process rather than membership target. For example, during the 2000s, Turkey started to follow a multi-dimensional foreign policy instead of European based foreign policy (Oğuzlu, 2010; Öniş, 2009; Mercan, 2015).

Economic crises, energy safety, combatting international terrorism, environmental issues, principles of democracy, human rights, rule of law, the construction of stability in neighbourhood were common issues which institutionalize the EU-Turkey relations. With the Arab Spring and Syrian Civil War, two parties needed to cooperate for solving the regional problems to promote stability. This was the reason of forming "Positive Agenda" for the EU-Turkey relations at the beginning of 2010s (Mercan, 2015).

Today's conditions create new functional and operational definition between two parties. Turkey might affect the future of European integration with new partnerships and new partnerships might affect Turkey's positions and choices in its favour. Covid-19 pandemic have become new functional and operational pillar between two sides and new promoter to institutionalize bilateral contributions under current conditions. The EU-Turkey cooperation on pandemic is based on experience sharing, vaccination process, healthcare supplies, and humanitarian supports predominantly. The EU is organizing some surveys to know national efforts in economic recovery, and how measures to contain the pandemic have affected citizens' lives in border regions (Ministry of Foreign Affairs, 2020). Number of tests, number of cases, number of patients, number of deaths, number of recoveries, travel restrictions, lifting restrictions, and collecting health data can be accepted as basic considerations between two parties in relation to Covid-19. Progress is limited to these for the time being.

Conclusion

This chapter has evaluated the impact of Covid-19 on the EU with special reference to the concept of Europeanization, politicization, governance and coordination. Europeanization includes national and international changes, common policies, regulations, and instruments in the EU. Common EU policies, laws, obligations, and instruments are accepted as independent variables. Europeanized agent is dependent variable. Although there are Europeanized transactions in national policies, there is not an absolute national incorporation for health issues in the EU. Considering Europeanization, two types of integration can be defined. These are positive and negative integrations. Positive integration includes common supranational policies and rules at the EU level, and regulatory pressure. Negative integration does not include national legislation to realize common EU policy and conformity with the EU rules. There is not a high level of regulatory pressure. EU polices may challenge national preferences and policies on health. If challenge level is high, adaptational pressure for common health policies rises for the EU members. Common health policies exhibit a shift from negative integration to positive integration thanks to Covid-19.

In the EU, there is a place for common health policy between the positions of pace-setting and foot-dragging as defined previously. Article 168 is basic reference for this inference. Although Article 168 requires intergovernmentalist view for Europeanization of health policies, spread of cooperation strengthens supranationalist rationale. For this inference, Article 152 is main reference point. The EU members do not want to lose sovereignty in health area. But there are some reasons to support Europeanization in health sector. Global crises like Covid-19 pandemic necessitate burden sharing at EU level. Benefits of burden sharing trigger Europeanization. The other factor which triggers Europeanization is politicization effect. There is a positive or negative contribution of politicization to Europeanization of health policies. Covid-19 has made politicization positive in the EU. There are also policy uploading and downloading processes in the EU. Most popular one is uploading process for the member states.

In terms of decision making in the EU, complexity perspective helps to explain agreements on treaties and secondary EU law. Low level of certainty about a subject raises different opinions and disagreements on that subject. But, differences and disagreements produce high politicization. High politicization triggers agreements on treaties and regulations at EU level. The cost of separation is tried to be eliminated by integration. The EU has become complementary to policies of the member states. Interaction and cooperation of the EU members against Covid-19 have given EU institutions an opportunity to be effective on health. The EU initiatives on health sector include some remarkable attempts and actions to combat Covid-19. Because Covid-19 turned into a global crisis, the EU's attempts and actions have become related with crisis management. Crisis management has increased role of the EU institutions and supranationalism. Economic conditions and security issues has become related with health under the conditions of this management. Rising Europeanization effect on health sector to combat Covid-19 reflects member states based bottom-up impact and institutions based top-down impact. The understanding of crisis management shifts former impact to the latter.

Lastly, Covid-19 created new option for the EU to support Turkey considering refugees and other vulnerable people in its society. The EU planned humanitarian projects before Covid-19 and these types of support became more important under Covid-19 conditions in the way of strengthening sustainable relations. Turkey has an intergovernmentalist view for health policies. Because Turkey is a candidate for the EU membership, Europeanization of health policies under the impact of the Covid-19 pandemic just remains a debate within the EU. Although Covid-19 is unavoidable for the EU-Turkey relations, hard foreign and security policy issues overshadowed pandemic related dimension of the relations.

References

Böhm, K., & Landwehr, C. (2014). The Europeanization of health care coverage decisions: EU-regulation, policy learning and cooperation in decision-making. *Journal of European Integration*, 36(1), 17–35.

Börzel, T. A. (2002). Member state responses to Europeanization. *JCMS: Journal of Common Market Studies*, 40(2), 193–214.

Börzel, T., & Risse, T. (2000). When Europe hits home: Europeanization and domestic change. *European Integration Online Papers*, 4(15).

Brooks, E., & Geyer, R. (2020). The development of EU health policy and the Covid-19 pandemic: Trends and implications. *Journal of European Integration*, 42(8), 1057–1076.

Bulmer, S. J., & Radaelli, C. M. (2004). The Europeanisation of National Policy? *Queen's Papers on Europeanisation*, 1, 1–18.

Cachia, J. C. (2021). The Europeanization of the Covid-19 pandemic response and the EU's solidarity with Italy. *Contemporary Italian Politics*, 13(1), 81–104.

Consolidated version of the Treaty on the Functioning of the European Union. (2008). *Official Journal 115*, https://eur-lex.europa.eu/legal-content/EN/TXT/?uri=CELEX%3A12008E168, Access date 18.05.2021.

European Commission. EU4Health 2021–2027-A vision for a healthier European Union. https://ec.europa.eu/health/funding/eu4health_en.

European Commission. Recovery Plan for Europe. https://ec.europa.eu/info/strategy/recovery-plan-europe_en.

European Council. (2020). European Council meeting-Conclusions. https://www.consilium.europa.eu/en/press/press-releases/2020/12/11/european-council-conclusions-10-11-december-2020/.

Featherstone, K., & Papadimitriou, D. (2008). *The limits of Europeanization: Reform capacity and policy conflict in Greece*. Palgrave Macmillan.

Featherstone, K., & Radaelli, C. M. (Eds.) (2003). *The Politics of Europeanization*. Oxford University Press.

Fleming, S. (2021). EU must prepare for 'era of pandemics', von der Leyen says. *Financial Times*, https://www.ft.com/content/fba558ff-94a5-4c6c-b848-c8fd91b13c16.

Földes, M. E. (2016). Health policy and health systems: A growing relevance for the EU in the context of the economic crisis. *Journal of European Integration*, 38(3), 295–309.

Genschel, P., & Jachtenfuchs, M. (2021). Postfunctionalism reversed: Solidarity and rebordering during the COVID-19 pandemic. *Journal of European Public Policy*, 28(3), 350–369.

Greer, S. L. (2006). Uninvited Europeanization: Neofunctionalism and the EU in health policy. *Journal of European Public Policy*, 13(1), 134–152.

Hill, P. S. (2011). Understanding global health governance as a complex adaptive system. *Global Public Health*, 6(6), 593–605.

Loss, R., & J. Puglierin. (2020). The Truth about European Solidarity during Corona. *ECFR Commentary.* https://www.ecfr.eu/article/commentary_the_truth_about_european_solidarity_during_corona

Mercan, S. (2015). The role of Turkey in EU policies in the 2000s: An examination of foreign policy partnership. *Research Turkey,* 4(2), 106–112.

Ministry of Foreign Affairs. (2020). Directorate for EU Affairs. The EU needs your story about COVID-19. https://www.ab.gov.tr/52008_en.html.

Mnich, C. (2019). Is there Europeanization of physical activity promotion? – A neofunctional approach. *Health Policy,* 123, 317–326.

OECD/European Union. (2020). *Health at a Glance: Europe 2020: State of Health in the EU Cycle.* OECD Publishing.

Oğuzlu, T. (2010). Turkey and Europeanization of foreign policy. *Political Science Quarterly,* 125(4), 657–683.

Öniş, Z. (2009). The new wave of foreign policy activism in Turkey drifting away from Europeanization? *DIIS Report. Danish Institute for International Studies.*

Pierru, F., Stambach, F., & Vernaudon, J., (2021). Vaccine fight against patents. *Le Monde Diplomatique Turkey,* 14, 1–6.

Radaelli, C. M. (2004). Europeanisation: Solution or Problem? *European Integration Online Papers,* 8(16).

Randall, E. (2000). European Union health policy with and without design: Serendipity, tragedy and the future of EU health policy. *Policy Studies,* 21(2), 133–164.

Rhinard, M. (2020). Assessing the European Union's performance in the Covid-19 pandemic. *LSE EUROPP Blog.* https://blogs.lse.ac.uk/europpblog/2020/03/26/assessing-the-european-unions-performance-in-the-covid-19-pandemic/.

Schmidt, V. A. (2020). Theorizing institutional change and governance in European responses to the Covid-19 pandemic. *Journal of European Integration,* 42(8), 1177–1193.

Siciliania, L., Wild, C., McKee, M., Kringos, D., Barry, M. M., Barros, P. P., Maeseneer, J. D., Murauskiene, L., & Ricciardi, W. (2020). Strengthening vaccination programmes and health systemsin the European Union: A framework for action. *Health Policy,* 124, 511–518.

Thompson, R. (2020). Ursula von der Leyen tells EU countries to share medical supplies. *Euronews.* https://www.euronews.com/2020/03/16/ursula-von-der-leyen-tells-eu-countries-to-share-medical-supplies.

Treaty Establishing the European Community (Nice consolidated version). (1997). *Official Journal C 325*, https://eur-lex.europa.eu/LexUriServ/LexUriS erv.do?uri=CELEX:12002E152:EN:HTML.

Wolff, S., & Ladi, S. (2020). European Union responses to the Covid-19 pandemic: Adaptability in times of permanent emergency. *Journal of European Integration*, 42(8), 1025–1040.

Part III Gender in Health Policies and Law

Ahu Sumbas

Veiled Impact of Gender Equality Policies on Gender Disparities in Self-Rated Health: The Case of Turkey

Introduction

Inequalities in health are resulted from many factors, including gender, race, ethnicity, class, level of education, quality of work, level of pay and living conditions, and so forth. Likewise, in the last decades, the number of studies on gender-based analysis of health inequalities have increased. Accordingly, various determinants of gender differences in health became the focus of much research which include the role of psychological (e.g. gender images and identities, chronic stressors), behavioural (smoking, drinking, eating, physical exercise), and social factors (e.g. social support, socioeconomic status) on women's and men's health. These studies demonstrated that gender disparities in health were for the most part socially and culturally produced, rather than biologically given (Annandale & Hunt, 2000). Several of these studies have also addressed the role of gender policies in eliminating gender inequalities in health. The main argument of these works is that gender inequalities in health are closely related to the socio-economic and political dimensions in which gender inequality is manifested in the world. As such they could be ameliorated and eradicated through gender equality policies. Since such studies are particularly limited for the Turkish context, this chapter aims to close this gap by focusing on the relation of gender equality policies and gender disparities in the self-rated health (SRH) index in Turkey based on the 2019 Turkey Health Interview Survey.

Health has been measured using different indicators such as SRH, mental health, psychological well-being, limiting longstanding illness or mortality rates. Among them, the SRH status of men and women is regarded as one of the essential indicators in measuring and understanding gender disparities and inequalities in health. SRH is measured based on the question of "how would you describe your health?" (Excellent, Very Good, Good, Fair, or Poor). This indicator generally presents the poorer health status of women compared to men and, thereby, can be considered as the evidence of the disadvantaged position of women in health worldwide (Schütte et al., 2013; Palencia et. al., 2014; OECD, 2019: 20). At this point, some scholars put a caveat on the argument of female poor SRH is the reflection of gender inequalities in health. They attributed to gender differences in symptom reporting and patterns of help-seeking. On the other hand, as Takahaski et al. (2020: 2) indicated that women are more exposed to various stressors over their life course relative to men due to gender roles, including gender-based discrimination and violence, workplace harassment, work-family conflicts, and caregiver burden. Cumulatively, these stressors help to account for the "gender paradox", whereby women live longer than men, but they also report higher morbidity. In a similar vein, recent research on gender and validity of SRH in Europe concludes that SRH was associated with physical and mental health problems and this indicator is useful for assessing gender inequalities in health (Baćak, & Ólafsdóttir, 2017).

According to the Gender Gap Index 2020 (GGI) of the World Economic Forum, Turkey is the 130th country out of 153 countries. Similarly, Turkey ranked as the 68th country out of 162 countries at the United Nations Gender Inequality Index 2020 (GII). Another gender index, the Gender Development Index 2019 (GDI), valued Turkey with 0,924 placing her into Group 4.[1] Along this line, the Gender Equality Report of UNFPA Turkey (GER) indicates that gender inequality persists in the labour market, political participation, and women's access to education. The labour force participation rate of women is 30 % and 70 % for men (TurkStat Labor Statistics, 2015). The unemployment rate of men is 9.7 % and 13 % for women. Every 4 women out of 10 are exposed to physical and sexual violence at least once in their lifetime as stated in the Domestic Violence Research of Hacettepe University in Turkey in 2014 (Yüksel-Kaptanoğlu et al., 2015). Women's political representation is around 17 % at the parliamentary level. This picture illustrates that Turkey which is the 17th biggest economy in the world is the 23rd last country in terms of gender equality.

Accordingly, this study aims to first present gender disparities in health in Turkey considering the health indicator of SRH on gender and the cross-analysis of this data with the socio-demographic variables of age, education, employment status, marital status, and household income. Second, benefiting from these data and their analysis, I intend to discuss the role of gender

---

1   The 2019 female HDI value for Turkey is 0.784 in contrast with 0.848 for males. Countries are divided into five groups by absolute deviation from gender parity in Human Development Index (HDI) values. Group 4 comprises countries with medium to low equality in HDI achievements between women and men (absolute deviation of 7.5–10 %) (Human Development Report Turkey, 2020: 5).

equality policies on the elimination of gender disparities in SRH in the case of Turkey. Recent data from the 2019 Turkey Health Interview Survey, were used for the analysis.

In conclusion, the scores and ranks of Turkey in GGI, GDI, GII and GER present that Turkey has failed to promote gender equality policies to advance women's well-being which is closely related to women's educational level, the participation of women in the labour market, and family policies, therefore it is argued that women's SRH condition is worse than men compared to other Western countries. Indeed, among OECD countries, Turkey has the second highest rates on SRH difference by gender (Etiler, 2016: 3) and is behind these countries in gender equality indexes. It is believed that scrutinizing the relationship between gender policies and gender disparities in health can contribute to identifying possible policy strategies to eliminate gender health gaps in Turkey.

I. Literature Review on Gender Equality Policies and Gender Disparities in Health

Health data show that women tend to live longer than men in all countries, except Kuwait, Bhutan, and Bahrain (Global Gender Gap Report, 2020: 15) but they often do it in worse health (Annandale and Hunt, 2000; Espelt et al., 2010; Van de Velde et. al., 2010; Wang et al., 2013; Dreger et al., 2016; OECD, 2019; 20). The data constitutes a ground to claim that gender is an important determinant of health studies.

Inequalities in power, status, and financial resources as well as the sex-based division of work sharpen gender differences in health. In other words, women's lower positions in families and societies, their vulnerabilities in welfare states and their inabilities to access health services, the gender gap in wages, the burden of paid and unpaid work are considered as the leading factors of gender disparities in health (Burrell et al., 2014; Palencia et al., 2014). In this sense, the detrimental effects of patriarchal structures and ideology do not only restrict women's access to social, political, and economic resources but also prevent women from feeling healthier. Gender disparities in health can therefore be eliminated by struggling with gender inequalities at social, political and economic levels. Indeed, a study of adolescent health found out that the gender gap in health complaints was lower in countries with a high Gender Empowerment Measure (GEM) (Torsheim et al., 2006).

Adoption and implementation of successful gender equality policies hold a critical role in the fight against the inequalities and disparities in health.

Accordingly, the World Health Organization (WHO) and the European Commission have stated that reducing gender inequalities is one of the strategies of eliminating health inequalities all around the world and in Europe. Strategies to eradicate gender inequalities in health must therefore involve efforts to improve the status of women and respond to the gender-based needs of women in society. For instance, in the Nordic countries, gender inequalities in health are smaller as the socio-economic position of women is better and their scores in gender equality indexes are the highest.

Gender equality policies address four main strategy areas; political representation, employment policies, income policies, care/family, and time-use policies. The studies on the effects of policies on gender disparities in health focus on a spectrum of policy areas, ranging from reproductive policies and violence-protection policies to welfare gender regimes and family support at the country level (Borrell et al., 2014). Among them, family policies, in this sense the welfare regime of a country, which are closely related with the gender equality policy approach of a government, play a critical role in health outcomes by gender (Backhans et al., 2012; Palencia et al., 2014; Borrell et al., 2014; Pinillos-Franco & Somarriba, 2018). For instance, according to the research of Palencia et al. (2014), women were found to be "reporting worse self-perceived health than men, in countries with family policies that were less oriented to gender equality". Similarly, Borrell et al. (2014) found that longer paid maternity leave in dual-earner Nordic social-democrat welfare regimes are generally associated with better mental health in women and thus, they promote women's health. Chandola et al. (2004) concluded that Finland's successful family-work reconciliation policies are contributing to better mental health among Finnish working women compared to working women in Japan. Backhans et al. (2012) found that for external cause mortality, the earner carer cluster countries had a lower gender gap than the male breadwinner cluster countries. This difference was related to several of the policies characteristic of the earner-carer cluster; generous maternity and reserved paternity leave, high social services expenditure, and high universal basic pensions. In other words, social democratic welfare states and universal career family models favour women, eliminating gender disparities in health resulted from the inequalities in education, income, power, and social status.

On the other hand, the research of Bambra et al. (2009) on the relationship between gender and SRH in 13 countries showed that women in the social democratic and Southern welfare states were more likely to report worse health than men, while women in the corporatist states were not. Women's dual roles and a sex-segregated labour market offering worse jobs for women in these social welfare states are considered as possible causes of the difference.

Consequently, studies on the effects of policy on gender disparities in health mostly agree that successful implementation of gender equality policies improved health outcomes for women or diminished gender inequalities in health through their effect on social, political and economic determinants of health, such as the distribution of power, income, paid and unpaid work, the use of free time, and the incidents of violence (Borrell et al., 2014; Palencia et al., 2014; Pinillos-Franco & Somarriba, 2018). Moreover, as Kawachi et al. (1999) concluded in their study that there is a strong correlation between women's empowerment and population health status. In other words, combatting gender inequalities in a society not only helps to eliminate gender disparities in health but also improves population health status as a whole.

II. Methodology

The data of Turkey Health Interview Surveys have been gathered since 2008 through 2019 by the Turkish Statistical Institute (TurkStat) via face-to-face interviews. In this study, the data were derived from the 2019 Turkey Health Interview Surveys of TurkStat. This survey is a national survey that uses representative samples of all persons aged 0 and over residing in private households in Turkey. Within the scope of the research, survey data covering those aged 15 and above was used for the analysis. The micro data set of the 2019 Turkey Health Interview Surveys were officially obtained from Turkstat, and the research was developed on further analysis of these data via Statistical Package for Social Sciences (IBM SPSS). The sample is based on the National Address Database which includes 17.084 respondents aged 15 and above. The study sample consisted of 7.784 men and 9.300 women.

The dependent variable is SRH and the main independent variable is gender. Since age, educational attainment, household income, job and marital status are important to understand the impact of socio-economic and environmental status on health, they are included as independent variables in the analysis of gender disparities considering SRH status.

For the analysis of data, IBM SPSS Statistics are used. Crosstables, chi-square test, and two-way ANOVA for independent samples test are applied as the main statistical tests to reveal the statistical relations and evaluate the research questions. The statistical significance level was p <0.5. IBM SPSS analysis of the data and evaluations of the results are made by the author.

III. Gendered Analysis of Self-Rated Health Status in the Case of Turkey

"Gender paradox" in health enunciates that women have a longer life expectancy at birth but worsened SRH compared to men in most of the democratic and richest countries. Turkey exhibits similar patterns with this gender paradox. First, life expectancy is 80,7 for women while it is 74,9 for men in Turkey, based on the UN Population Division 2019 Data. The countries with the highest score of gender empowerment measure have life expectancies of over 80 years (Takahaski et. al., 2020: 1) and a lower gender gap in SHR. Turkey follows these countries in life expectancies at birth as the second highest rate category, yet lag behind most other developed countries concerning to the gender gap in SRH and indices of gender equality. Women consistently report a higher prevalence of poor health compared to men in Turkey Health Interview Surveys between 2008–2019 as illustrated at Tab. 1. The gender gap (F/M) in poor SRH was 1,88 in 2008; 1,95 in 2010; 1,75 in 2012; 1,82 in 2014; 1,69 in 2016, and 1,72 in 2019. This gap ranks Turkey among the countries with the worst scores in terms of the prevalence of poor SRH in women to men. According to OECD Data, the gender gap was 1,51 (F/M) in Turkey with one of the highest levels compared to other OECD countries (Etiler, 2016: 3). In New Zealand, Canada, and Australia, the proportion of women to men was almost equal (OECD, 2019: 62).

Tab. 1: The percentage of SRH status by sex, 2008–2016, Turkey Health Interview Surveys

SRH	2008			2010			2012			2014			2016			2019		
Total	Total	Male	Female	Total	Male	Female	Total	Male	Female	Total	Male	Female	Total	Male	Female	Total	Male	Female
Good/Very good	63,6	71,9	55,5	64,9	73,5	56,7	70,7	77,1	64,5	61,2	68,8	53,8	63,5	69,8	57,5	60,9	68,1	53,9
Bad/Very bad	10,1	7,0	13,2	10,0	6,7	13,1	7,2	5,2	9,1	11,5	8,1	14,8	10,7	7,9	13,4	10,4	7,6	13,1

Ahu Sumbas

Table 2 illustrates the responses of men and women on their SRH status in 2019 Health Survey in detail.

Tab. 2: The percentage of SHR status by sex, the 2019 Turkey Health Interview Survey

			Self-Rated Health			Total
			Fair	Very good/Good	Bad/Very bad	
Gender	Male	Count	2019	5124	641	7784
		% sex	25.9 %	65.8 %	8.2 %	100.0 %
	Female	Count	3195	4864	1241	9300
		% within sex	34.4 %	52.3 %	13.3 %	100.0 %
Total		Count	5214	9988	1882	17084
		% within sex	30.5 %	58.5 %	11.0 %	100.0 %

Tab. 3: Chi-square tests on the relation of sex and self-rated health

Chi-Square Tests			
	Value	df	Asymptotic Significance (2-sided)
Pearson Chi-Square	331.379[a]	2	<.001
Likelihood Ratio	334.269	2	<.001
Linear-by-Linear Association	77.844	1	<.001
N of Valid Cases	17084		

Notes: (a) 0 cells (0.0 %) have expected count less than 5. The minimum expected count is 857.50.

These tables demonstrate that 13,3 % of women reported bad/very bad health conditions whereas only 8,2 % of men rated their health bad/very bad. Along this line, the percentage of women reporting good SRH (52,3 %) is lower than men (65,8 %). The responses of men and women on SRH status are also compared by using the chi-square test (see table 3). The result of the chi-square test shows that there is a statistical difference in the distribution of the responses to SRH among men and women (χ^2 =331,37, p < 0.5). These data and results are coherent with the literature on gender and health and reveals that women have poorer SRH in Turkey than men.

This finding also corresponds to the percentage of main diseases/health problems declared by individuals in the last 12 months by sex, based on the 2019 Turkey Health Survey. As Tab. 4 illustrates, women have health problems more than men, as the sole exception is stroke. This existing asymmetry in having main health problems can not only be explained by biological differences in sexes but also it can be elucidated by socio-cultural and behavioural differences owing to gender. In this regard, the reflections of gender identity, roles, and relations on health can be taken into account in assessing gender disparities in health in the context of Turkey.

Tab. 4: The percentage of main diseases/health problems declared by individuals in the last 12 months by sex, the 2019 Turkey Health Survey

[15+ age]	2019		
Disease/health problem	Total	Male	Female
Low back disorders (lumbago, back hernia, other back defections)	29,7	22,6	36,6
High blood pressure (hypertension)	16,4	11,9	20,8
Neck disorders (neck pain, neck hernia, other neck defections)	20,5	12,8	27,9
Allergy, such as rhinitis,eye inflammation, dermatitis, food allergy or other (allergic asthma excluded)	12,3	8,9	15,6
Diabetes	10,2	8,2	12,2
Asthma (allergic asthma included)	8,9	5,8	12,1
Coronary heart disease (angina pectoris, chest pain, spasm)	7,2	6,6	7,7
Chronic obstructive pulmonary disease (Chronic bronchitis, emphysema)	7,1	5,2	9,0
Urinary incontinence,problems in controlling the bladder	7,8	5,3	10,4
Depression	9,0	5,7	12,2
Myocardial infarction (heart attack)	2,2	2,5	1,9
Stroke (cerebral haemorrhage, cerebral thrombosis)	0,8	0,7	0,8
Cirrhosis of the liver, liver dysfunction	1,6	1,5	1,7
Arthrosis	11,2	7,6	14,6
Kidney Problems	5,7	4,9	6,4
Alzheimer (Alzheimer was evaluated for individuals in the 65+ age group.)	6,0	6,0	6,0
High blood lipids (high cholesterol or triglycerides)	10,1	7,7	12,5

Given that the variables of age, education, household income, employment status, and marital status are the significant determinants of socioeconomic and environmental status of women, they are assumed to be key determinants to measure health disparities by gender. Furthermore, it is believed that assessing the impacts of such variables on gender and SHR may allow us to scrutinize the role of gender equality policies in reducing gender gap in SHR. Thus, the following analysis of the data tries to explain the relations and differences of these variables with gender and SRH. Tables 5–7 exhibit the relation between gender, age, and SRH.

Tab. 5: The percentage of SRH by sex and age, the 2019 Turkey Health Interview Survey

SRH			15–24	25–34	35–44	45–54	55–64	65–74	75+	Total
Good/ Very Good	Male	Count	1162	1144	1130	781	564	271	72	5124
		% within sex	22.7 %	22.3 %	22.1 %	15.2 %	11.0 %	5.3 %	1.4 %	100.0 %
		% of Total	11.6 %	11.5 %	11.3 %	7.8 %	5.6 %	2.7 %	0.7 %	51.3 %
	Female	Count	1176	1282	1088	690	411	163	54	4864
		% within sex	24.2 %	26.4 %	22.4 %	14.2 %	8.4 %	3.4 %	1.1 %	100.0 %
		% of Total	11.8 %	12.8 %	10.9 %	6.9 %	4.1 %	1.6 %	0.5 %	48.7 %
	Total	Count	2338	2426	2218	1471	975	434	126	9988
		% within sex	23.4 %	24.3 %	22.2 %	14.7 %	9.8 %	4.3 %	1.3 %	100.0 %
		% of Total	23.4 %	24.3 %	22.2 %	14.7 %	9.8 %	4.3 %	1.3 %	100.0 %
Bad/ Very Bad	Male	Count	14	33	59	113	133	139	150	641
		% within sex	2.2 %	5.1 %	9.2 %	17.6 %	20.7 %	21.7 %	23.4 %	100.0 %
		% of Total	0.7 %	1.8 %	3.1 %	6.0 %	7.1 %	7.4 %	8.0 %	34.1 %
	Female	Count	24	54	125	235	272	288	243	1241
		% within sex	1.9 %	4.4 %	10.1 %	18.9 %	21.9 %	23.2 %	19.6 %	100.0 %
		% of Total	1.3 %	2.9 %	6.6 %	12.5 %	14.5 %	15.3 %	12.9 %	65.9 %
	Total	Count	38	87	184	348	405	427	393	1882
		% within Gender	2.0 %	4.6 %	9.8 %	18.5 %	21.5 %	22.7 %	20.9 %	100.0 %
		% of Total	2.0 %	4.6 %	9.8 %	18.5 %	21.5 %	22.7 %	20.9 %	100.0 %
		F/M in % of total	1,53	1,61	2,12	2,08	1,48	1,48	1,62	-

Tab. 6: Two-way ANOVA For Independent Samples Test, Gender, Age, SRH

Descriptive Statistics

Dependent Variable: Self-Rated Health

Gender	Age	Mean	Std. Deviation	N
Male	15–24	5.71	.905	1305
	25–34	5.61	1.057	1366
	35–44	5.33	1.306	1553
	45–54	5.15	1.477	1302
	55–64	4.92	1.592	1158
	65–74	4.88	1.695	729
	75+	5.20	1.840	371
	Total	5.30	1.390	7784
Female	15–24	5.54	1.109	1425
	25–34	5.38	1.264	1704
	35–44	5.04	1.492	1842
	45–54	4.86	1.644	1616
	55–64	4.71	1.735	1355
	65–74	4.91	1.851	861
	75+	5.28	1.898	497
	Total	5.10	1.556	9300
Total	15–24	5.62	1.020	2730
	25–34	5.48	1.181	3070
	35–44	5.18	1.418	3395
	45–54	4.99	1.577	2918
	55–64	4.81	1.673	2513
	65–74	4.89	1.781	1590
	75+	5.25	1.873	868
	Total	5.19	1.486	17084

Tab. 7: Tests of Between-Subjects Effects

Dependent Variable: Self-Rated Health

Source	Type III Sum of Squares	df	Mean Square	F	Sig.
Corrected Model	1624.805[a]	13	124.985	59.099	<.001
Intercept	370454.221	1	370454.221	175168.273	.000
Gender	80.486	1	80.486	38.057	<.001
Age	1395.595	6	232.599	109.984	<.001
Gender * Age	50.657	6	8.443	3.992	<.001
Error	36100.450	17070	2.115		
Total	498712.000	17084			
Corrected Total	37725.256	17083			

Note: (a) R Squared = .043 (Adjusted R Squared = .042)

Table 5 shows that that poor SRH increases with older age for both men and women, particularly after age 45 and 55. One of the reasons of this correlation particularly stems from the increasing number of chronic conditions and diseases at old ages. However, the tables also indicate that there is gender inequality in poor SRH depending on age differences. According to the two-way ANOVA for independent samples test, as expected, SRH is relational with gender and age at the same time [F=3,99, p<001]. The gender gap in poor SHR is marked almost at all ages but mostly worse in women between the ages of 15 and 54. This period is mostly the childbearing years and/or working ages for women in Turkey. Women in Turkey mostly have their first babies at the ages of 20–29 (TurkStat, 2019). Women face difficulties both at home and in the labour market due to traditional division of gender roles (cleaning, cooking, and caring responsibilities, lack of power in family relations), gender discrimination (glass ceilings in hiring & promotion, gender wage gaps), and maintaining work-family balance. Turkey is mostly categorized under the corporatist welfare regimes which adopts traditional family policies. The policies on care mostly target women as the main carrier in the family and influence women's labour participation negatively (Sumbas, 2019). The pressure of work combines with the heavy burden of caring responsibilities at home due to the lack of publicly supported free daycare centres and co-responsibility of both parents (Sumbas, 2018; 2019). Indeed, the employment rate of women aged between 25 and 49 with child/ren under 3 years old is 26,7 % whereas this ratio is 52,8 % for women without a child in Turkey (TurkStat, 2019). Hence, gendered inequalities of work and family life as well as lack of agency and power in family relations might trigger the emotional stress and physical work of most women which might cause poor SRH in

Turkey. Indeed, studies looking at different health indicators such as depression, have also found that gender differences were greater in Eastern and Southern European Countries which have traditional family models and the smallest in Nordic countries with dual-earner family types (Van de Velde et al., 2010).

The findings on the relation of employment status, gender, and SRH clear up the aforementioned explanation on SHR. As Tab. 8 indicates, 45,9 % of individuals who reported poor SRH were unpaid female care workers at home. Along this line, as the second highest percentage in reporting poor SHR among women were the paid female workers with 5,1 % when we exclude disability and retirement ages. Thus, it is possible to claim that the lack of gender equality perspective in family/society and workplace policies in addition to the strategies of women's labour participation triggers women's poor SRH status in Turkey. This finding is coherent with the literature, as the recent scholarly works found that women feel healthier in countries with egalitarian family policies and under social-democratic welfare regimes (Backhans et al., 2012; Borrell et al., 2014; Chandola et al., 2004; Palencia et al., 2014; Pinillos-Franco & Somarriba, 2018).

Based on the analysis of the data on employment status and SHR by gender (see Tables 8–10), there is a gender gap in reporting SRH. Two-way Anova for independent sample test (Table 10) indicates a statistical relation of gender and employment status on SRH at the same time [F=3,55, p<001]. The most significant difference between women and men in reporting poor SRH is marked between unpaid care worker and retired categories. 45,9 % of individuals who reported poor SRH were unpaid female care workers at home whereas only 0,7 % of individuals in this employment category with poor SRH were male. On the other hand, men with poor SRH were mostly retired. 15,6 % of individuals with poor SHR were retired men whereas only 4,8 % of responders with poor SHR were retired women. One of the reasons for this gender gap in SRH by employment status is closely related to the traditional division of labour. Existing traditional socio-cultural and economic structures in Turkey mostly oblige women to serve as unpaid care workers at home whereas men are accepted as the main breadwinners with secure jobs. Indeed, most of the respondents who are retired (10,1 % male, 3,1 % women) and employed at a paid job (19,5 % men, 9,2 % women) were men whereas almost all unpaid care workers at home were women (32,2 % women, 0,3 % men). Such gendered expectations do not only disadvantage women but also men in health. For instance, unemployment might cause more emotional stress and depression in men as they are considered the main breadwinners. Thus, unemployed men (2,1 %) reported worse health than unemployed women (0,7 %) in Turkey. These findings emphasize not only the significance of policies on women's labour participation but also the critical role of gender equality policies aiming to value women and men as equals in the care job and labour market.

Tab. 8: The percentage of SRH by sex and employment status, the 2019 Turkey Health Interview Survey

SRH			Employment Status[a]										Total
			11	12	13	21	22	24	25	231	232		
Good/Very Good	Male	Count	2521	700	74	512	587	5	25	692	8		5124
		within Sex	49.2 %	13.7 %	1.4 %	10.0 %	11.5 %	0.1 %	0.5 %	13.5 %	0.2 %		100.0 %
		of Total	25.2 %	7.0 %	0.7 %	5.1 %	5.9 %	0.1 %	0.3 %	6.9 %	0.1 %		51.3 %
	Female	Count	1107	89	153	213	562	3	2535	190	12		4864
		within Sex	22.8 %	1.8 %	3.1 %	4.4 %	11.6 %	0.1 %	52.1 %	3.9 %	0.2 %		100.0 %
		of Total	11.1 %	0.9 %	1.5 %	2.1 %	5.6 %	0.0 %	25.4 %	1.9 %	0.1 %		48.7 %
	Total	Count	3628	789	227	725	1149	8	2560	882	20		9988
		within Sex	36.3 %	7.9 %	2.3 %	7.3 %	11.5 %	0.1 %	25.6 %	8.8 %	0.2 %		100.0 %
		of Total	36.3 %	7.9 %	2.3 %	7.3 %	11.5 %	0.1 %	25.6 %	8.8 %	0.2 %		100.0 %
Bad/Very bad	Male	Count	111	67	4	39	4	72	14	294	36		641
		within sex	17.3 %	10.5 %	0.6 %	6.1 %	0.6 %	11.2 %	2.2 %	45.9 %	5.6 %		100.0 %
		of Total	5.9 %	3.6 %	0.2 %	2.1 %	0.2 %	3.8 %	0.7 %	15.6 %	1.9 %		34.1 %
	Female	Count	63	9	37	14	7	96	864	90	61		1241
		within sex	5.1 %	0.7 %	3.0 %	1.1 %	0.6 %	7.7 %	69.6 %	7.3 %	4.9 %		100.0 %
		of Total	3.3 %	0.5 %	2.0 %	0.7 %	0.4 %	5.1 %	45.9 %	4.8 %	3.2 %		65.9 %
	Total	Count	174	76	41	53	11	168	878	384	97		1882
		within sex	9.2 %	4.0 %	2.2 %	2.8 %	0.6 %	8.9 %	46.7 %	20.4 %	5.2 %		100.0 %
		of Total	9.2 %	4.0 %	2.2 %	2.8 %	0.6 %	8.9 %	46.7 %	20.4 %	5.2 %		100.0 %

Notes: (a) 11 – Paid Workers; 12 – Employer; 13 – Unpaid family worker; 21 – Unpaid care worker; 22 – Unemployed; 22 – Student; 24 – Unpaid care worker at home; 25 – Disabled; 231 – Retired; 232 – Old to work

Tab. 9: Two-way ANOVA for Independent Samples Test, Employment Status, Gender and SRH

Descriptive Statistics

Dependent Variable: Self-Rated Health

Gender	Employment Status	Mean	Std. Deviation	N
Male	11- Paid Workers	5.41	1.248	3323
	12 -Employer	5.23	1.405	1063
	13- Unpaid family worker	5.62	1.093	91
	21-Unemployed	5.45	1.254	690
	22-Student	5.73	.880	652
	24- Unpaid care worker at home	5.50	1.911	121
	25-Disabled	5.34	1.610	56
	231-Retired	4.89	1.669	1724
	232- Old to work	5.63	1.813	64
	Total	5.30	1.390	7784
Female	11- Paid Workers	5.27	1.351	1577
	12 -Employer	4.86	1.535	163
	13- Unpaid family worker	4.96	1.589	310
	21-Unemployed	5.22	1.384	313
	22-Student	5.63	1.006	651
	24- Unpaid care worker at home	6.07	1.675	128
	25-Disabled	5.01	1.619	5508
	231-Retired	4.74	1.695	535
	232- Old to work	5.43	1.878	115
	Total	5.10	1.556	9300
Total	11- Paid Workers	5.36	1.283	4900
	12 -Employer	5.18	1.428	1226
	13- Unpaid family worker	5.11	1.515	401
	21-Unemployed	5.38	1.300	1003
	22-Student	5.68	.945	1303
	24- Unpaid care worker at home	5.80	1.812	249
	25-Disabled	5.01	1.619	5564
	231-Retired	4.85	1.676	2259
	232-Old to Work	5.50	1.852	179
	Total	5.19	1.486	17084

Ahu Sumbas

Tab. 10: Tests of Between-Subjects Effects

Dependent Variable: Self-Rated Health

Source	Type III Sum of Squares	df	Mean Square	F	Sig.
Corrected Model	1165.383[a]	17	68.552	32.000	<.001
Intercept	101411.701	1	101411.701	47338.570	.000
Gender	28.095	1	28.095	13.115	<.001
Employment Status	689.838	8	86.230	40.252	<.001
Gender * Employment Status	60.944	8	7.618	3.556	<.001
Error	36559.873	17066	2.142		
Total	498712.000	17084			
Corrected Total	37725.256	17083			

Note: (a) R Squared = .031 (Adjusted R Squared = .030)

Education is another important demographic determinant in assessing both gender and health inequalities. Thus, observing the impact of education level on gender disparities in SRH may help us to understand the role of gender equality strategies focusing on women's education in the elimination of health disparities by gender. Tables 11–13 explains that, as expected, both women and men with lower education levels reported poor SRH. According to two-way ANOVA for independent samples test, gender and education have no significant effect on SRH at the same time [F=3,42, p>01]. But having said that, the results of crosstables on gender, education, and SHR (Tab. 11), demonstrates that the percentage of women who reported poor SRH is higher (87,5 % in total of illiterate-49,2 % and primary education- 38,3 %) compared to men (69,4 % in total of illiterate- 20,9 % and primary level- 48,5) who have a low level of education. Accordingly, women with high school or graduate degrees mostly likely do not report bad/very bad health (4,5 % and 3 % respectively, and 7,5 % in total). Women with lower education levels are more vulnerable in terms of poverty, social security and insurance coverings,[2] and psychical works they carry. They marry and have babies at earlier

---

2 Since Turkey is a welfare state with state funded health insurance, 92.1 % of survey responders indicated that they have a state funded health insurance. It is therefore difficult to discuss the role of insurance type on SRH by gender based on 2019 Health Interview Survey. However, it is possible to say that medium social service expenditures and low universal basic pensions mostly punish women in society as the dependents of husbands or unregistered/informal employers in the context of Turkey.

ages compared to educated women (Durgun, 2020). Along this line, the number of children mostly correlates with the level of education in women. The number of gravidities and children is most likely to affect women's SRH status negatively. On the other hand, women with higher education are probably finding higher status jobs with higher wages in the labour market. They may be able to afford child-caring support and thus, reduce family-work conflict and the burden of child-rearing. Additionally, as the 2019 Health Survey ascertained, women with higher education routinely exercise and they may probably get enough nutrition to protect their health. Since the higher education level of women is 18,5 while it is 23,1 for men in Turkey (TurkStat, 2019) the poor SRH status of women can be considered as one of the reflections of gender inequalities in accessing higher education and higher income.

Tab. 11: The percentage of SRH status by sex and education, 2019 Turkey Health Interview Surveys

Self-Rated health			Illiterate	Primary	Secondary	High School	Graduate & Over	Total
		Count	**139**	**1260**	**1175**	**1298**	**1252**	**5124**
Good/ Very good	Male	% within sex	2.7 %	24.6 %	22.9 %	25.3 %	24.4 %	100.0 %
		% of Total	1.4 %	12.6 %	11.8 %	13.0 %	12.5 %	51.3 %
	Female	Count	441	1254	954	1083	1132	4864
		% within sex	9.1 %	25.8 %	19.6 %	22.3 %	23.3 %	100.0 %
		% of Total	4.4 %	12.6 %	9.6 %	10.8 %	11.3 %	48.7 %
	Total	Count		5223	2129	2381	2384	9988
		% of Total		52,3 %	21.3 %	23.8 %	23.9 %	100.0 %
Bad/ Very Bad	Male	Count	134	311	76	75	45	641
		% within sex	20.9 %	48.5 %	11.9 %	11.7 %	7.0 %	100.0 %
		% of Total	7.1 %	16.5 %	4.0 %	4.0 %	2.4 %	34.1 %
	Female	Count	610	475	63	56	37	1241
		% within sex	49.2 %	38.3 %	5.1 %	4.5 %	3.0 %	100.0 %
		% of Total	32.4 %	25.2 %	3.3 %	3.0 %	2.0 %	65.9 %
	Total	Count		786	139	131	82	1882
		% of Total		41.8 %	7.4 %	7.0 %	4.4 %	100.0 %

Tab. 12: Two-way ANOVA For Independent Samples Test, Gender, Education, and SRH

Descriptive Statistics
Dependent Variable: Self-Rated Health

Gender	Education	Mean	Std. Deviation	N
Male	1-İllitarate	5.43	1.661	392
	2-Primary	5.00	1.579	2508
	3-Secondary	5.40	1.277	1595
	4-High School	5.45	1.233	1711
	5-Graduate and Over	5.49	1.173	1578
	Total	5.30	1.390	7784
Female	Education	5.09	1.806	1802
	1-İllitarate	4.82	1.661	3104
	2-Primary	5.27	1.356	1370
	3-Secondary	5.26	1.347	1535
	4-High School	5.38	1.255	1489
	5-Graduate and Over	5.10	1.556	9300
Total	Education	5.15	1.785	2194
	1-İllitarate	4.90	1.627	5612
	2-Primary	5.34	1.315	2965
	3-Secondary	5.36	1.292	3246
	4-High School	5.44	1.215	3067
	5-Graduate and Over	5.19	1.486	17084

Tab. 13: Tests of Between-Subjects Effects

Dependent Variable: Self-Rated Health

Source	Type III Sum of Squares	Df	Mean Square	F	Sig.
Corrected Model	949.142[a]	9	105.460	48.962	<.001
Intercept	358273.219	1	358273.219	166335.053	.000
Sex	117.432	1	117.432	54.520	<.001
Education	765.842	4	191.461	88.889	<.001
Sex * Education	13.708	4	3.427	1.591	.174
Error	36776.114	17074	2.154		
Total	498712.000	17084			
Corrected Total	37725.256	17083			

Note: (a) R Squared = .025 (Adjusted R Squared = .025)

Previous studies found out that marital status is relational with SRH. Married/coupled people are expected to report good SRH compare to unmarried people, but marriage quality affects women more than men in reporting good SRH (Palencia et al., 2014). One explanation is derived from the protective effect of marriage on women. First, marriage provides higher and expectable social status for women as well as powerful positions for them over unmarried or younger women in most traditional societies. Second, the institution of marriage might require income and health security for the nonworking housewife in most state regulations. A cumulation of these factors most probably affects the physiological and physical health of women in a good manner. However, we cannot reach similar findings in the context of Turkey. Table 14 indicates that 42,1 % of individuals who reported poor SRH were married women whereas % 27,4 of them were married men. The percentage of unmarried women reporting poor health is solely 2,9 %. Additionally, the most marked difference in responses was between widowed men (3 %) and women (18,1 %) reporting poor SRH. On the other hand, such difference is not observed in divorced women and men. Since women are more dependent on their partners in terms of income and social insurance in Turkey, this might be explained by the low widow allowance and lower household income of widow women in Turkey. Indeed, the crosstable analysis of gender, household income, and marital status shows that %97,5 of widow women have low household income. But having said that, the two-way ANOVA for independent sample test (Tables 15 and 16) does not show any significant effect of marital status and gender on SRH at the same time [F=1,32, p>01]. Moving from these limited data, it is difficult to discuss the role of marital status as a social determinant affecting women's social and economic status on SRH. However, deriving from the above data and the literature, it is possible to say that psychical and emotional gendered burden of care and family responsibilities, as well as lack of power in marriage relations, might make women feel worse compared to unmarried women and married men in Turkey. Moreover, the Research on Domestic Violence in Turkey (Yüksel-Kaptanoğlu et al, 2015) reveals that married women are more exposed to violence than unmarried or single women in Turkey. The presence of violence affects one's emotional and physical health badly. Since violence against women is one of the pivotal reflections of unequal power relations between men and women, gender equality policies combatting violence against women would contribute to women's good health conditions.

Tab. 14: The percentage of SRH by sex and marital status, the 2019 Turkey Health Interview Surveys

Self-Rated Health			Marital Status				Total
			1-Unmarried	2-Married	3-Divorced	4-Widow	
Good/ very good	Male	Count	1693	3268	106	57	5124
		% within Sex	33.0 %	63.8 %	2.1 %	1.1 %	100.0 %
		% of Total	17.0 %	32.7 %	1.1 %	0.6 %	51.3 %
	Female	Count	1291	3207	189	177	4864
		% within Sex	26.5 %	65.9 %	3.9 %	3.6 %	100.0 %
		% of Total	12.9 %	32.1 %	1.9 %	1.8 %	48.7 %
	Total	Count	2984	6475	295	234	9988
		% of Total	29.9 %	64.8 %	3.0 %	2.3 %	100.0 %
Bad/Very Bad	Male	Count	43	516	25	57	641
		% within Sex	6.7 %	80.5 %	3.9 %	8.9 %	100.0 %
		% of Total	2.3 %	27.4 %	1.3 %	3.0 %	34.1 %
	Female	Count	54	793	54	340	1241
		% within Sex	4.4 %	63.9 %	4.4 %	27.4 %	100.0 %
		% of Total	2.9 %	42.1 %	2.9 %	18.1 %	65.9 %
	Total	Count	97	1309	79	397	1882
		% of Total	5.2 %	69.6 %	4.2 %	21.1 %	100.0 %

Tab. 15: Two-Way Anova for Independent Samples Test, SHR, Gender, Marital Status

Descriptive Statistics

Dependent Variable: SHR

Gender	Marital Status	Mean	Std. Deviation	N
Male	1-Unmarried	5.66	.996	1974
	2-Married	5.18	1.473	5448
	3-Divorced	5.36	1.444	177
	4-Widow	5.16	1.751	185
	Total	5.30	1.390	7784
Female	1-Unmarried	5.50	1.176	1636
	2-Married	5.04	1.571	6278
	3-Divorced	4.97	1.605	397
	4-Widow	4.91	1.860	989
	Total	5.10	1.556	9300
Total	1-Unmarried	5.59	1.084	3610
	2-Married	5.10	1.527	11726
	3-Divorced	5.09	1.567	574
	4-Widow	4.95	1.845	1174
	Total	5.19	1.486	17084

Tab. 16: Tests of Between-Subjects Effects

Dependent Variable: Self-Rated Health

Source	Type III Sum of Squares	Df	Mean Square	F	Sig.
Corrected Model	839.353[a]	7	119.908	55.510	<.001
Intercept	108777.696	1	108777.696	50357.664	.000
Gender	54.526	1	54.526	25.242	<.001
Marital Status	630.496	3	210.165	97.294	<.001
Gender * Marital Status	8.594	3	2.865	1.326	.264
Error	36885.903	17076	2.160		
Total	498712.000	17084			
Corrected Total	37725.256	17083			

Note: (a) R Squared = .022 (Adjusted R Squared = .022)

Previous studies argue that household income correlates with poor and good health and gender. But contrary to this expectation, the data analysis (table 17-18) could not reveal any statistical relationship between gender, household income, and SRH at the same time (two-way ANOVA for independent samples test, F=0,84, p>01). At this point, it is important to emphasize a limitation to evaluate the data. 92,7 % of respondents in the survey declared low household income (below 2.656 TL). The percentage is 94.3 % for women respondents and 92.2 % for men. It is therefore difficult to understand the impact of income on SRH by gender. However, all female respondents with higher income -8.913 TL and over- (18 women-8.3 %) reported good/very good SRH whereas no women in this income category reported poor health. Although it does not illustrate a statistical significance, it is possible to read such findings as a reflection of high income on women's SRH.

Tab. 17: The percentage of SRH status by sex and household income, 2019 Turkey Health Interview Surveys

SRH			Household Income			
			1 (0-2656 TL)	2 (2657–8912 TL)	20 (8913+TL)	Total
Good/Very Good	Male	Count	873	30	59	962
		% within sex	90.7 %	3.1 %	6.1 %	100.0 %
		% of Total	74.1 %	2.5 %	5.0 %	81.7 %
	Female	Count	196	2	18	216
		% within sex	90.7 %	0.9 %	8.3 %	100.0 %
		% of Total	16.6 %	0.2 %	1.5 %	18.3 %
	Total	Count	1069	32	77	1178
		% of Total	90.7 %	2.7 %	6.5 %	100.0 %
Bad/Very bad	Male	Count	165	4	4	173
		% within sex	95.4 %	2.3 %	2.3 %	100.0 %
		% of Total	53.9 %	1.3 %	1.3 %	56.5 %
	Female	Count	131	2	0	133
		% within sex	98.5 %	1.5 %	0.0 %	100.0 %
		% of Total	42.8 %	0.7 %	0.0 %	43.5 %
	Total	Count	296	6	4	306
		% of Total	96.7 %	2.0 %	1.3 %	100.0 %

Tab. 18: Two-way ANOVA for Independent Samples Test, Sex, Household Income and SRH

Dependent Variable: SRH				
Source	Type III Sum of Squares	Df	Mean Square	F	Sig.
Corrected Model	16.758[a]	5	3.352	1.415	.216
Intercept	5212.509	1	5212.509	2200.170	.000
Sex	3.820	1	3.820	1.612	.204
Household Income	10.960	2	5.480	2.313	.099
Sex * Household Income	3.982	2	1.991	.840	.432
Error	5204.999	2197	2.369		
Total	63873.000	2203			
Corrected Total	5221.757	2202			

Note: (a) R Squared = .003 (Adjusted R Squared = .001)

Consequently, moving from the above data and analysis, it is possible to claim that gender inequalities in education, labour market, income, social status, and family care work sharpen health inequalities in Turkey, similar to the conventional pattern observed in other countries. As expected, women with low educational attainment, unpaid female care workers, and widow women were more likely to report poor SRH in Turkey. Additionally, all women with high-income levels in the survey reported good/very good SRH. This picture exhibits the significance of gender policies aiming to eliminate gender inequalities in education, labour market, poverty, and home-family.

Conclusion

The main argument of this study is that the better the gender equality policies of a state in advancing the socio-economic position of women, the smaller the gender inequalities in health. In this sense, gender inequalities and disparities in health are mostly considered avoidable. Gender equality policies refer to the policies aiming to eliminate gender inequalities in the labour market, political sphere, social and power relations, and family. Previous research shows that implementation of gender equality perspective in family, education, and labour market policies provides a ground in eliminating gender inequalities and disparities in health in general, in SRH in particular, through their effect on social, political, and economic determinants of health, such as the distribution of power, income, paid and unpaid work (Pinillos-Franco & Somarriba, 2018; Palencia et al., 2014).

The analysis of the data based on 2019 Turkey Health Interview Survey, reveals that there is a strong relationship between gender and SRH in Turkey. Women reported worse SRH than men. Over and above, this is the case starting from the collection of these data back to 2008. Along this line, the research takes age, education, employment status, household income, and marital status as the critical socio-economic variables in determining women's socioeconomic position in society into account to elucidate the gender gap in SRH in the context of Turkey. It is found that women aged between 15–55, women with low educational attainment, low income, unpaid female care workers, and widow women were more likely to report poor SRH in Turkey.

Moving from these results and benefitting from the aforementioned literature on gender inequalities in health, it is possible to claim that empowering women in education, in the labour market, within family-society, and combatting female poverty, ameliorate women's SRH status. The countries with the highest score of gender empowerment measure have higher life expectancies and better SRH status in women. Owing to Turkey's low scores of GGI, GDI, GII, and GER, Turkey needs to strengthen the institutional capacities of its state mechanisms in the pursuit of gender equalities. Particularly, the adoption of a gender equality approach in formulating family and care policies as well as family and work reconciliation policies at the labour market might be critical to improve women's SRH status in Turkey and thereby eliminate gender disparities and inequalities in health. For instance, adopting dual-earner family policies and integrating gender perspective into employment policies can reduce the gender difference in SRH indicators. Furthermore, adopting and implementing such gender equality policies not only favour women by enhancing their social and economic status in society but also contribute to strengthening state capacity to minimize health costs and provide a healthier life for its citizens as a whole.

References

World maps of political regimes over 200 years. https://ourworldindata.org/democracy

Annandale, E., & Hunt, K. (Eds.). (2000). *Gender inequalities in health.* Buckingham: Open University Press.

Baćak, V., & Ólafsdóttir, S. (2017). Gender and validity of self-rated health in nineteen European countries. *Scandinavian Journal of Public Health*, 45(6), 647–653.

Backhans, M., Burström, B., de Leon, A. P., & Marklund, S. (2012). Is gender policy related to the gender gap in external cause and circulatory disease mortality? A mixed effects model of 22 OECD countries 1973–2008. *BMC Public Health*, 12(1), 1–12.

Bambra C, Pope D, Swami V, Stanistreet D, Roskam A, Kunst A., & Scott-Samuel. (2009). A: Gender, health inequalities and welfare state regimes: A cross-national study of 13 European countries. *Journal of Epidemiology and Community Health*, 63, 38–44.

Borrell, C., Palència, L., Muntaner, C., Urquía, M., Malmusi, D., & O'Campo, P. (2014). Influence of macrosocial policies on women's health and gender inequalities in health. *Epidemiologic reviews*, 36(1), 31–48.

Chandola, T., Martikainen, P., Bartley, M., et al. (2004). Does conflict between home and work explain the effect of multiple roles on mental health? A comparative study of Finland, Japan, and the UK. *International Journal of Epidemiology*, 33(4), 884–893.

Dreger, S., Gerlinger, T., & Bolte, G. (2016). Gender inequalities in mental well-being in 26 European countries: Do welfare regimes matter? *European Journal of Public Health*, 26, 872–876.

Durgun, D. (2020). Eğitim düzeyinin bireylerin evlenme davranışlarında nasıl bir rolü var? https://haberler.boun.edu.tr/tr/haber/egitim-duzeyinin-bireyle rin-evlenme-davranislarinda-nasil-bir-rolu-var. Access date 19.05.2021.

Etiler, N. (2016). Gender differences in self-rated health and their determinants in Turkey: A further analysis of Turkish health survey. *Türkiye Halk Sağlığı Dergisi*, 14(3), 152–163.

Global Gender Gap Report 2020 (2020). Switzerland, Geneva: World Economic Forum. http://www3.weforum.org/docs/WEF_GGGR_2020.pdf Access Date 19.04.2021

Human Development Report Turkey (2020). http://hdr.undp.org/sites/default/ files/Country-Profiles/TUR.pdf Access date 21.05.2021.

Kawachi, I., Kennedy, B. P., Gupta, V., & Prothrow-Stith, D. (1999). Women's status and the health of women and men: A view from the States. *Social Science & Medicine*, 48(1), 21–32.

OECD. (2019). Health at Glance 2019. https://www.oecd-ilibrary.org/docserver/ 4dd50c09-en.pdf?expires=1618837542&id=id&accname=guest&checksum= 9124033C3456F7BB4D466DCE4EDBC9CD Access Date 11.05.2021

Palència, L., Malmusi, D., De Moortel, D., Artazcoz, L., Backhans, M., Vanroelen, C., & Borrell, C. (2014). The influence of gender equality policies on gender inequalities in health in Europe. *Social Science & Medicine*, 117, 25–33. http:// dx.doi.org/10.1016/j.socscimed.2014.07.018

Pinillos-Franco, S., & Somarriba, N. (2018). Examining gender health inequalities in Europe using a Synthetic Health Indicator: The role of family policies, *The European Journal of Public Health*, 29(2), 254–259.

Schütte, S., Chastang, J. F., Parent-Thirion, A., et al. (2013). Social differences in self-reported health among men and women in 31 countries in Europe. *Scandinavian Journal of Public Health*, 4, 51–7.

Sumbas, A. (2018). Toplumsal Cinsiyet Eşitlik Politikası Olarak Ebeveyn İzni. *Hacettepe Hukuk Fakültesi Dergisi*, 8(2), 167-194.

Sumbas, A. (2019). A Policy Response to the Gendered Childcare in Turkey: Transformative Role of Egalitarian Parental Leave. in *Public Policy Analysis in Turkey Past, Present and Future*, edit. O. Kulaç, E. Akman & C. Babaoğlu, Berlin, Peter Lang.

Torsheim, T., Ravens-Sieberer, U., Hetland, J., Välimaa, R., Danielson, M., & Overpeck, M. (2006). Cross-national variation of gender differences in adolescent subjective health in Europe and North America. *Social Science & Medicine*, 62, 815–827.

TurkStat. (2015). Labor Statistics. https://data.tuik.gov.tr Access Date 21.04.2021

TurkStat. (2019). İstatistiklerle Kadın. https://data.tuik.gov.tr/Bulten/Index?p= Istatistiklerle-Kadin-2020-37221 Access Date 20.04.2021

UN Population Division. (2019). Data, https://ourworldindata.org/life-expectancy. Access Date 20.05.2021

United Nations Gender Inequality Index. (2020). http://hdr.undp.org/en/content/gender-inequality-index-gii Access Date 29.04.2021

Van de Velde, S., Bracke, P., Levecque, K., & Meuleman, B. (2010). Gender differences indepression in 25 European countries after eliminating measurement bias in the CES- D 8. *Social Science Research*, 39, 396–404.

Wang, H., Dwyer-Lindgren, L., Lofgren, K. T., et al. (2013). Age-specific and sex-specific mortality in 187 countries, 1970–2010: A systematic analysis for the Global Burden of Disease Study 2010. *Lancet*, 380 (9859), 2071–2094.

Yüksel-Kaptanoğlu, I., Çavlin, A. & Akadlı Ergöçmen, B. (2015). *2014 Research on Domestic Violence against Women in Turkey*. Ankara: Elma Teknik Matbaacılık.

Ezgi Sevinçhan

Fiscal Justice for Women: Suggestions for Turkey on Menstrual Hygiene Products' Taxation

Introduction

The word "tampon tax", which is an umbrella word, refers to any menstrual product[1] that is subject to sales tax or value-added tax (VAT). Menstruation, a natural biological phenomenon that does not indicate a lack of health but is a requirement, is not excluded from the tax.

The aim of this study is to demonstrate that, since women for biological reasons, a tax on menstrual products is discriminatory, and that there is an urgent need for us to recognize menstrual products as necessities. While examining the subject, it is crucial to state that the tampon tax (even more generally, any paid access to menstrual goods) is an economic limitation with a gender-discriminatory basis that discriminates against women. The tampon tax demonstrates how legal and ostensibly impartial systems, such as the tax system, are profoundly embedded in gender discrimination. Instead of compensating women for previous economic disadvantages, the tax tends to harm them financially. And it sends the message that products that enable women to leave the house and engage in society are luxuries rather than necessities. As a result, tax reform can be seen as a critical mechanism for promoting gender equality and improving civil rights.

While many other countries have abolished or reduced the tax on menstrual hygiene products, in Turkey these products are still taxed at 18 % like other luxury products. Although the definition of "luxury" is nebulous and varies from year to year in the same country and from country to country at the same time, it appears clear that women's sanitary protection products are not luxurious but necessary. Being taxed for a biological need as a woman, rather than as a human or a citizen, is discrimination. Besides, the size of tax revenue makes states reluctant to abolish this tax. However, this would be the ideal solution within the framework of the welfare state. This article aims to show that these products are basic

---

1 Menstrual pads, tampons, cups and any other menstrual product.

necessities for women's health and the tax on them should be removed, or the rate should be reduced at least.

In this sense, first, pink tax, which is strongly related to tampon tax, will be examined. Before detailing the problems and solutions about tampon tax, menstrual taboo would be clarified and comparative examples around the world will be pointed out. Afterwards, the current situation in Turkey will be mentioned and suggestions will be made.

I. Gender Approach to Taxation: Pink Tax, Menstrual Taboo and Tampon Tax

The tampon tax should be framed within the broader "pink tax" debate. The pink tax, unlike the tampon tax, is not a literal tax but has come to refer to gender-based price disparity with economic consequences in general (Herman, 2021). Even when they transcend all social, economic, and psychological barriers, work in high-skilled occupations, and provide services that are perceived to be of "equal" quality to those provided by men, women earn less in worldwide. The *"gender wage gap"* is a term used to describe this phenomenon (Yazıcıoğlu, 2018). Besides this wage gap, *pink tax* and *tampon tax* are closely related terms which refer additional costs charged by women to buy goods and services that are equivalent to those purchased at lower rates by men, as well as the consumption tax levied on women's sanitary hygiene products, which are considered "luxury objects."

Pink is widely perceived as a symbol of femininity all throughout the world, with an obviously discriminating approach. However, pink tax is not only applied to pink products. Since it impacts items that are usually targeted at women, this effect is known as the "pink tax" (Ricci, 2020). It can be imposed on all female-targeted items. For example, the study, titled "From Cradle to Cane: The Cost of Being a Female Consumer," found that women's goods are 7 % more expensive than men's products (Bessendorf, 2015). Indeed, the pink tax demonstrates how even seemingly insignificant details, such as the cost of shampoo, will reveal a story of inequity. These disparities represent how men and women are viewed differently, and they are caused by institutional indifference as well as social and economic processes and mechanisms.

A survey shows that women are charged up to $5.20 more per shirt than men. A men's shirt cost $2.06 to dry clean on average, while a women's shirt cost $3.95. (Duesterhaus, Grauerholz, Weichsel, & Guittar, 2011). This is, obviously, gender-based pricing and it can be defined as "the practice of charging different prices for goods or services based on the consumer's gender" (Vermont the Office of the Attorney General and the Human Rights Commission, 2016). As a side note, it is not a fair solution to buy men's products. We would be overlooking other critical issues if we proposed such a solution. The dry-cleaning example above demonstrates how prices vary. Individual behaviours would not be enough to overcome it. It can only be escaped to a limited extent by collective efforts. It is a problem that needs to be solved by governments. If we live in countries where government intervention is thought to be essential to advance social justice, we would expect such governments to use the tax system to reduce socioeconomic inequality among individuals (Ricci, 2020). Above all, it would be not only an economic but also a political support for women.

Before explaining the tampon tax, it will be useful to address the menstrual taboo since the taboo surrounding menstruation explains not just why the tax has gone unnoticed, but also why it has remained invisible after it has been identified. Menstruation has been viewed as taboo or toxic for decades, and these attitudes have persisted in today's cultural debate and social activities. This widespread and ancient understanding has undeniably influenced our current viewpoints. Even in industrialized capitalist cultures, dominant traditions affirm that women should be able to do all that men can do, but they also compel women to hide their menstruation (Ricci, 2020). For example, the Apple Watch Health-Kit, which was introduced in 2014, allowed users to monitor anything from height, weight, and BMI to sodium intake, medication usage, and blood alcohol content. However, despite assurances by the company's technology executive that it would monitor something of interest to customers, it initially did not provide a period tracker (Hunter, 2016). Menstruation is more than a stigma in certain countries; society members demonize this common occurrence. In Nepal, for example, women are forced to stay in hazardous, dilapidated sheds during their period for fear of infecting others. (Scaramella & Fagan, 2016). Menstruation also has a major effect on women's wellbeing around the world, but it is not generally recognized. In any given day, there are 800 million menstruating women on the planet, with at least 500 million of them without basic services, services, education, and support for handling their cycles (Barron, 2017).

"If Men Should Menstruate", a brilliant exploration of what it takes to turn the tables on sexism and inequality, was written by Gloria Steinem for Ms. Magazine in 1978, at the height of ERA organizing. "So what would happen if suddenly, magically, men could menstruate and women could not?" Steinem believes: "Clearly, menstruation would become an enviable, worthy, masculine event" (Weiss-Wolf, 2019). Instead, every month, millions of women around the

world are subjected to a painful cycle, humiliation, discomfort, anxiety, and isolation as a result of economic disadvantage, period insecurity, a lack of access to
menstrual products and adequate and hygienic services and a fear of revealing
menstruation.

Following the above-mentioned study's[2] release, the term "pink tax" became
highly popular, resulting in numerous newspaper and magazine and social
media. After that, the discussion quickly moved on to another tax, the so-called
"tampon tax."

In 2016, the world was swept up in a whirlwind of feminist activism centred
on the burdens of menstruation. The United States-centric movement's goal
was straightforward: repeal the tax on tampons and other feminine hygiene
products. Time Magazine declared 2016 the "Year of the Period," and a New York
Times editorial headline screamed, "End the Tampon Tax." In Europe, feminist activists lobbied the European Commission to repeal the VAT on tampons
(Ooi, 2018). The issue is defined as follows by Laura Coryton, the founder
of the global change.org movement against the tampon tax: "…Tampon tax
needs to end. Period." (Coryton, ret. 2021). Currently, LOLA, a menstrual care
company whose tampons and liners are made entirely of recycled cotton, is an
outspoken supporter of tampon tax repeal. Seventh Generation (an Unilever
company) made similar investments as part of the "Generation Good" initiative (Herman, 2021).

While the campaign is getting bigger, the tampon tax debate inextricably
turned into a discussion of current sex inequality, particularly in terms of parliamentary representation. Barack Obama, the former president of the United
States, repeated this sentiment, saying: "I have no idea why states would tax these
[tampons] as luxury items. I suspect it's because men were making the laws when
those taxes were passed. I think it's pretty sensible for women […] to work to get
those taxes removed" (Rhodan, 2106).

Women who cannot afford tampons are not as uncommon as one would
imagine. 22 year-old Beth claiming "I usually skip my placebo week to avoid
having periods at all. I've asked a couple of doctors and nurses and had no clear
answer on what the long term health effects might be but, at the end of the day,
the pill is free and tampons aren't" (Preskey, 2015). Like Beth, menstrual products
cost a higher proportion of a person's income for those living at or below the
poverty line, forcing some to choose food over tampons (Perciva, 2020). For

---

2   From Cradle to Cane: The Cost of Being a Female Consumer.

instance, homeless women cannot afford sanitary products. In a survey, a homeless woman said that her shelter had only 2 pads per cycle, while the average woman uses approximately 20 tampons/pads per cycle. Her only choices were toilet paper, re-used cloths, or ruining her only pair of underwear (Parillo & Feller, 2017). These examples can be expanded.

While the "unfairness" of the tampon tax has been highly publicized and argued, its economic impact has also attracted attention. The opposition to repealing local, federal, and national taxes on feminine hygiene products (as in Canada and France) is based on two main arguments: First, that feminine hygiene products are not necessities, and second, that states cannot afford to reduce the guaranteed revenue from tampon taxes. Although every woman is different, a recent study reported that the average woman spends approximately 2280 days (6.25 years) of her life menstruating. Given variations in use and price, the average woman could spend between $70486 and $200087 on tampons and pads alone (excluding any tax) over her lifetime (Crawford & Gold Waldman, The Unconstitutional Tampon Tax, 2019). The average woman would have about 450 cycles in her lifetime (Hartman, 2017). Basically, this is really huge tax revenue for governments. Correlatively, in France, he government opposed the proposal in October 2016 for reasons close to those offered by California Governor Jerry Brown when he vetoed proposed legislation: Argued that if the amendment had passed, tax revenues would have declined by 55 million Euros (63 million USD) (BBC News, 2015).

It is obvious that there isn't a single rational criterion that can be used to explain gender-based pricing or the tampon tax. In addition to this, there is no equivalent tax on any sex-based medical product which is predominantly consumed by men. (Giokaris & Pouliasi, 2020) The reasons for the lack of government involvement seem to be somewhat close to the reasons for the long-standing failure to reform or repeal the window tax[3] which was kept in place due to financial reasons, even after the significant public health risk it posed became evident (Yazıcıoğlu, 2018). On the other hand, it is the government's responsibility to balance the effect of the taxation mechanism on various groups in society in the public interest.

---

3 For further information about window tax: https://www.parliament.uk/about/living-heritage/transformingsociety/towncountry/towns/tyne-and-wear-case-study/about-the-group/housing/window-tax/

A. Taxation as a Discrimination Instrument

United Nations General Assembly adopted the Universal Declaration of Human Rights[4] on December 10, 1948, stating[5] for the first time in history that everyone is entitled to human rights "without distinction of any kind, such as race, colour, sex, language, religion, political or other opinion, national or social origin, property, birth or other status". Since menstrual hygiene and affordable access to menstrual hygiene products are inextricably linked to rights to health, sanitation, education, dignity, and employment, among other rights, the tampon tax is a human rights problem (Crawford & Spivack, 2019). This is also a welfare state requirement and solutions should not be left to the initiative of civil society organizations, the women's movement or the market. It is a necessity for the *welfare state* that all states make their own regulations to abolish tax or reduce rates.

Pink tax and tampon tax should be classified as cases of overt "sex discrimination" because it specifically targets women based on their gender. Most constitutions contain a particular provision relating to gender equality and/or a non-discrimination clause enumerating a list of prohibited grounds, which usually includes sex. For example, article 10 of Constitution of the Republic of Turkey claims that "Everyone is equal before the law without distinction as to language, race, colour, sex, political opinion, philosophical belief, religion and sect, or any such grounds." In contrast with this article (and in most other countries) consumption taxes are not always sex neutral in Turkey.

To prove tampon tax is a gender-based price discrimination Ooi uses the example of two taxpayers, Amy and Ben, who make the same amount of money and are "equally well off in the no-tax universe" to demonstrate that it is unjust to redistribute the results of menstrual product taxes among men and women. When there is a tax on period products, Amy should pay more in taxes than Ben so she has no choice but to purchase those products. As a result, a tax on menstrual products puts an extra burden on Amy simply because she needs them. Amy and Ben don't have the same consumption and saving opportunities. If the consumption tax is supposed to be fair to savers, it isn't fair to women who can't save instead of consume. Also the tax would violate horizontal equity in this situation (Ooi, 2018).

---

4   Also the UN General Assembly adopted the Convention on the Elimination of All Forms of Discrimination against Women (CEDAW) in 1979, which is a rich source of universal human rights for women in particular.
5   Art. 2.

B. Tampon Tax-legal Analysis

The concept of a tax is malleable. Both the definition of tax and its functionalities have evolved over time, based on a variety of factors such as the state-individual relationship. While different countries place different emphasis on different aspects of taxation, the basic concept of taxation remains the same: compulsion (Yazıcıoğlu, 2018). As OECD's definition, tax is "a compulsory unrequited payment to the government" (OECD). In addition to that the following can be said as primary characteristics of taxes: They are compulsory, unrequited, regulated by public law and collected by government (or a government-controlled entity). While the primary goal of taxation has historically been to collect funds for government expenditures, other political, social, and economic objectives may also be important (Yazıcıoğlu, 2018).

OECD examines the consumption tax as following: "… generally consist of general taxes on goods and services (taxes on general consumption) and taxes on specific goods and services. Taxes on general consumption comprise value added tax (VAT) and its equivalent in several jurisdictions (goods and services tax, or GST), sales taxes, and other general taxes on goods and services"(OECD, 2020). Generally, consumption taxes generate significant revenue for the states that levy them. For example, in the USA, states collected more than $430 billion in sales taxes in 2015, but just slightly more than $338 billion in income taxes (Crawford & Spivack, 2019).

Consumption tax may be "hidden". A hidden tax may be classified as either "partially" or "completely" hidden, depending on the extent of taxpayer ignorance. In reality, before being able to adjust their behaviour in response to a tax (elasticity), taxpayers must first be aware of the tax (Yazıcıoğlu, 2018). By lowering tax salience, hidden taxes reduce visibility. It could be argued that when retail prices include VAT, as they do in the EU and Turkey, VAT becomes a partly hidden tax. Since high-income individuals are able to save a greater percentage of their income, low-income individuals will almost always pay a larger portion of their income in sales taxes/VAT than higher-income individuals. It not only has a disproportionate effect on lower-income earners as a result of their consumption and savings habits, but also applies to all consumers of taxable goods and services regardless of wealth, gender, or age (Do, Hodgson, & Wilson-Rogers, 2017).

As mentioned above, the pink tax cannot be classified as a tax in legal terms. While the pink tax does not meet fully of the legal requirements to be classified as a tax, it does meet the two conditions that cause taxes to have an economic impact: being compulsory and unrequited. More significantly, their customer base is the same: women. (Yazıcıoğlu, 2018). The pink tax, which is more of a social and economic norm than a tax, represents a common trend of price disparity against a certain group of individuals, with women paying more.

For tampon tax, it is a bit different. It is an "actual tax" and has all requirements above. Consumption taxes are mostly levied on luxury products. However, some goods and services are deemed "necessary," meaning they must be purchased regardless of budget in order to live a dignified life, and in some cases, simply to survive. Specific to tampon tax, it has important and undesirable results to not to buy sanitary products to avoid paying the tax. As a result, depending on the national VAT/GST scheme, the unfair treatment of basic needs goods may be questioned under both constitutional law and (international) human rights provisions. (Rüll, 2020).

C. Sanitary Products: Luxury or Essential?

Despite these concerns, some might argue that, in order to escape the pink tax, women should choose less costly products from among those produced for men. In the case of the tampon tax, though, the same point would fall flat since such a tax cannot be avoided. The tampon tax is a tax on menstrual products, which means it is a tax on anything that women cannot choose whether or not to purchase, just as they cannot choose whether or not to menstruate. Maintaining a tampon tax clearly means that we do not consider menstrual products to be necessities.

A "necessity" is a term that has no clear meaning. Furthermore, determining what constitutes "necessity" is often subjective. Individuals also consider menstrual products to be "luxuries" rather than "necessities" due to subjectivity in assessing need (Perciva, 2020). However, a product that allows a woman to completely participate and work in society is not a luxury. A woman menstruating who does not have access to tampons and pads is unable to engage in her society since her only options are to remain at home or to menstruate openly.

Scientifically, safe menstrual cycles include the use of sanitary hygiene items (Parillo & Feller, 2017). During this time, a woman's body is most susceptible to infections. Owing to a lack of suitable materials, poor hygiene raises the risk of infection. Skin rashes, urinary tract infection, genital infection, tubal obstructions, miscarriage, and worsening of existing diseases are all medical effects of not having access to enough sanitary products (WWSC & UN Women, 2015). As a result, it can be said that infections and poor health-related quality-of-life have been linked to poor menstrual hygiene.

It's worth noting that during the public debate about the tampon tax, women's sanitary care products were often compared to "men's personal care products," such as razors and shaving cream. The logic behind this analogy is incomprehensible while men who shave with natural soap rather than shaving cream or with an electric shaver that does not need shaving cream do not experience any health issues or disruptions in their daily activities (Yazıcıoğlu, 2018). It should also mean that women's need for menstrual products is far from elastic.

Women who spend money on period products do not improve their overall wellbeing. Instead, they return to their previous level. It must be differentiated between options and requirements. Whatever angle we take at the claim, it will always be real: menstrual products are a necessity as long as there are women who menstruate (Ricci, 2020). As a matter of fact menstrual hygiene care is a vital requirement for all women and should be considered a fundamental women's right. (Kuhlmann, Peters Bergquist, Danjoint, & Wall, 2019).

II. Comparative Examples for Taxing Sanitary Products around the World

A. VAT on Women's Sanitary Products in Turkey

Most, if not all, tax codes[6] exempt certain essential items, such as groceries and clothes. Turkey's tax codes have some exempts too. However, there is not an exempt for women's sanitary products, women's sanitary products are not considered as necessities and being taxed while diamonds are exempted. The standard rate of 18 % VAT is applied to these products in Turkey (Revenue Administration).

In 2019, Istanbul Deputy Sera Kadıgil Sütlü made a proposal (as of May 2020, the proposal is still waiting in the commission) to reduce the 18 % VAT on hygiene products such as pads or tampons to 5 % during menstruation. She said "We do not want to pay taxes because we have menstruation" (NTV, 2019). However, despite this proposal and the increasing call of women, feminine hygiene products are still taxed at 18 %, while products such as Viagra and

---

6   Before beginning any analysis, it is important to categorize the term "tampon tax." We can define it broadly to include the VAT in Europe, the sales tax in the United States, as well as GST and other equivalent taxes in some countries levied on menstrual hygiene products.

condoms are taxed at 8 %. According to the information contained in the proposal (Kadıgil Sütlü, 2019), a study shows that, in 2016, 1.5 billion sanitary pads, 550 million daily pads and 18 million tampons were consumed annually. The total market value of all these products is 500 million Turkish Liras according to the data of the same year. The size of the market gives us a clue about the size of the tax revenue. It is clear that this tax income arises from a biological need and that women are obliged to pay taxes due to this need.

B. Relevant Practices around the World

During the Great Depression, the USA imposed a sales tax as a new source of state revenue. By 1947, sales taxes had become the most important source of income for governments. With the exception of five states, all states now tax some sort of sales tax. Each state creates its own set of sales tax laws and exemptions. Most states allow cities and counties to raise revenue by levying a sales tax, but any exception provided at the state level also extends to counties and cities. (Perciva, 2020). Currently 13 states have removed the tax on tampons and sanitary pads in the USA (Doris, 2021).

The majority of goods and services subject to VAT have a standard rate that is applied to them. Most countries[7] choose to have exceptions to this general rule in their VAT systems. Reduced rates, zero rates, and exemptions are among the variations. Menstrual hygiene products are taxed at the standard VAT/GST rate in the majority of countries.

1. Exemption

Bhutan, Colombia, India, Jamaica, Kenya, Lebanon, Malaysia, Nicaragua, Rwanda, South Korea, Nigeria, Saint Kitts and Nevis all have an exception for menstrual hygiene products. Exempting products from VAT/GST has ramifications beyond the final sale of a product or service to a customer. Exemption has an effect on the entire supply chain because it prevents all participants from recovering production taxes. As a result, the VAT/GST that manufacturers have already paid for the raw materials they used cannot be reclaimed. As a result, the price discount that customers can expect is determined by the normal VAT rate as well as the cost of raw materials (Rüll, 2020).

---

7   For further information about VAT rates applied in the Member States of the European Union, following link can be visited: https://ec.europa.eu/taxation_customs/sites/taxation/files/resources/documents/taxation/vat/how_vat_works/rates/vat_rates_en.pdf

2. Zero-Rating

To some extent, the zero rate and exemption practices are identical. Consumers do not have to pay VAT on the products or services in question under either mechanism. The distinction is in the deductibility of input VAT. The exemption method would not allow the supplier to credit the input VAT under the zero rate scheme (Yazıcıoğlu, 2018). Australia, Canada, Ireland, Lesotho, the Maldives, Mauritius, South Africa, Uganda, the United Kingdom, and Trinidad and Tobago have chosen the course of no taxation on the supply of menstrual hygiene products thus allowing for input tax recovery (Rüll, 2020).

3. Reduced Rates

Belgium, Cyprus, Estonia, France, Germany, Italy,[8] Luxembourg, the Netherlands, Poland, Portugal, the Slovak Republic, Spain and Vietnam are the countries that using reduced rates (Rüll, 2020). The majority of these are EU member states, and their decision to use a lower rate is governed by EU law: Since this field of law is harmonized in the European Union, member states' flexibility in shaping VAT laws is restricted. The VAT Directive restricts the number of exemptions and zero-rated transactions that can be created. As a result, under the VAT Directive, neither an exemption nor a zero-rating of menstrual hygiene products is possible since the reduced rate cannot be less than 5 %, according to Art. 99 (1) of the VAT Directive.

However, if a Member State already applied a zero-rating or other reduced rate on January 1, 1991, it is permitted to do so under Article 110 of the VAT Directive. Ireland is an example of this. As a result, Ireland is the only EU member state that allows menstrual hygiene goods to be taxed at zero percent. Luxembourg was able to extend a "super-reduced rate" of 3 % to menstrual hygiene products under the same clause since it already favoured pharmaceutical products (Rüll, 2020).

It also can be argued that the VAT directive violates the EU's charter of fundamental rights because it requires member states to impose at least 5 % VAT on sanitary products, implying that the domestic law enforcing the directive would therefore violate the Charter of Fundamental Rights of the European Union

---

8   For both menstrual cups and for items certified to be compostable or washable, Italy applies a discounted rate of 5 %. It can be said that combining preferential treatment for menstrual hygiene products with the possibility of more sustainable consumer action is a valuable idea to consider.

(Giokaris & Pouliasi, 2020). It is obvious that gender equity has a major connection to human rights. According to Articles 2 and 3(3) of the Treaty on European Union, equality between men and women is one of the EU's aims. Furthermore, this fundamental value is protected under the Charter, which prohibits any form of sex discrimination, whereas Article 8 of the Treaty on the Functioning of the European Union (TFEU) mandates that the EU take measures to eliminate discrimination and promote gender equality, and Article 19 of the TFEU provides for the necessary authorization for the EU to take active measures to combat any form of discrimination, including sex discrimination.

Suggestions and Conclusion

The solution to this so-called cultural and epistemic problem is not easy, but it is critical. If we accept that taxes are the price we pay for living in a civilized society, there would be a problem from this viewpoint: some taxes, like tampon tax, are simply unfit for a civilized society. In the contrary, they lead to the perpetuation of injustice and inequality (Kuhlmann, Peters Bergquist, Danjoint, & Wall, 2019). According to Article 1 of the Constitution of the Republic of Turkey, Turkey is a social state.[9] Tax is also a concept that is highly related to the welfare state. The tax levied by the state on menstrual hygiene products is quite high considering the size of the market. The abolition of this tax, of course, causes a loss of income for the state, but it should be considered as a necessity of the welfare state.

When it comes to the precise wording of provisions that give a favourable taxation to menstrual hygiene goods, there are three major approaches: A detailed list of privileged goods, a general clause and a hybrid of the two, consisting of a general clause and an illustrative list of privileged goods. The detailed listing of privileged goods is the most frequently used method. Both sanitary pads and tampons are usually used. Just a few countries, such as Germany, have comprehensive lists that contain items such as sponges and period pants (Rüll, 2020). However, when innovations arise, there would be still a need to amend the legislation. A general provision, on the other hand, is applicable to a wide range of goods but does not have the most legal certainty. As a proposal for this problem, combination of the general clause with an outstanding list of privileged products can be suggested.

---

9   Here, the "social state" is given as a literal translation as it appears in the Constitution. The concept of "welfare state" can also be used instead.

Furthermore, government intervention is important to discuss this problem on a political level since abolishing the tampon tax will send a powerful message to society that menstruating people's needs are significant and should not be ignored. Also, ending the taxes that being a burden to women would be much more easier than eliminating the wage gap (Bennett, 2017).

In free market, manufacturers could increase the price of tampons by the amount of the tax break, so that the customer pays the same amount as before the repeal (Ooi, 2018). An optimal tax incidence study describes the impact of a tax reform on customers' utility levels, taking into account not only market changes but also any opportunity costs associated with achieving the prices currently charged. Prices for a given product, for example, may vary between retailers, and different customers may buy at different stores (Cotropia & Rozema, 2018). As a result, taxes can be passed on to consumers at various rates, often within the same product.

Consequently, we all must accept that these products are essential. If legal substructures allow it, a zero-rate application with an overarching general provision would be ideal for Turkey rather than an exemption. In addition to tax solutions, the provision of sanitary products free of charge can be offered as an option within the framework of welfare programs. This suggestion can be preferable that low-income women will need financial assistance with their periods and the effect of a tax break is unlikely would be meaningful for them.

If organizations and policymakers really want to promote equity and fairness, they must change the mechanisms that contribute to system inequality. Although removing the tampon tax seems to be a simple way to eliminate the economic disadvantage, there is still a long way to go. As we know, the tampon tax is not the only cause of the structural disadvantages that women and girls face, removing this tax should only be considered as a step. In other words, attempts to repeal the tampon tax can be seen as part of a wider plan to reduce or eliminate gender discrimination.

References

Barron, T. (2017, October 11). *800 Million Women and Girls are on Their Period Right Now - Let's Talk about It*. Retrieved March 21, 2021, from https://www.ibtimes.co.uk/800-million-women-girls-are-their-period-right-now-lets-talk-about-it-1642606. Accesd date 22.05.2021.

BBC News. (2015, October 15). *France Rejects 'Tampon Tax' Change*. Retrieved March 29, 2021, from https://www.bbc.com/news/world-europe-34538672

Bennett, J. (2017). The Tampon Tax: Sales Tax, Menstrual Hygiene Products, and Necessity Exemptions. *The Business, Entrepreneurship & Tax Law Review, 1* (8), 183–215.

Bessendorf, A. (2015). *From Cradle to Cane: The Cost of Being a Female Consumer A Study of Gender Pricing in New York City.* Retrieved April 21, 2020, from https://www1.nyc.gov/assets/dca/downloads/pdf/partners/Study-of-Gender-Pricing-in-NYC.pdf

Coryton, L. (n.d.).(Retrieved April 12, 2021). https://www.change.org/m/end-the-sexist-and-illogical-tax-on-tampons-sanitary-pads-and-mooncups-period#about-movement

Cotropia, C., & Rozema, K. (2018, September). Who Benefits from Repealing Tampon Taxes? Empirical Evidence from New Jersey. *Journal of Empirical Legal Studies,* 620–647.

Crawford, B., & Gold Waldman, E. (2019). The Unconstitutional Tampon Tax. *University of Richmond Law Review, 53* (2), 439–490.

Crawford, B., & Spivack, S. (2019). Human Rights and the Taxation of Menstrual Hygiene Products in an Unequal World. In P. Alston, & N. Reisch, *Tax, Inequality, and Human Rights.* Oxford University Press.

Do, C., Hodgson, H., & Wilson-Rogers, N. (2017). The Tax on Feminine Hygiene Products: Is This Reasonable Policy. *Australian Tax Forum, 32* (3), 521–540.

Doris, A. (2021, March 23). *What happened when a US state scrapped the 'tampon tax'.* Retrieved April 11, 2021, from https://review.chicagobooth.edu/economics/2021/article/what-happened-when-us-state-scrapped-tampon-tax

Duesterhaus, M., Grauerholz, L., Weichsel, R., & Guittar, N. (2011). The Cost of Doing Femininity: Gendered Disparities in Pricing of Personal Care Products and Services. *Gender Issues, 28* (4), 175–191.

Giokaris, I., & Pouliasi, M. (2020). To Tax or Not to Tax? Tampon Taxes and Gender (In)Equality: The Cyprus Case-Study. *The Cyprus Review, 32* (1), 257–278.

Hartman, V. (2017). End the Bloody Taxation: Seeing Red on the Unconstitutional Tax on Tampons. *Northwestern University Law Review, 112* (2), 313–354.

Herman, S. (2021). A Blood-Red-Herring: Why Revenue Concerns Are Overestimated in the Fight to End the "Tampon Tax". *Fordham Urban Law Journal Journal, 48* (2), 596–624.

Hunter, L. (2016). The "Tampon Tax": Public Discourse of Policies Concerning Menstrual Taboo. *Hinckley Journal of Politics, 17* (1), 11–18.

Kadıgil Sütlü, S. (2019, January 19). Retrieved May 16, 2021, from https://www2.tbmm.gov.tr/d27/2/2-1576.pdf

Kuhlmann, A., Peters Bergquist, E., Danjoint, D., & Wall, L. (2019). Unmet Menstrual Hygiene Needs Among Low-Income Women. *Obstetrics & Gynecology, 133* (2), 238–244.

NTV. (2019, February 15). Retrieved March 3, 2021, from https://www.ntv.com. tr/turkiye/chpli-kadigil-regl-oldugumuz-icin-vergi-odemek-istemiyoruz,-BDjS5-NVUuClALyFl5Cyw

OECD. (n.d.). Retrieved April 15, 2020, from https://www.oecd.org/ctp/glossaryoftaxterms.htm#T

OECD. (2020). *Consumption Tax Trends 2020*. Paris: OECD Publishing.

Ooi, J. (2018). Bleeding Women Dry: Tampon Taxes and Menstrual Inequity. *Northwestern University Law Review, 113* (1), 109–154.

Parillo, A., & Feller, E. (2017). Menstrual Hygiene Plight of Homeless Women, a Public Health Disgrace. *R I Med J (2013), 100* (12), 14–15.

Perciva, A. (2020). California's Tampon Tax: Will the Third Time be the Charm? *University of the Pacific Law Review, 52* (2), 429–446.

Preskey, N. (2015, February 16). *There's Nothing Luxurious about My Periods, So Why Is the Government Taxing Tampons as if There Is?* Retrieved May 1, 2021, from https://www.independent.co.uk/voices/comment/there-s-nothing-luxurious-about-my-periods-so-why-government-taxing-tampons-if-there-10045629.html

Revenue Administration. (n.d.). Retrieved April 8, 2021, from https://www.gib.gov.tr/node/108756

Ricci, N. (2020, June). Menstrual Experience and Structural Injustice: Why Menstruation Should Be a Political Matter (Unpublished Master Thesis). Utrecht University.

Rhodan, M. (2016). Retrieved from https://time.com/4183108/obama-tampon-tax-sanitary/

Rüll, D. (2020). How to Abolish Indirect Taxes on Menstrual Hygiene Products. *Copenhagen Business School Law Research Paper Series, 20–28* (III), 1–23.

Scaramella, N., & Fagan, J. (2016). *Rutgers University Libraries*. Retrieved May 3, 2021, from https://rucore.libraries.rutgers.edu/rutgers-lib/51726/

Vermont the Office of the Attorney General and the Human Rights Commission. (2016, June). *Guidance on the Issue of Gender in Pricing of Goods and Services.* Retrieved April 20, 2021, from https://hrc.vermont.gov/sites/hrc/files/gender-based%20pricing%20guidance.pdf

Weiss-Wolf, J. (2019). *ERA Campaign and Menstrual Equity* (pp. 168–174). New York: New York University School of Law.

Window Tax. (n.d.). Retrieved April 13, 2021, from UK Parliament: https://www.
parliament.uk/about/living-heritage/transformingsociety/towncountry/
towns/tyne-and-wear-case-study/about-the-group/housing/window-tax/

WWSC, & UN Women. (2015). *Menstrual Hygiene Management: Behaviour And
Practices In The Kedougou Region, Senegal* . WWSC and UN Woman.

Yazıcıoğlu, A. (2018). *Pink Tax and the Law Discriminating against Woman
Consumers*. Oxon: Routlege.

Ayça Zorluoğlu Yılmaz

Surrogate Motherhood in Turkey

Introduction

Surrogate motherhood is carrying a fertilized embryo, belonging to a person who has medical problems related to childbearing, in the womb of another woman and also being born by this woman. Surrogacy is one of the assisted reproductive technologies used when women are unable to have children because they cannot carry a child in their uterus, have infertility problems due to another reason, has health conditions that prevent her from becoming pregnant or may be reluctant to conceive.

In surrogacy process, the embryo obtained by fertilization of the egg belonging to the genetic mother, surrogate mother or other donor is carried in the uterus of the surrogate mother and delivered to the intended parents after birth (Corradi, 2008; Gruenbaum, 2012; Şensöz Malkoç, 2014, 2015; Ateş, 2016; Ekşi, 2016). There are many applications in different legal systems regarding surrogacy. While in some legal systems surrogacy is permitted in exchange of money, some legal systems do not allow this. Performing surrogacy in return for money is called commercial surrogacy, and performing surrogacy without a monetary compensation is called non-commercial or altruistic surrogacy. In traditional surrogacy, the surrogate mother is also the genetic mother of the child. In this method, surrogate mother agrees to give the child to the intended parents after birth. In this technique, mostly the genetic father is the intended father. In gestational surrogacy, also known as the host method, the surrogate mother is not the biological mother of the child. The surrogate mother becomes pregnant via the transfer of embryo. In this technique, both of the intended parents might be genetic parents or the child may be conceived via egg, sperm or embryo donation (Pasayat, 2008; Brunet, et al., 2013; Hakeri, 2015; Turgut, 2016; Voskoboynik, 2016; Savaş, 2019).

In accordance with the principle of "mater semper certa est", that is "mother is always certain", which is the basic principle adopted since Roman law, the rules regarding determining the mother in legal systems are based on the principle of accepting the person who gives birth as the mother. However, advances in science and medicine have increased access to and benefit from advanced reproductive health services. Infertility is increasing in Turkey. The increase in infertility also leads to more use of surrogacy at the international level. It is inevitable that parents who desire to have a child want to benefit from a medically possible opportunity. The law must also adopt appropriate regulations. While there is such a medical development, legally ignoring it does not prevent such application, on the contrary, it causes the law to be circumvented. Couples who want to have children through surrogate mothers apply for surrogacy tourism (Gruenbaum, 2012; Şensöz Malkoç, 2014; Ateş, 2016; Ungan Çalışkan, 2016; Parlak Börü, 2019; Ağaoğlu, 2020) and this does not protect the surrogate mothers, the families who use this route, nor the children born. The uncertainties in the legal systems regarding surrogacy and the application of surrogacy practices in other countries by the citizens of countries that do not allow surrogacy may cause problems at the international level. For example; when the delivery time comes, the surrogate mother can avoid surrendering the child by using the legal gaps in the country's legislation, or situations may arise where families do not want to take the child due to the child's illness or disagreements between the parents. Problems are not limited to these. Since surrogacy is not allowed in their own country, couples who have a child through surrogate mother in another country cannot obtain a passport when they want to take the child to their homeland, or even if they bring the child to their homeland, they are not legally accepted as parents, cannot take their own children under their name, the child is accepted as stateless and taken away from the family and given under State protection. (Şensöz Malkoç, 2015; Parlak Börü, 2019; Ağaoğlu, 2020). In this case, parents try to register their children under their name by circumventing the law, such as adopting their own children.

The legal prohibition of this method deprives only intended parents, children born in this way and surrogate mothers from legal protection. Instead of this approach, the law should keep up with the pace of technology and this issue should be legally regulated in accordance with the rules of public order, fundamental rights and freedoms, family and inheritance law within the legal order. For this, possible problems related to surrogacy should be taken into consideration and the issue should be addressed in ethical, economic and policy aspects as well as legal.

I. Literature Review and Theoretical Discussions

A. Historical Background and Cases

In order to better understand the problems related to surrogacy, the cases that are considered the cornerstone in this area should be looked at.

1. Baby Cotton Case (Re C (A Minor) (Wardship: Surrogacy) [1985] FLR 846)

The legal disputes regarding surrogacy started in 1985 with the Baby Cotton case. The embryo, which was formed as a result of the combination of the egg of the surrogate mother and the sperm of the American father, was born by the surrogate mother for 6500 Pounds in the incident. After the child was born, the surrogate mother did not deliver the child, and the family applied to the English courts with the allegation of child abduction. The court ultimately ruled that the child had been abducted and allowed the couple to take the child to the USA. (Latey, 1985; Gamble & Ghevaert, 2009; Şensöz Malkoç, 2014; Turgut, 2016; Parlak Börü, 2019; Savaş, 2019).

2. Baby M. Case (Matter of Baby M (1988, N J) 537 A2d 1227)

In this case, there was a dispute between the surrogate mother and the intended parents regarding the delivery of the child. According to the contract, the surrogate mother, who became pregnant through artificial insemination using the plaintiff's sperm, agreed to hand over the child to the intended parents after birth and to waive all maternal rights for the intended family to adopt the child for $ 10,000.00. Despite the contract, the surrogate mother did not deliver the baby on the grounds that she would not live without the baby after birth. The New Jersey Supreme Court decided that the contract for surrogacy was unethical on the grounds that a child could not be sold in exchange for money and annulled the contract, but decided to retain custody of the child in accordance with the best interests of the child (In re Baby M - 109 N.J. 396, 537 A.2d 1227 (1988), 1988; Younger, 1988; Sanger, 2007; Şensöz Malkoç, 2014, 2015; Prinz, 2015; Voskoboynik, 2016;Parlak Börü, 2019; Savaş, 2019; Thapa, 2019).

3. W and B v H Case (W and B v H (Child Abduction: Surrogacy) [2002] 1 FLR 1008)

According to the contract between the American couple and the British surrogate mother, it was decided that the birth should take place in California in order to avoid any problems in terms of the child's parentage. Because when the child is born in America, the child can become an American citizen, and when the birth takes place in California, as surrogate motherhood is accepted in California, the parentage between the intended parents and the child can be established without any dispute. However, when the pregnancy progressed, it was understood that the surrogate mother was expecting twin babies, and there was a conflict between the parties. Thereupon, the surrogate mother gave birth in England and refused to give the children to the American couple. Intended parents applied to the California Supreme Court to request the return of the child in accordance with The Hague Convention on Civil Aspects of International Child Abduction of 1980. The Court, on the other hand, held that in international surrogacy cases, this Convention was not applicable with regard to the return of the child. This decision is important in that the American Courts change their case law in child abduction cases related to surrogacy (Setright, 2002; Clissmann & Hutchinson, 2005; Fiorini, 2012; Şensöz Malkoç, 2014; Laurie, Harmon, & Porter, 2016).

4. Baby Donna Case (Rechtbank Groningen, 20 July 2004, Rechtbank Utrecht, 26 October 2005, Rechtbank Utrecht, 24 October 2007, Rechtbank Utrecht, 7 May 2008, Gerechtshof Amsterdam, 25 November 2008, Rechtbank Utrecht, 10 June 2009, Gerechtshof Amsterdam, February 2, 2010)

A Belgian couple made a surrogacy contract with a surrogate mother, also from Belgium, for € 10,000. According to this contract, the embryo formed with the sperm of the intended father and the egg of the surrogate mother was placed in the uterus of the surrogate mother. After a while, the surrogate mother notified the intended parents that the child had fallen. But this was a lie. The surrogate mother entered into a second surrogacy contract with a Dutch couple and pledged to give the child to the Dutch couple for € 15,000. After the birth, the Dutch couple adopted the child. But the genetic father found out about the situation 2 years later. The DNA test also proved the situation. The genetic father sued the Dutch Court for the return of the child. Under Dutch law, blood ties are also essential, however, since the child was adopted by the Dutch couple and had lived in a family relationship with the Dutch couple since the child was born, the child remained in the Dutch couple under the principle of the best interests of the child, and the genetic father obtained only the right to communicate with the child. The Utrecht District Court decided that before Donna started school, the Dutch couple have to inform her that they were not biological parents (Vonk, 2010; Brunet, et al., 2013; Şensöz Malkoç, 2014).

5. Baby Manji Case (Baby Manji Yamada v. Union of India, AIR 2009 SC 84; (2008) 13 SCC 518)

A Japanese couple hired an Indian surrogate mother to have a child through surrogacy. Pregnancy occurred through fertilization of the egg of the surrogate mother with the sperm of the genetic father. During the pregnancy, the Japanese couple got divorced. When the child was born, the genetic father applied to the Japanese Consulate in India to take the child to Japan. However, the Consulate did not give the child a passport on the grounds that the child cannot obtain Japanese citizenship. The Indian Law stipulates that the child should be adopted immediately before the intended parents leave the country, while it also prohibits the adoption of a single father. The Japanese father had to take the custody of the child by filing a lawsuit with the Indian Courts (Pasayat, 2008; Darnovsky, 2009; Points, 2011; Şensöz Malkoç, 2014; Thapa, 2019).

6. Buzzanca Case (In re Marriage of Buzzanca - 61 Cal. App. 4th 1410, 72 Cal. Rptr. 2d 280, 1998)

The Buzacca couple signed a surrogacy contract with the surrogate mother, and the embryo, which was obtained entirely by donor, ie genetically not belonging to the Buzacca couple, was placed in the surrogate mother. Later, the Buzacca couple divorced. Intended father claimed that he was not the legal and genetic parent of the child. The California Supreme Court accepted the Buzacca couple as the child's family because they wanted him to be born, even though they did not have genetic ties to the child. This case means that couples who want to have a baby through a surrogate mother in California will be considered directly as the family of the child (In re Marriage of Buzzanca, 1998; Cohen, 2014; Şensöz Malkoç, 2014; Turgut, 2016).

7. X&Y Case (Re X and Y (Foreign Surrogacy) [2009] 1 FLR 733)

In this case, a British couple had twins through commercial surrogacy in Ukraine. The Ukrainian mother does not have a genetic link with the children, moreover, the surrogate mother is married. In Ukraine, the intended parents are registered as parents for birth certificates, but English law does not recognize this and does not grant children the right of British nationality. Because according to English law, it is the mother who gave birth to the child. At this point, English law accepts the woman who gives birth as a legal mother, regardless of the genetic link between the children and the mother. Moreover, since the surrogate mother is married, the husband is also considered the father of the children, whereas the genetic father is the intended father. According to this, the family of the twins is English couple according to Ukrainian law and Ukrainian couple according to English law. After a long legal struggle, it was decided to keep the children in England due to the DNA results, but again, the twins were not directly considered British citizens. According to English law, if this contract is a commercial surrogacy, it is invalid pursuant to the principle of public order.

Even if the contract is made in countries that accept commercial surrogacy, it is not considered valid under English law. The only way out is to adopt children, which means going a long way (Şensöz Malkoç, 2014; Wade, 2017; X & Y (Foreign Surrogacy) [2008] EWHC 3030 (Fam), 2008; Gamble & Ghevaert, 2009; Grusic, 2015; Gruenbaum, 2012).

The situation is similar in terms of Turkish law. Even if a Turkish couple is signed the contract in a country that legally recognizes surrogacy, this contract is invalid under Turkish law, as it is against public order, also against the mandatory rules and morality. In addition, in terms of Turkish law, since the woman who gave birth to the child is accepted as the mother, it is extremely possible in terms of Turkish law to have an event similar to the one in this case and to experience problems.

B. The Regulation of Surrogate Motherhood in Turkey

The first legislation regarding artificial insemination in Turkish law is the Invitro Fertilization Embryo Transfer Centres Regulation dated 1987. This regulation was amended in 1996, 1998 and 2005 and eventually this regulation was repealed in 2010 with a new regulation. The regulation dated 2010 was also implemented until 2014.

One of the legislations in force regarding surrogacy is the Regulation on Assisted Reproductive Treatment Practices and Assisted Reproduction Treatment Centres published in the Official Gazette on 30.09.2014. Surrogacy is prohibited with this regulation. The provision prohibiting surrogacy is regulated in row no 4 in Annex 17 of the Regulation. According to this regulation, only their own reproductive cells are applied to the spouses. It is forbidden for people who want to have children to use donors in any way, to obtain embryos using donors, to carry the embryo formed by the eggs and sperms taken from the intended parent by the surrogate mothers, and to get pregnant with the eggs or sperm taken from the donors.

Moreover, as a result of the addition made to the Law on Organ and Tissue Removal, Storage, Vaccination and Transplantation numbered 2238 with article 16 of the Law dated 05.12.2018 and numbered 7151, having a child through the reproductive cells taken from one or both spouses and the application of the embryo obtained from these cells to other people and surrogate motherhood is prohibited. As a result of this provision, surrogacy is prohibited in Turkish legal system.

Another source that can be applied for surrogacy in Turkish law is the Convention on the Protection of Human Rights and Human Dignity in terms of the Application of Biology and Medicine: Human Rights and Bio-medicine Convention, which entered into force on 01.11.2004. Surrogacy is considered to be contrary to Articles 2 and 14 of this Convention. Accordingly, it is accepted that surrogacy is contrary to the principle of human primacy contained in this Convention, that the surrogate mother cannot renounce it once she has signed this Convention, which is contrary to human rights and dignity. In Article 14, it is claimed that the sex of the baby cannot be determined with medically assisted procreation techniques, however, many surrogacy companies show this among their services. In addition, the Turkish Civil Code finds application to the extent that it is appropriate. Since surrogacy is prohibited in Turkish law, if a contract has been established in this regard, evaluations regarding the outcome of this contract are made within the framework of the Turkish Civil Code and the Turkish Code of Obligations.

Couples, surrogate mother, husband of the surrogate mother, donors or those who mediate this activity with one of the prohibited assisted reproductive methods are prosecuted for the offense of changing their lineage pursuant to Article 231 / I of the Turkish Penal Code. As a result, they can be punished with a penalty binding freedom of 1–3 years. In addition, the activities of treatment centres that use prohibited assisted reproductive techniques are also suspended and their licenses are cancelled and they are prevented from providing reproductive assistance services again. With these regulations, it is aimed to deter couples who want to have babies through surrogacy(Şensöz Malkoç, 2015; Şensöz Malkoç, 2014).

II. Research and Methods

An interdisciplinary non-systematic literature review and legal analysis of existing journal articles, books, laws, cases, regulations and policy related to surrogate motherhood in Turkey have been followed. The article is focused on papers that are related to domestic and international law, regulations, policy and governance about commercial and non-commercial surrogacy. WoS, Ulakbim, Google Scholar for Turkish and English-language articles related to surrogate motherhood are queried, resulting from the inclusion of the keywords "surrogacy" and "surrogate motherhood", in combination with "legal framework", "regulations", "court order", "public policy" and "economic analysis". In order to reveal the need for surrogacy, the most recent fertility rate statistics published by Turkish Statistical Institute (TurkStat), which is a research institution affiliated to the Ministry of Treasury and Finance of the Republic of Turkey and provides official data, are reviewed.

III. Findings and Discussion

Surrogate motherhood is a complex and global issue with many controversial aspects. In my opinion, the subject should be handled in policy, legal and economic aspects in order to come up with a useful solution on this issue.

A. Policy Aspect

Surrogacy is not only a social practice but also a public debate. It is a controversial issue shaped around the different suggestions put forward by different interest groups in the society based on their own perspectives, family structures, interpretation of fundamental rights and freedoms, their perspective on the principle of the best interests of the child, and their value judgements regarding the use of technology on the human body (Bandelli, 2021). It is possible to see the effects of these approaches in legal systems. While some systems completely reject and prohibit surrogacy, some systems try to regulate, and some systems remain completely silent. With TCC Art 282, the Turkish legal system has adopted the Roman law principle of "the woman who gives birth to a child is the mother" and banned surrogacy completely.

According to the view that the woman who gives birth should be accepted as a mother, this method is extremely pragmatic and simple, since the woman who gave birth to the child is known first, more advanced technologies such as genetic testing are not needed. Secondly, a woman establishes an intense and strong physical and psychological bond with the child by carrying a child for 9 months and giving birth to him/her. (Gruenbaum, 2012). But nowadays, with the development of technology, adopting only this approach in determining motherhood has become far from meeting the need.

According to TurkStat data, there are increasing infertility rates in Turkey. This situation is clearly seen with the fertility rates remaining below the population renewal rate. Married couples have more difficulty in having children than in the past. For this reason, couples who want to have children apply for a wide variety of infertility treatments. Couples who cannot have children with other infertility treatments apply to clinics abroad to have a child through surrogacy. While there is surrogacy technology, it is natural for couples to want to use this method.

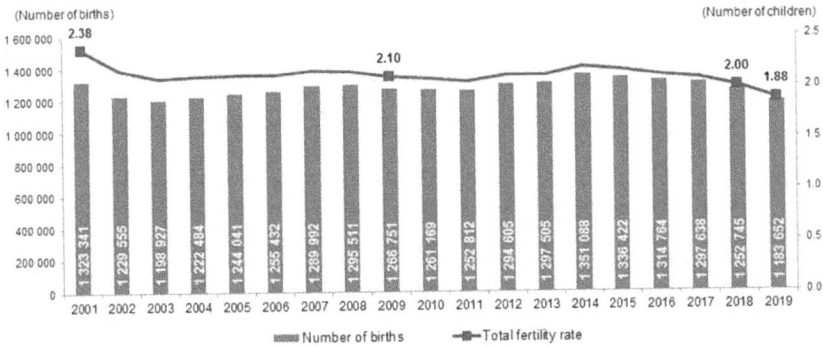

(Number of births) | (Number of children)

Number of births — Total fertility rate

Fig. 1: Number of births and total fertility rate, 2001–2019

Source: TurkStat, Birth Statistics, 2019

General Directorate of Civil Registration and Citizenship Affairs

Note: Total fertility rate is calculated as follows: TFR = Σ (Bi / Pi) (i=15,...,49)

TFR: Total fertility rate, B_i Number of births at age i, P_i Mid-year female population at age i. Those of unknown age were distributed to other ages by weighting method and age-specific fertility rates and total fertility rates were calculated over the ages with weighting.

Total fertility rate shows the average number of children a woman can give birth in the 15–49 age group, when she is fertile. The total fertility rate in Turkey fell from 2.38 children in 2001 to 1.88 children in 2019. In other words, the average number of children a woman can give birth during her fertile period remained at 1.88 in 2019. This indicates that fertility is below 2.10, which is the population's replacement level (Fig.1.).

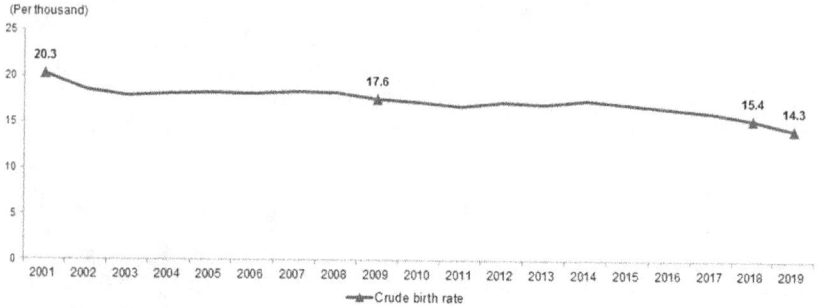

Fig. 2: Crude Birth Rate, 2001–2019
Source: TurkStat, Birth Statistics, 2019–
General Directorate of Civil Registration and Citizenship Affairs

Note: Crude birth rate is calculated as follows: CBR $= \dfrac{B}{P} \times 1000$

CBR: Crude birth rate, B: Number of births, P: Mid-year population.

Crude birth rate refers to the number of live births per thousand population. While the crude birth rate was 20.3 per thousand in 2001, it was 14.3 per thousand in 2019. In other words, while there were 20.3 births per thousand population in 2001, this rate decreased to 14.3 births in 2019 (Fig. 2).

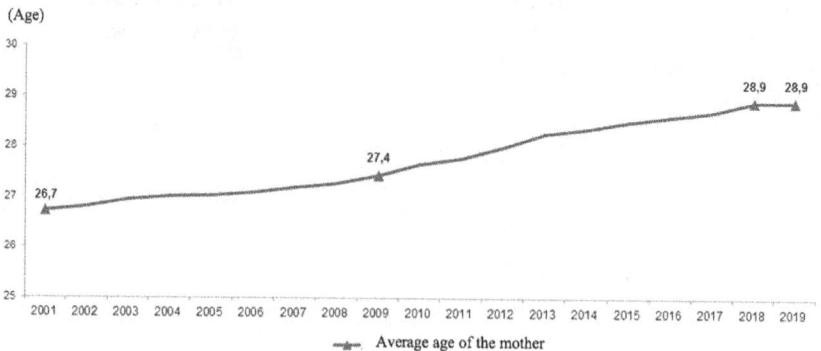

Fig. 3: Average age of the mother, 2001–2019
Source: TurkStat, Birth Statistics, 2019
General Directorate of Civil Registration and Citizenship Affairs

While the average age of mothers who gave birth in 2001 was 26.7, it increased to 28.9 in 2019. Moreover, the average age of mothers who had their first birth in 2019 was determined to be 26.4 (Fig. 3).

Tab. 1: Basic Fertility Indicators, 2001–2019

[Date as of 31/03/2020]			Total fertility rate	Adolescent	
		Crude birth rate		fertility rate	Average age
Year	Number of births	(‰)	(Number of children)	(‰)	of mother
2001	1 323 341	20,3	2,38	49	26,7
2002	1 229 555	18,6	2,17	43	26,8
2003	1 198 927	17,9	2,09	40	27,0
2004	1 222 484	18,1	2,11	40	27,0
2005	1 244 041	18,2	2,12	41	27,0
2006	1 255 432	18,1	2,12	40	27,1
2007	1 289 992	18,4	2,16	40	27,2
2008	1 295 511	18,2	2,15	39	27,3
2009	1 266 751	17,6	2,10	37	27,4
2010	1 261 169	17,2	2,08	34	27,7
2011	1 252 812	16,9	2,05	32	27,8
2012	1 294 605	17,2	2,11	31	28,0
2013	1 297 505	17,0	2,11	29	28,3
2014(r)	1 351 088	17,5	2,19	28	28,4
2015(r)	1 336 422	17,1	2,16	26	28,5
2016(r)	1 314 764	16,6	2,11	24	28,6
2017(r)	1 297 638	16,2	2,08	22	28,7
2018(r)	1 252 745	15,4	2,00	19	28,9
2019	1 183 652	14,3	1,88	17	28,9

Source: TurkStat, Birth Statistics, 2019
General Directorate of Civil Registration and Citizenship Affairs
(r) Birth data were revised with updated administrative records.

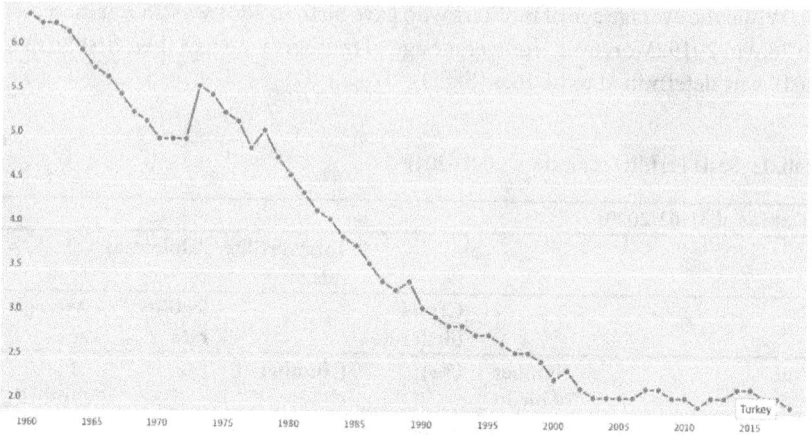

Fig. 4: Fertility rates Total, Children/woman, 1960 – 2018
Source: OECD (2021), Fertility rates (indicator). doi: 10.1787/8272fb01-en (Accessed on 05 May 2021).

As can be clearly seen from TurkStat and OECD data, the total fertility rate in Turkey is constantly falling (Fig. 4 and Tab. 1). As of 2019, this ratio was 1.88. Even though official data for 2020 have not been announced yet, the fertility rate is expected to decline further to 1.73–1.75 in 2020 (News, 2021). This is the lowest fertility level in the history of the Republic. Besides, the data show that the average age of becoming a mother for women is gradually increasing. In the light of all these data, it can be said that Turkey will have to apply more to artificial reproduction technology in the coming years. Again, in connection with this, it is not difficult to predict that Turkish citizens will increasingly resort to surrogate motherhood practices.

B. Legal Aspect

Approaches evaluating surrogacy agreement in terms of violation of personality rights (Altunkaya, 2007; Şıpka, 2007; Corradi, 2008; Kalkan Oğuztürk, 2011; Erol, 2012; Gruenbaum, 2012; Şensöz Malkoç, 2014), surrogacy is a contract against personality rights and human dignity as it commodifies the woman's body and uterus, and therefore null and void in accordance with Article 27 of the Turkish Code of Obligations (TCO). At the same time, according to TCC Art. 23, no one can give up their personal rights or restrict them unethically. Due to these approaches, the surrogate mother's obligation to deliver the child to the intended parents after birth is seen as the limitation of her personality rights unethically (Andrews, 1995; Kırkbeşoğlu, 2006; Şıpka, 2007; Kalkan Oğuztürk, 2011; Ateş, 2016; Turgut, 2016). In addition, there are criticisms that surrogacy also commodifies the female body in terms of ethics. However, against these criticisms, it has been argued that women can use their reproductive rights as they wish, and preventing this would be against the equality of women and men (Hatzis, 2009; Şensöz Malkoç, 2015; Turgut, 2016; Parlak Börü, 2019; Vertommen & Barbagallo, 2021). Surrogacy actually carries great risks in many respects. First of all, physically surrogate mothers can even face death in this process. Moreover, the surrogate mother may regret this decision after the process begins and may suffer psychologically and emotionally. It is possible to see this in the examples of surrogate mothers who avoid giving the child to intended parents. According to this approach, surrogacy should be banned because of such risks (Andrews, 1995; Armstrong, 2021).

Surrogacy is extremely attractive as it provides the opportunity to have children of their own genetically to couples who cannot have children naturally. However, the society is distant from surrogacy for reasons such as it can enable same-sex people, who are considered badly by the majority of the society, to become parents or single people to have children in this way (Parlak Börü, 2019). Surrogacy is not welcomed, worrying that this situation will harm the moral structure of the society and shake the concept of family.

According to the opinions regarding the surrogacy contract in terms of immorality, the contract between the surrogate mother and the intended parents is against general morality. Because, in accordance with the surrogacy contract, the surrogate mother is under the obligation to deliver the child to the intended parents after birth, and such a contract is immoral, even if it is demanding or not, just because it includes child transfer (Aytaç, 2002; Kırkbeşoğlu, 2006; Ateş Karaman, 2007; Kalkan Oğuztürk, 2011; Gruenbaum, 2012; Şensöz Malkoç, 2015; Turgut, 2016). Another opinion (Nomer, 2000; Kırkbeşoğlu, 2006; Şıpka, 2007; Hatzis, 2009; Erol, 2012; Şensöz Malkoç, 2015; Parlak Börü, 2019; Vertommen & Barbagallo, 2021) separates surrogacy as commercial and non-commercial and claims that only commercial surrogacy contracts should be considered as unethical. According to this approach, non-commercial surrogacy contracts are not immoral. Since non-commercial surrogacy is an assisted reproductive technique that is applied after all other alternatives are consumed and ultimately serves the public good, this procedure is not unlawful (Nomer, 2000; Şensöz Malkoç, 2015; Ateş, 2016; Yakuppur, 2019). According to Turkish law, a contract that is against personal rights and general morality is absolutely invalid and cannot be made valid later in legal life (Şensöz Malkoç, 2015; Ateş, 2016).

Another problem arising as a result of this situation is that if the surrogate mother refrains from delivering the child after birth in commercial surrogacy, whether this monetary compensation can be claimed or not. As a rule, in accordance with Article 81 of the TCO, money given for the realization of a result contrary to law or morality in Turkish law cannot be reclaimed. However, in terms of commercial surrogacy contracts, an exception should be accepted at this point and in such a case, it should be decided that the surrogate mother should return the monetary amount (Şensöz Malkoç, 2015; Ateş, 2016; Turgut, 2016; Serozan, 2017; Kırkbeşoğlu, 2006; Parlak Börü, 2019).

A different issue regarding to surrogacy arises at the point of the lineage of the child According to Turkish law, the parties cannot make changes regarding lineage based on the contract between them. Due to public order, regulations regarding lineage can only be made by law. Legal parentage can only be changed by a court decision in the event of adoption(Şensöz Malkoç, 2015; Yakuppur, 2019). The determination of lineage has consequences in many areas, from family law, marriage barriers, even determination of inheritance status.

According to TCC article 282 /I, it is the mother who gave birth to the child. It is accepted that the parentage between the mother and child will be established by birth, and there is no other regulation regarding the determination of the maternity (Ateş, 2016). The paternity between the father and the child is established by marriage with the mother of the child, recognition or court decision (Ateş, 2016; Ekşi, 2016). Although TCC was a new law adopted in 2002 at the point of determining the maternal linage with her child, it seems to ignore the implications of medical developments. If a woman other than the genetic mother is recorded as the mother in the population records, the genetic mother cannot file an action for rejection of hereditary maternity, but can only resort to correcting the population records. Whereas, TCC grants the genetic father the right to file an action for denial of lineage in such a case (Ateş, 2016; Hakeri, 2015). The gravity of this situation in terms of surrogacy is as follows: For intended parents who have no other choice but to apply to surrogacy, it is not possible to receive this treatment in Turkey. In this case, intended parents apply for surrogacy tourism, but due to many legal gaps in this regard, neither the surrogate mother, the intended parents nor the child receive the necessary and sufficient legal protection (Şensöz Malkoç, 2015; Savaş, 2019; Uyanık, 2019; Yakuppur, 2019; Ağaoğlu, 2020). This situation brings with it many legal, ethical and family problems. For example, when the surrogate mother gives birth in a hospital, a birth certificate is automatically issued by the hospital and only the name of the surrogate mother is written as the mother on this birth certificate. In this case, the genetic mother is forced to undertake a great legal struggle in order to be included in the population records as the mother of the child. Due to the legal prohibition of surrogacy, the genetic mother's hand is tied before the judiciary. At this point, if the surrogate mother is willing to give the child, the intended parents undergo the adoption procedure of their genetic child. Moreover, the procedure for the adoption of a minor in Turkish law is also a very long and difficult task (Ateş, 2016). It is the new born who is in great need of care and attention that suffers the most from this process. Adoption also causes major problems in terms of inheritance. As per TCC Art. 500, while the adopted and his descendant become inheritors to the person who adopted him / her, the adopters and their relatives cannot be inheritors to their adopted. In other words, the adoption of the child acquired through surrogacy causes new problems in Turkish law in terms of inheritance law for the intended parents. Intended parents, although they may also be the parents of the child genetically and therefore should be the heirs of the child, if they adopt the child, they cannot be the inheritor of the child and the child's inheritance is inherited by the surrogate mother. Another side of the problem shows itself as follows. What should happen if the surrogate mother refuses to deliver the child after birth? According to Turkish law, since the person who is accepted as a mother is a surrogate mother, it becomes almost impossible for the genetic family to take the child from her. At this point, the intended parents must prove that the surrogate mother mistreated the child. Even in the presence of such a situation, the child is not directly delivered to the genetic family, is placed under State protection and the intended parents are still unable to reach their child. With the progress of this process, the child gradually grows and is subjected to emotional and psychological violence with the stress of not knowing who his real family is, he is almost pulled from one place to another between the intended parents and the surrogate mother.

C. Economic Aspect

Surrogate motherhood also has an economic dimension. Due to the increased ease of mobility and the prohibition of surrogacy in some countries, the citizens of these countries have led to the formation of a new sector called "surrogacy tourism". This situation carries surrogacy to an international dimension that transcends borders (Parlak Börü, 2019; Uyanık, 2019; Armstrong, 2021). Since the early 2000s, surrogacy, which was previously small scale and extremely intimate, helping someone else to have children without any financial interest, has rapidly evolved into an extremely popular and profitable frontier industry. The market has reached the level of $ 20 Mn by 2019 and it is projected to reach $ 41 Mn by 2026 (Data Bridge Market Research, 2019). This baby business is a big branch of activity that includes surrogacy companies, fertility clinics, genetic consultants, law firms specializing in family and immigration law, shipping and logistics companies, hospitality services (hotel, restaurant, tourist attractions), egg-sperm-embryo donors and surrogate mothers, nurses, nannies, drivers etc. As a result of the fact that surrogacy is not regulated properly or banned in legal systems, this line of business paves the way for women in poor countries to become surrogate mothers at low wages and commodifies the body of women every day (Armstrong, 2021; Vertommen & Barbagallo, 2021). Studies show that there is an obvious social inequality and power imbalance among the actors of surrogacy. Wealthy couples' resort to surrogacy as intended parents, while low-educated poor women, even from vulnerable communities such as immigrant or indigenous groups, are employed as surrogate mothers (Bandelli, 2021). This situation reveals more clearly why surrogacy should be legally regulated without ignoring it, because every actor of surrogacy needs protection in their own way and this issue is too important to be left to the mercy of private companies.

Conclusion

Infertility is gradually increasing in Turkey. As a result of this, the demand for advanced reproductive technology is also increasing. Having a child through a surrogate mother is considered illegal in Turkish Law. However, this situation cannot prevent couples from using surrogate motherhood. Since there is surrogacy method that couples can apply to acquire the child, who they long for, it is very natural that they resort to this technology. The prohibition of this method only deprives the actors of this procedure of the legal protection they need.

Legal systems often lag behind technology. But TCC is a relatively new law, since it was adopted in 2002. It was not difficult to predict these artificial reproduction technology developments in the years when the Turkish Civil Code was passed, but the lawmaker ignored these technological developments and found it appropriate to accept an almost archaic rule. This provision, which defines lineage only in terms of men and cannot adapt to technological developments, should be changed. Because there is surrogacy as a result of technological developments, and although it is illegal, people who do not have the opportunity to have biological children other than surrogacy apply to this medical technique. This paves the way for filling this gap, which is not regulated by the law, by circling the law.

The current legislation is insufficient to solve the problems caused by surrogacy, and may even lead to more unfair results. At this point, first of all, the legal regulation that prohibits the surrogacy should be abolished. With the abolition of this regulation, the criticism that the contract between the surrogate mother and intended parents is impossible due to the ban or that it is against the law or morality will be removed and the necessary legal protection will be provided in case of violation of this contract. For example, if the surrogate mother has received some money and refrained from giving the child, both the delivery of the child to the intended parents and the refund of the money should be provided. It is currently not possible. Through these regulations, a tight inspection opportunity would be obtained as well. For example, in the legal system, surrogacy can be arranged as a reproductive technique to be used as a last resort in cases where all other reproductive techniques are used and a solution cannot be reached. In this way, surrogacy can be used as an auxiliary reproductive technique instead of being seen as a commercial activity. So only altruistic or gestational surrogacy might be adopted. When this issue is arranged in detail, the contract between the surrogate mother and the intended parents can be established under the supervision of the relevant governmental institutions in a way that both the interests of the surrogate mother, the intended parents and the best interests of the child are taken into account, and immediately after the birth of the child, it can be transferred to the personal records of the intended parents. This solution also removes concerns about public policy (Gamble & Ghevaert, 2009; Şensöz Malkoç, 2014; Ateş, 2016; Parlak Börü, 2019; Yakuppur, 2019). Even more ideal at this point would be to establish an order in which national laws and international regulations are compatible with each other, due to the transnational character of surrogacy practices. The solutions provided by national laws to the problems related to transnational surrogacy are different from each other. In addition, there are differences between court decisions regarding surrogacy. A legal relationship valid in one country may be invalid in the other country. This creates limping legal relationships. The legal regulation and policy harmonisation of surrogacy, designed to align with public health and human rights principles, can ensure that the fertility agencies and clinics that mediate these procedures are brought under control and inspection, which requires cooperation in the international arena. This cooperation will only be effective if it has a broad participation. The Hague International Private Law Conference has prepared a preliminary report and project on this issue (Gruenbaum, 2012; The Permanent Bureau t. C., 2012; The Permanent Bureau H. C., 2015; Ekşi, 2016).

Secondly the current regulations related to lineage in TCC shall be amended and more gender equal provisions should be adopted. Archaic assumptions that only accept the woman who give birth as a mother and remain behind medical technology can thus be left behind. A child born through a surrogate mother must be tied to the intended mother in terms of lineage. This can be done by court order. At this point, if the rule "the woman who gives birth is the mother" is not abandoned, the surrogate mother should be given the opportunity to reject the lineage of the child and the intended mother to recognize the child. (Oktay Özdemir & Tek, 2013; Hakeri, 2015; Parlak Börü, 2019; Savaş, 2019). With the adoption of a detailed law regulating surrogacy, all three pillars of this legal relationship - surrogate mother, intended parents, child - can be protected as it should be, and the child can develop in a peaceful environment as it should be.

It is observed that the legal perspective regarding surrogacy in European law has changed and became more moderate after ECHR's Mennesson v. France and Labassee v. France cases. In these cases, the attachment of children born via surrogacy in the US to the intended parents in France was denied due to French law. The common feature of both cases is that the parent-child relationship, which is recognized abroad, is not recognized in France, against the best interests of the child. The ECHR found that, in fact, the purpose of the French authorities in doing this was to prevent French citizens from having children by resorting to a method of reproduction prohibited within France. After the decisions of ECHR in these cases, even in European countries that ban the surrogacy method, the establishment of a legal relationship between the child and the intended parents has begun to be facilitated, taking into account the principle of the best interests of the child (The Permanent Bureau, 2015; Ekşi, 2016; Basın Birimi, 2017). In my opinion, a similar attitude should be adopted by Turkish law.

All kinds of legal and policy harmonization in the field of surrogacy can also provide the supervision and control of commercial surrogacy and surrogacy tourism, which has turned into a highly exploited industry. Because despite the existence of a growing transnational market for commercial surrogacy, lawmakers turn their backs on this technology and ignore it as if it were not there or prefer to ban it. It should not be overlooked that this sector has an economic as well as a legal aspect. The baby industry is in a state of oppressing and exploiting surrogacy mothers who have low income and have no income source other than surrogacy. The uncertainties in this area mostly harm the actors of the surrogacy procedure who are in need of protection and benefit commercial companies.

References

Ağaoğlu, C. (2020). Cross-Border Surrogacy Motherhood in Comparative Law and the Problem of Legal Parenthood. *Public and Private International Law Bulletin*, 437–480.

Altunkaya, M. (2007). Tabii Olmayan Yollarla Çocuk Sahibi Olmanın Soybağına Etkisi, Organ ve Doku Naklinde Tıp Etiği ve Tıp Hukuku Sorunları. *I. Uluslararası Tıp Etiği ve Tıp Hukuku Kongresi Bildiri Kitabı* (pp. 99–118). İstanbul.

Andrews, L. B. (1995). Beyond Doctrinal Boundaries: A Legal Framework for Surrogate Motherhood. *Virginia Law Review*, 2343–2375.

Armstrong, S. (2021). Surrogacy: Time we Recognized it as a job? *Journal Of Gender Studies*, 1–5.

Ateş, B. (2016). *Soybağı ve Soybağı Alanında Oluşabilecek Hukuksal Problemler*. İstanbul, Turkey.

Ateş Karaman, D. (2007). *Borçlar Hukuku Sözleşmelerinde Genel Ahlaka Aykırılık*. Ankara: Turhan Yayınevi.

Aytaç, İ. (2002). Yardımcı Üreme Tekniklerinin Nesep Hukuku Açısından İncelenmesi. *Adalet Bakanlığı Dergisi*, 183– 199.

Bandelli, D. (2021). Gestational Surrogacy: Transnational Procreative Practice and Work for Women in Contemporary Society. *Current Sociology*, 146–157.

Basın Birimi, A. İ. (2017). *Tematik Bilgi Notu – Taşıyıcı Annelik*. Retrieved from European Court of Human Rights: https://www.echr.coe.int/Documents/FS_Surrogacy_TUR.pdf, Access date 19.10.2021

Brunet, L., King, D., Carruthers, J., Marzo, C., Davaki, K., & McCandless, J. (2013). *A Comparative Study on the Regime of Surrogacy in EU Member States*. European Parliament Directorate General For Internal Policies Policy Department C: Citizens' Rights And Constitutional Affairs.

Clissmann, I., & Hutchinson, P. (2005). The Hague Convention and the habitual residence of newborn infants. *The Bar Review*, 75–79.

Cohen, I. G. (2014). *In re Marriage of Buzzanca*. Retrieved from H2O: https://h2o.law.harvard.edu/collages/8862

Corradi, L. (2008). Redefining "Reproductive Rights": An Ecofeminist Perspective on In Vitro Fertilization, Egg Markets and Surrogate Motherhood. In M. Texler Segal, & V. Demos, *Advancing Gender Research from the Nineteenth to the Twenty-First Centuries (Advances in Gender Research, Vol. 12)* (pp. 245–273). Bingley: Emerald Group Publishing Limited.

Darnovsky, M. (2009). *Complications of Surrogacy: The Case of Baby Manji*. Retrieved from Center For Genetics and Society: https://www.geneticsandsociety.org/biopolitical-times/complications-surrogacy-case-baby-manji, Access date 01.08.2021

Data Bridge Market Research. (2019). Retrieved from Fertility Services Market crosses USD 20 Mn with growing CAGR of 9% and expected to reach USD 41 Mn by 2026: https://www.globenewswire.com/news-release/2019/11/22/1951516/0/en/Fertility-Services-Market-crosses-USD-20-Mn-with-growing-CAGR-of-9-and-expected-to-reach-USD-41-Mn-by-2026.html, Access date 10.08.2021

Ekşi, N. (2016). Legal Problems Arising from International Surrogacy in the Court Decisions. *Public and Private International Law Bulletin*, 1–51.

Erol, Y. (2012). *Yapay Döllenme Yöntemleri ve Taşıyıcı Annelik*. Ankara: Yetkin Yayınları.

Fiorini, A. (2012). Habitual Residence And The Newborn – A French Perspective. *International and Comparative Law Quarterly*, 530–540.

Gamble, N., & Ghevaert, L. (2009). *The Chosen Middle Ground: England, Surrogacy Law and the International Arena*. Retrieved from https://www.ngalaw.co.uk/: https://www.ngalaw.co.uk/uploads/docs/535faf6133845.pdf

Gruenbaum, D. (2012). Foreig n Surrogat e Motherhood: Mater semper certa erat. *The American Journal Of Comparative Law*, 475–505.

Grusic, U. (2015). The Difficulty of Enforcing Surrogacy Regulations. *The Cambridge Law Journal*, 34–37.

Hakeri, H. (2015). Taşıyıcı Annelik. In H. Hakeri & C. Doğan, *Uluslararası Sağlık Hukuku Sempozyumu* (pp. 83–93). Ankara: Türkiye Barolar Birliği Yayınları.

Hatzis, A. N. (2009). From Soft to Hard Paternalism and Back: The Regulation of Surrogate Motherhood in Greece. *Portuguese Economic Journal*, 205–220.

In re Baby M – 109 N.J. 396, 537 A.2d 1227 (1988), 109 N.J. 396, 537 A.2d 1227 (1988) (1988).

In re Marriage of Buzzanca, 61 Cal. App. 4th 1410, 72 Cal. Rptr. 2d 280 (1998) (1998).

Kalkan Oğuztürk, B. (2011). *Türk Medeni Hukuku'nda Biyoetik Sorunlar*. İstanbul: Vedat Kitapçılık.

Kırkbeşoğlu, N. (2006). *Soybağı Alanında Biyoetik ve Hukuk Sorunları*. İstanbul: Vedat Kitapçılık.

Latey, J. (1985). *RE C (A MINOR) (Wardship: Surrogacy) – [1985] FLR 846*. Retrieved from Family Law Reports: https://www.lexiswebinars.co.uk/legal/family-law/update-on-surrogacy-2020/supporting-materials/Re-C-A-Minor-Surrogacy-Wardship-1985.PDF, Access date 01.07.2021

Laurie, G. T., Harmon, S., & Porter, G. (2016). *Mason and McCall Smith's Law and Medical Ethics*. Oxford: Oxford University Press.

News, M. (2021). 2020'de Türkiye'de doğum oranları sert bir şekilde düştü. Mepa

Nomer, H. N. (2000). Suni Döllenme Dolayısıyla Ortaya Çıkabilecek Nesep Problemleri. In N. Barlas, A. Kendigelen, & S. Sarı, *Prof. Dr. M. Kemal Oğuzman'ın Anısına Armağan* (pp. 545– 594). İstanbul: Beta Basım Yayın.

Oktay Özdemir, S., & Tek, G. S. (2013). Türk Hukukunda Tıp Bilimindeki Gelişmelerin Soybağına Etkileri. In P. D. Öğüz, *Prof. Dr. Mustafa Dural'a Armağan* (pp. 909–931). İstanbul: Filiz Kitabevi.

Parlak Börü, Ş. (2019). A Difficult Turning Point in Family Law: The Current Developments on Surrogate Motherhood with a Comparative Law Perspective. *Public and Private International Law Bulletin*, 63–110.

Pasayat, A. (2008). *Baby Manji Yamada vs Union Of India & Anr on 29 September, 2008 in the Supreme Court of India Civil Original Jurisdiction Writ Petition (C) NO. 369 OF 2008*. Retrieved from Supreme Court of India: https://indiankanoon.org/doc/854968/?__cf_chl_jschl_tk__=77489dbdf3fdf887c52e47cc66c02f3aa9c78ff6-1619374152-0-AX9q8NwutfJcfGr4WFsTwB0KDlnIMa-cJjd0XKQrs4_7PM4r1YYR_9xbf1Y8hyD_MxVVVqB0_Ld-h0SYT5ac7DF0TSUggYayCgrkVRDpbtQo61A7Q-hZI7Y-Qv8adIXr8bRe NKIk58aMULan, Access date 17.08.2021

Points, K. (2011). *Commercial Surrogacy and Fertility Tourism in India – The Case of Baby Manji*. Retrieved from The Kenan Institute For Ethics at Duke University – Case Studies in Ethics: https://kenan.ethics.duke.edu/wp-content/uploads/2018/01/BabyManji_Case2015.pdf, Access date 10.07.2021

Prinz, D. (2015). *In the Matter of Baby M*. Retrieved from https://scholar.harvard.edu/: https://scholar.harvard.edu/files/dprinz/files/in_the_matter_of_baby_m.pdf, Access date 09.06.2021

Sanger, C. (2007). Developing Markets in Baby-Making: In the Matter of Baby M. *Harvard Journal of Law and* Gender, *67*, 67–97.

Savaş, E. (2019). *Tıp Hukukunda Taşıyıcı Annelik*. Retrieved from http://earsiv.medeniyet.edu.tr, Access date 13.07.2021

Şensöz Malkoç, E. (2014). *Sağlık Düşüncesi ve Tıp Kültürü Platformu, Milletlerarası özel hukukta boşluk: Taşıyıcı annelik*. Retrieved from sdplatform.com: http://www.sdplatform.com/Dergi/676/Milletlerarasi-ozel-hukukta-bosluk-Tasiyici-annelik.aspx, Access date 01.08.2021

Şensöz Malkoç, E. (2015). Applicable Law to the Disputes Arising from International Surrogacy Agreements. *Public and Private International Law Bulletin*, 13–49.

Serozan, R. (2017). *Çocuk Hukuku*. İstanbul: Vedat Kitapçılık.

Setright, H. (2002). *W and B v H (2002)*. Retrieved from 4pb for Family: https://www.4pb.com/case-detail/w-and-b-v-h-2002/, Access date 13.04.2021

Şıpka, Ş. (2007). *Taşıyıcı Annelik Ve Getirdiği Hukuki Sorunlar*. Retrieved from turkhukuksitesi.com: https://www.turkhukuksitesi.com/makale_537.htm, Access date 05.06.2021

Thapa, J. D. (2019). The 'Babies M': The Relevance of Baby Manji Yamada V. Union of India (Uoi) and in the Matter of Baby "M". *Journal of Indian Law And Society*, 83–112.

The Permanent Bureau, H. C. (2015). *Preliminary Document No 3A of February 2015 for the attention of the Council of March 2015 on General Affairs and Policy of the Conference, The Parentage / Surrogacy Project: An Updating Note*. Retrieved from Hague Conference on Private International Law General Affairs and Policy: https://assets.hcch.net/docs/82d31f31-294f-47fe-9166-4d9315031737.pdf, Access date 04.04.2021

The Permanent Bureau, t. C. (2012). *A Preliminary Report On The Issues Arising From International Surrogacy Arrangements*. Retrieved from Preliminary Document No. 10 of March 2012 for the attention of the Council of April 2012 on General Affairs and Policy of the Conference: https://assets.hcch.net/docs/d4ff8ecd-f747-46da-86c3-61074e9b17fe.pdf, Access date 06.04.2021

Turgut, C. (2016). *Yapay Döllenme Taşıyıcı Annelik ve Soybağına İlişkin Hukuki Sorunlar*. İstanbul: On İki Levha Yayıncılık.

Ungan Çalışkan, H. (2016). Bırakınız Taşısınlar: Taşıyıcı Anneliğe Güncel Bakış. *Marmara Üniversitesi Hukuk Fakültesi Hukuk Araştırmaları Dergisi*, 489–510.

Uyanık, A. (2019). Fertilite Turizminin Hukuki Arka Planı. In Z. Ö. Üskül Engin, *Toplumsal Cinsiyet ve Hukuk* (pp. 1–22). İstanbul: On İki Levha Yayıncılık.

Vertommen, S., & Barbagallo, C. (2021). The In/Visible Wombs of the Market: The Dialectics of Waged and Unwaged Reproductive Labour in the Global Surrogacy Industry. *Review of International Political Economy*, 1–23.

Vonk, M. (2010). Maternity for Another: A Double Dutch Approach. *Electronic Journal of Comparative Law*, 1–12. Retrieved from Netherlands Comparative Law Association: https://www.ejcl.org/143/art143-22.pdf, Access date 03.05.2021

Voskoboynik, K. (2016). Clipping The Stork's Wings: Commercial Surrogacy Regulation and its Impact on Fertility Tourism. *Indiana International & Comparative Law Review*, 336–382.

Wade, K. (2017). The Regulation of Surrogacy: A Children's Rights Perspective. *Child and Family Law Quarterly*, 113–131.

X & Y (Foreign Surrogacy). (2008). [2008] EWHC 3030 (Fam), FD08P01466 (in the High Court of Justice Family Division 12 09, 2008).

Yakuppur, S. (2019). VI. Türk Hukuku Açısından Taşıyıcı Annenin Doğurduğu Çocuğun Soybağının Kim İle Kurulacaği Sorunu. In Z. Ö. Üskül Engin, *Toplumsal Cinsiyet ve Hukuk Cilt I* (pp. 273– 299). İstanbul: On İki Levha Yayıncılık.

Younger, J. T. (1988). What the Baby M Case Is Really All About. *Minnesota Journal of Law & Inequality*, 75–82.

Part IV Legal and Public Policy Perspective to Vaccination Application

Nazmiye Tekdemir

Pelin Varol İyidoğan

To Be Vaccinated or Not? An Assessment on the Vaccination Attitude Profile in Turkey

Introduction

In Turkey, the first official case of Covid-19 appeared on March 11, 2020. After this, Turkey, like all the other countries in the world, has taken serious measures that may disrupt in economic and social life. Examples included various restrictive measures such as social distancing measures, curfews, travel bans, quarantines for citizens returning from abroad, and closing schools/universities, shops, and entertainment venues. However, despite all these measures, it is a known fact that the pandemic will only come to an end when a large part of the world population becomes immune to the virus. It is widely accepted that the safest way to achieve this is by vaccination.

Vaccines have been used as effective tools to end many diseases throughout history. In this context, the failure to find an effective treatment method for Covid-19 suggests that vaccination is the most effective solution and inevitable. As studies show that people perceive Covid-19 as a threatening disease, demand for vaccines against the disease is expected to be high. However, in some cases, concerns about vaccination may become riskier than the disease itself. As in many examples throughout history, there are anti-vaccine discourses as well as those that embrace vaccines. It is very important to understand the causes of people's hesitancy regarding the Covid-19 vaccine as it can help increase vaccine acceptance because increasing vaccine acceptance seems to be the most effective way to control the spread of the disease for now. Research indicate that vaccine acceptance is a complex decision-making process influenced by a wide range of factors (Karlsson, et al., 2021). However, generally it is possible to say that risk perceptions and demographic characteristics of people and societies are the most prominent factors that influence attitude to vaccination (Fridman, Gershon, & Gneezy, 2020).

In this framework, our study aimed to explain the factors affecting the attitudes to the Covid-19 vaccine in Turkey. Thus, we planned to present an impression of the public policies to be followed by the government, which constitutes the supply-side of vaccination policies due to being a merit good. Based on this motive, our study consisted of four parts. First, there is a comprehensive discussion on attitude to vaccination in the context of supply and demand side approaches. The second part presents the literature aiming to measure the attitude to the Covid-19 vaccine in a summary table. The third part analyses the data obtained in the survey conducted with a study group of 838 people with various statistical tests. Finally, there are various policy recommendations to increase efficiency based on the findings on attitude to vaccination.

I. Addressing Attitude to Vaccination from the Supply and Demand Perspective

The goods produced for effectiveness are also expected to be the demanded goods both in the market economy and public economy. In other words, reaching an optimum result is linked to the balance between supply and demand. In this context, the effectiveness of vaccination, which is considered a merit good and supplied by the government, is also linked to how much it is demanded by the public.

The concept of merit good was first introduced into public finance literature in 1959 by Richard Musgrave. According to this, merit goods, like some private goods, have positive externalities on other people and society as a whole. Musgrave essentially claimed that the goods in this category tend to be less consumed and therefore cannot be left to the free market economy as the value given to this good by each consumer is different. For this reason, the government should encourage the consumption of these goods by pursuing people's interests more than people (Brennan & Lomasky, 1983; Mendoza, 2011). So, the government acts with a paternalistic motive in such situations where consumer sovereignty is left aside (Basu, 1976; Desmarais-Tremblay, 2016). As mentioned before, one of the most important examples of these goods with positive externality and high social benefits is the vaccination service.

However, providing a vaccine does not imply that the problem has been solved. The government also has the responsibility to inform the public about vaccines and persuade them to be vaccinated. Ideally, vaccinating a sufficiently large part of the population will protect the unvaccinated population by providing herd immunity. For Covid-19, vaccine uptake would need to be between approximately 67 % and 80 % to reduce its spread, i.e. to make the vaccination policy successful (Graffigna et al., 2020; Robertson et al., 2021). However, vaccine hesitancy among the public is one of the biggest obstacles to efforts to control Covid-19. Therefore, the government should try to minimize vaccine hesitancy and increase the demand for vaccines with various policies.

According to WHO (2021), vaccine hesitancy arises in two ways. These are reluctance to be vaccinated and strict refusal of vaccination. *Vaccine Hesitancy* is a situation that varies according to the content, time, and place of vaccines. In this context, people accept some vaccines, refuse some vaccines or accept them with delay. *Vaccine Refusal* is the most advanced level of vaccine hesitancy. These people are extremely against vaccination. They do not accept any vaccine administration. Even if scientific evidence is presented, their opinions on this subject do not change (Özen, 2020). In short, vaccine hesitancy reflects concerns about the decision to vaccinate oneself or one's children (Salmon, Dudley, Glanz, & Omer, 2015).

Opposing and hesitant attitudes to vaccination are as old as the history of vaccines. After Edward Jenner introduced the concept of vaccine to the medical community, widespread vaccination started in the early 1800s, and vaccination became mandatory in England as a result of vaccination movements between 1840 and 1853. E. Massey, a religious scholar at the time, claimed that diseases were inflicted on people by God as a punishment and that trying to prevent them was synonymous with opposing God, and described vaccination attempts as following devil (Alben, 2019, p. 43). Anti-Vaccination League, established in London in the same years, formed a core structure for vaccine opponents. Through organizations, books, leaflets, and magazines, anti-vaccination activists disseminated their anti-vaccine arguments. In times and geographies where they were successful, people suffered from serious epidemics (Kutlu & Altındiş, 2018).

While vaccine hesitancy, which often does not have a scientific basis, has existed in every period of history, it has become more widespread today with the effect of increasing communication networks. Therefore, it is possible to say that vaccine hesitancy mostly emerges in developed countries today. The most important cause of vaccine hesitancy in these countries is the concerns about the content and reliability of vaccines. However, this does not mean that vaccine hesitancy is not a problem in low- and middle-income countries. For example, boycotts were made against vaccination because people thought that the polio vaccine sterilized Muslim children in 2003–2004 in Nigeria (Kennedy, 2020). In 2019, the 13th General Program of Work (2019–2023) of the WHO explained 10 threats to global health as follows: air pollution and climate change, non-communicable diseases, global influenza pandemic, fragile and vulnerable settings, antimicrobial resistance, Ebola, and other high-threat pathogens, weak primary health care, Dengue, HIV and vaccine hesitancy (https://www.who.int/news-room/spotlight/ten-threats-to-global-health-in-2019, 2021). In other words, vaccine hesitancy is considered an important agenda item. It is viewed as a threat because it may threaten to reverse the progress made in the fight against vaccine-preventable diseases.

Table 1 presents some possible reasons for vaccine hesitancy.

Tab. 1: Possible Reasons for Vaccine Hesitancy

Vaccines contain mercury, aluminium, ether, antibiotics, and many chemicals and these cause autism and similar diseases.

Vaccine-producing companies can be a malicious "Market" because they make a lot of money.

Better immunity is gained by undergoing a disease instead of vaccination.

Complementary and alternative medicine is more effective and has fewer side effects.

Children's immune systems are not yet fully developed, and vaccinations damage the immune system.

There are no studies proving the efficacy and safety of vaccines.

There are studies reporting the side effects of vaccines.

Some "people with religious and philosophical influence" and some "doctors" say that vaccines are harmful and do not have their children vaccinated.

Source: (Bozkurt, 2018)

The table shows that there can be many reasons for vaccine hesitancy. It is possible to group them into three overall groups. The first is those who do not find the benefit/damage relationship sufficient. The main objections of this group are the side effects of vaccines and the long-term damage of the ingredients of the vaccine. Therefore, the reactions of this group are mostly directed towards the ingredients. The other two groups are those who do not feel it is necessary because they think they are not at risk and those who object on religious, philosophical, or conspiracy grounds (Ataç & Aker, 2014). Regardless of the reason, vaccine hesitancy is one of the major barriers to immunization programs and goals (Sonawane, Troisi, & Deshmukh, 2021).

II. Literature on Attitudes to Covid-19 Vaccine

Since the initiation of efforts to develop the Covid-19 vaccine, various surveys have tried to evaluate the public's perception and acceptance of the vaccine because vaccination is considered one of the most effective methods to end the pandemic. Therefore, analysing the factors that affect the attitude of the public to vaccination and determining the reasons behind it will increase the effectiveness of turning public policies into action. Table 2 indicates the various studies conducted for this along with their main findings.

Tab. 2: Review of Literature on Measuring the Attitude to Covid-19 Vaccine

Study	Sample and Method	Findings
Sherman et al., 2020	A survey was made with 1500 adults in the UK.	64 % of participants reported being very likely to be vaccinated against Covid-19, 27 % were unsure, and 9 % reported being very unlikely to be vaccinated. The effect of sociodemographic factors stands out in attitudes to vaccination.
Pogue et al., 2020	A survey was administered to 316 respondents across the United States. Structural equation modelling was used to analyse the relationships of several factors with attitudes to vaccination.	Approximately 68 % of all respondents were supportive of being vaccinated. However, there were serious concerns about the side effects and efficacy of the vaccine.
Dror et al., 2020	A survey was made with 1941 people including 828 healthcare staff and 1112 members of the general population in Israel.	Healthcare staff involved in the care of Covid-19 positive patients, and individuals considering themselves at risk of disease, had positive attitudes to vaccination. However, healthcare staff not caring for positive patients and other people expressed higher levels of vaccine hesitancy.
Wang et al., 2020	A cross-sectional survey was made with 2058 participants aged 18 and above in China in 2020.	Study results showed that 91.3 % of participants would accept the Covid-19 vaccine in China. Among them, 52.2 % wanted to get vaccinated as soon as possible, while the remaining 47.8 % would delay the vaccination until the vaccine's safety was confirmed.
Akarsu et al., 2020	A survey was conducted with 749 participants aged 18 and above in Turkey. Data were analysed by various statistical methods.	8.6 % of participants stated that they did not want to get Covid-19 vaccine while 35.9 % were indecisive. 14.8 % stated that they would not get their children vaccinated for the Covid-19 while 43.2 % were indecisive. Participants had more vaccine hesitancy for their children compared to themselves.
Graffigna et al., 2020	A survey was made with 1004 people in Italy. Data were analysed by various statistical methods.	Approximately 15 % of participants stated that they would refuse the vaccine, while 26 % stated that they were hesitant. The majority of the hesitant group was composed of young people. Furthermore, the study revealed psychological factors that affected Covid-19 vaccine hesitancy.

(continued on next page)

Tab. 2: Continued

Study	Sample and Method	Findings
Ward et al., 2020	Four online surveys were made with 5018 participants aged 18 and above in France.	The study found that almost a quarter of respondents would not get vaccinated. The main reason for this reticence was the idea that this vaccine would not be safe. Moreover, the political structure in the country was an effective factor.
Edwards et al., 2021	A survey was made with 3061 adults to examine the attitude to Covid-19 vaccine in Australia.	59 % of participants would get the vaccine, 29 % had low levels of hesitancy, 7 % had high levels of hesitancy and 6 % were resistant. In addition, females, those who had lower levels of household income and those living in disadvantaged areas, were more likely to be hesitant or resistant.
Robertson et al., 2021	A survey was made with 12,035 participants in the UK.	82 % of participants were willing to take up a Covid-19 vaccine while 18 % were hesitant. Marked differences existed across population subgroups. In particular, as older age and being male were the strongest drivers of risk of Covid-19 death, their vaccine hesitancy was very low. The main reasons for vaccine hesitancy were concerns over the unknown future effects of a vaccine (42.7 %). The main reasons for being willing to take up a vaccine were to avoid catching Covid-19 or becoming ill from the disease (54.6 %) and to allow social and family life to get back to normal (12.5 %).
Karlsson et al., 2021	Surveys were made with three sample groups in Finland. The first group had the parents of small children (825), the second one had the individuals living in an area with suboptimal vaccination coverage (205), and the third one had Facebook users (1325).	The study explored the role of two of the key factors affecting the Covid-19 vaccine acceptance (perceived risk of disease and perceived vaccine safety). All three groups perceived Covid-19 as a severe disease and worried about transmitting it to others. ¾ of respondents reported that they trusted a vaccine recommended by authorities to be safe.
Murphy et al., 2021	A survey was made with the participants from Ireland (1041) and the UK (2025) to understand Covid-19 vaccine hesitancy.	Vaccine hesitancy was 35 % (vaccine hesitancy: 26 % + resistance: 9 %) in Ireland and 31 % (vaccine hesitancy: 25 % + resistance: 6 %) in the UK. Three demographic factors were significantly associated with vaccine hesitance or resistance in both countries: sex, age, and income level.

Tab. 2: Continued

Study	Sample and Method	Findings
Shekhar et al., 2021	A survey was made with 3479 respondents in the United States to assess healthcare workers' attitude to Covid-19 vaccination.	8 % of respondents did not plan to get vaccinated. 36 % were willing to take up the vaccine while 56 % were not sure or would wait to review more data. Vaccine acceptance increased with increasing age, education, and income level. Furthermore, safety (69 %), effectiveness (69 %), and speed of development/approval (74 %) were noted as the most common concerns regarding Covid-19 vaccination.
Sallam et al., 2021	A survey was made with a total of 3414 respondents from Jordan (2173), Kuwait (771), and Saudi Arabia (154) to assess their attitudes to Covid-19 vaccines using the Vaccine Conspiracy Belief Scale (VCBS).	Jordan and Kuwait had high rates of vaccine hesitancy compared to other Arab countries. The main reasons for vaccine hesitancy were Covid-19 misinformation and conspiracy beliefs. Social media was the main source of spreading those beliefs. Moreover, 59.5 % of participants thought that Covid-19 was man-made.
Sonawane et al., 2021	This theory-based study cited the results of a study by Paul et al. in The Lancet Regional Health-Europe.	An online survey was made with 32.361 adult participants in the UK to examine the negative attitude to Covid-19 vaccine. About 16 % of the participants expressed a high level of mistrust of vaccines. More than one-third of the participants reported unwillingness or uncertainty. However, in general, a large majority of the population has a favourable perception regarding vaccines. In addition, building vaccine trust among undecided individuals was possible through effective communication strategies.

Source: Compiled by the authors.

III. Analysis: Attitude to Covid-19 Vaccine in Turkey

A. Data and Methods

In our cross-sectional-descriptive study,[1] we reached the target audience and data using the maximum diversity sampling method. The maximum diversity method aims to discover and define the main themes covering many differences related to the event or phenomenon studied (Baltacı, 2018). In this respect, we planned to reach different stakeholders in the 12-NUTS region, which reflected different characteristics and dynamics. Our study group consisted of 838 people. The distribution of the participants according to regions was as follows: Istanbul Region-TR1 (27– 3.2 %), Western Marmara Region-TR2 (15– 1.8 %), Aegean Region-TR3 (33– 3.9 %), Eastern Marmara Region-TR4 (47–5.6 %), Western Anatolia Region-TR5 (374–44.6 %), Mediterranean Region-TR6 (88–10.5 %), Central Anatolia Region-TR7 (80–9.5 %), Western Black Sea Region-TR8 (39–4.7 %), Eastern Black Sea Region-TR9 (94–11.2 %), North-eastern Anatolia Region-TRA (10–1.2 %), Middle Eastern Anatolia Region-TRB (912–1.4 %), and South-eastern Anatolia Region-TRC (19–2.3 %). The survey consisted of three parts. The first part was for approving voluntary participation in the survey. The second part focused on the socio-demographic characteristics of the participants. The third part questioned their knowledge about health and vaccination about the pandemic.

Statistical Package for Social Sciences (IBM SPSS v22.0) package software was used to evaluate the data obtained in the study. Survey data were shown in charts with numbers and percentages for survey responses. Independent Groups T-test and one-way analysis of variance (ANOVA) test were used to analyse the data. In addition, the confidence interval for all data was 95 %. The statistical significance level was $p < 0.05$.

We asked the participants[2] "*Would you consider being vaccinated for Covid-19 if you have not been vaccinated yet?*" to determine attitude to vaccination. Based on this, we statistically analysed whether attitude to vaccination differed significantly according to age, gender, and education level, which are the main socio-demographic characteristics.

---

1 Ethical approval of the study was taken from the Ethics Committee of Hacettepe University on 25 May 2021 with the document number 1572418.

2 At the time when we applied the survey on Covid-19 vaccine opinions, the vaccination of the group aged 75 years was ongoing. In this framework, those who were vaccinated received 1 point. Those considering vaccination positively (whose answer is "yes") received 2 points; those who either hesitate or refuse to be vaccinated (whose answer is "indecisive" or "no") received 3 and 4 points, respectively.

1. Findings

Table 3 illustrates the basic information obtained from the study group with the survey.

Tab. 3. Main socio-demographic Characteristics of the Participants

	n	%
Age (n= 838)	370	44,1
19–25	280	33,4
26–40	167	19,9
41–64	21	2,5
65 and above		
Gender (n= 838)	509	60,7
Female	329	39,3
Male		
Marital Status (n=838)	339	40,5
Married	467	55,7
Single	21	2,5
Divorced/separated	11	1,3
Widowed		
Education level-degree (n=838)	8	1
Uneducated	32	3,8
Elementary school	34	4,1
Middle school	273	32,6
High school	63	7,5
College	340	40,6
University (Bachelor's degree)	71	8,5
Master's degree	17	2
Ph.D.		
Ongoing education level (n=838)	462	55,1
None	74	8,8
High school	24	2,9
College	221	26,4
University	34	4
Master's degree	23	2,8
Ph.D.		
Monthly income (n=838)	460	54,9
0–3000 TL	230	27,4
3001–6000 TL	100	11,9
6001–10.000 TL	31	3,7
10.001–15.000 TL	17	2
15.001 TL and above		
Job status (n=838)	434	51,8
Not working	356	42,5
Wage-earner/salaried /casual worker	20	2,4
Employer	28	3,3
Self-employed		

Table 3 details the socio-demographic characteristics of 838 participants of the survey in detail. It is also worth noting the issues that are not specified in the table. Eight of 434 people, who reported that they did not work, stated that they were laid off during the pandemic; seven of them quitted their jobs voluntarily during the pandemic process; 46 of them stated that they could not find a job due to the economic crisis caused by the pandemic. The remaining 373 people stated the reasons for not working currently as being retired, student, housewife, unwilling to work, and unable to find a job.

Our study focused on the variables of gender, age, and education level as socio-demographic factors to measure the participants' attitude to vaccination. In this framework, Table 4 presents the results of the Independent Groups T-test examining the effect of gender on attitude to vaccination.

Tab. 4. Results of the Independent Groups T-test Regarding the Attitudes to Vaccination by Gender

Gender	N	$\bar{X}$	Ss	T	P
Female	509	2.72	0.980	1.888	0.059
Male	329	2.59	0.968	1.893	0.059

The results in the table showed that men had lower mean scores (= 2.59) and were more prone to the Covid-19 vaccine than women (= 2.72), but the t-test result reveals that this difference is not significant. Therefore, we concluded that gender is not a determinant in the vaccination attitude.

We used one-way analysis of variance (ANOVA) to measure the effect of age on participants' attitude to vaccination. Descriptive statistics on attitudes to vaccination by age show that the 19–25 (= 2.79) age group had the highest mean and the most negative attitude. This was followed by the 26–40 age group (= 2.67). The lowest average belonged to those aged 65 and above (= 1.14). Table 5 presented the information on the change in attitude to vaccination by age.

Tab. 5: Results of the ANOVA Test Regarding the Attitudes to Vaccination by Age

Source of Variance	Sum of Squares	Sd	Mean of Squares	F	P
Between groups	67.353	4	16.838	19.177	0.00
In-group	731.402	833	0.878		
Total	798.755	837			

According to Tab. 5, attitude to vaccination shows a significant difference between groups according to age. Bonferroni test was conducted to determine the source of the mean difference between groups under the assumption that variances are homogeneous. Bonferroni test was preferred because the number of participants in the groups was not equal. Table 6 illustrates the findings regarding the test.

Tab. 6: Results of Paired Group Comparison Regarding the Attitudes to Vaccination by Age

Groups		Mean difference
19–25	26–40	0.120*
	41–64	0.279*
	65 and above	1.645*
26–40	19–25	-0.120
	41–64	0.159
	65 and above	1.525*
41–64	19–25	-0.279*
	26–40	-0.159
	65 and above	1.366*
65 and above	19–25	-1.645*
	26–40	-1.525*
	41–64	-1.366*

Note: Values with * indicate that the difference between the relevant age groups is significant.

The results in the table demonstrate that attitude to vaccination of the 19–25 age group, which had the highest average score, was significantly negative compared to other higher age groups. People aged 65 and above, who had the lowest average score, were significantly more prone to get the Covid-19 vaccine compared to other age groups. Analysis results revealed that vaccine resistance was relatively high in younger age groups

The effect of education level, which is another socio-demographic factor, on attitude to vaccination was also measured by one-way analysis of variance (ANOVA). Descriptive statistics on attitude to vaccination according to education level demonstrated that the group with the most negative attitude to vaccination (hence the highest average) was high school graduates (=2.85). Among the groups, the group with the most positive attitude to vaccination (hence the lowest average) was the postgraduate group (=2.47).

Tab. 7: Results of the ANOVA Test Regarding the Attitudes to Vaccination by Education Level

Source of Variance	Sum of Squares	Sd	Mean of Squares	F	P
Between groups	15.359	3	5.120	5.450	0.001
In-group	783.396	834	0.939		
Total	798.755	837			

According to Tab. 7, attitude to vaccination showed a significant difference between groups according to education level. Bonferroni test was conducted to determine the source of the mean difference between groups under the assumption that variances are homogeneous. Table 8 illustrates the findings regarding the test.

Tab. 8: Results of Paired Group Comparison Regarding the Attitudes to Vaccination by Education Level

Groups		Mean difference
Before High School	High School	-0.326
	University	-0.093
	Postgraduate	0.061
High School	Before high school	0.326
	University	0.233*
	Postgraduate	0.388*
University	Before high school	0.093
	High School	-0.233*
	Postgraduate	0.154
Postgraduate	Before high school	-0.061
	High School	-0.388*
	University	-0.154

Note: Values with * indicate that the difference between the relevant age groups is significant.

The results in the table demonstrate that, among high school graduates, who had the highest average score, attitude to vaccination was significantly negative compared to university and graduate groups. The postgraduate group, who had the lowest average score, was significantly more prone to get the Covid-19 vaccine compared to high school graduates. According to Tab. 3, which includes sociodemographic characteristics, 245 of 273 high school graduates continue their college or university education. In this case, it is possible to say that, in our study, the most negative attitude to vaccination was among the students who were currently studying at university.

Finally, Tab. 9 shows the statistics of the survey's third section, which questioned the participants' general knowledge about health and the Covid-19 vaccine.

Tab. 9: Knowledge about Health and Vaccine

	Yes n (%)	Indecisive n (%)	No n (%)
Covid-19 vaccine studies draw my attention.	587 (70)	133 (15,9)	118 (14,1)
I trust the Covid-19 vaccine chosen by the government.	334 (39,9)	329 (39,3)	175 (20,9)
I generally trust the healthcare system.	444 (53)	243 (29)	151 (18)
I think the vaccination policy implemented by the government is successful.	285 (34)	294 (35,1)	259 (30,9)
I think Covid-19 is not as risky as it is exaggerated so the vaccine is not necessary.	70 (8,4)	123 (14,7)	645 (77)
I'd rather get Covid-19 than its vaccine.	46 (5,5)	83(9,5)	709 (85)
I think the vaccine is not administered under proper health and hygiene conditions.	115 (13,7)	192 (22,9)	531 (63,4)
I do not trust the ingredients of the vaccine.	203 (24,2)	326 (38,9)	309 (36,9)
I fear that the side effects of the vaccine will be more than its benefits.	257 (30,7)	226 (27)	355 (42,4)
I believe the vaccine may cause other diseases (infertility, cancer, etc.).	207 (24,7)	291 (34,7)	340 (40,6)
I avoid getting vaccinated because of the negative news about the vaccine in (social) media.	149 (17,8)	185 (22,1)	504 (60,1)
Since the vaccine is supplied from abroad, I avoid getting vaccinated.	162 (19,3)	180 (21,5)	496 (59,2)
Since the ingredients of the vaccine are not suitable for my religious beliefs, I avoid getting vaccinated.	53 (6,3)	79 (9,4)	706 (84,2)
I think the government should inform the public more about vaccines.	679 (81)	65 (7,8)	94 (11,2)

Note: The cumulative total for all questions is n = 838 people

Based on Tab. 9, it is possible to say that the sample group had high awareness (70 %) of vaccination studies in particular. There is trust in the health system on the whole (53 %). In addition, the study group perceives Covid-19 as a serious disease (70 %) and the participants prefer to get vaccinated (85 %). However, in general, trust in the vaccine chosen by the government (its content, side effects, etc.) and vaccination policies is relatively low.

There are some additional points made by survey participants. They are as follows:

- *I think that vaccination is unnecessary because I do not have any chronic disease and my immune system is strong.*
- *Vaccination should not be mandatory for everyone.*
- *More preferences should be offered to the public regarding the available vaccines.*
- *I am afraid of the long-term side effects of the vaccine.*
- *I think more detailed information should be given about the content of the vaccine.*
- *Covid-19 is caused by a man-made virus. I think the vaccination process that comes after is also a part of this.*
- *I think vaccination should be done primarily to the working population, especially the education sector rather than the elderly population, and I find the process slow.*
- *I want to get the local vaccine.*

Conclusion and Suggestions

Vaccination is one of the most successful and cost-effective health interventions to prevent infectious diseases. Therefore, vaccines are thought to be very important to prevent and control Covid-19. In this respect, vaccine studies for Covid-19 are increasing rapidly after its emergence all over the world. However, uncertainties and difficulties regarding the vaccine's acceptability by the public are among the biggest barriers to vaccination policies. The main reason why vaccine acceptance or vaccine hesitancy varies a lot between countries is the risk perception originating from cultural, political, and social factors.

In this framework, our study aimed to reveal the attitudes to vaccination and its determinants in Turkey. It questioned the determining effect of certain socio-demographic factors such as age, gender, and education level. Our analysis found that gender did not have a significant effect on attitude to vaccination for our study group. On the other hand, our findings showed that age and education level had a determining effect on attitude to vaccination. Regarding the age groups, we found that the most negative attitude to vaccination was in the age group of 18–25 and among high school graduates, i.e., those who were mostly currently continuing their university education (245 of 273 high school graduates reported that they were studying at college or university) according to education groups. This point indicates that more studies should be conducted on this group to achieve success in vaccination policies and attain higher rates in vaccination.

Moreover, as Tab. 9 indicates, our study group had a high awareness of vaccines; trusted the healthcare system in Turkey; perceived Covid-19 as a serious disease; and preferred to get vaccinated. However, there are hesitations about the Covid-19 vaccine in use. For this reason, people thought that the government should inform the public more about vaccines (81 %). In this framework, the state is expected to support the research and development in vaccination and carry out activities to increase the demand for vaccination. It should also be noted that media, public health workers, and other actors influential in the public have more responsibilities in the process of conveying scientific information to the public. Considering that vaccine hesitancy has always existed throughout the history of the vaccine, the importance of raising public awareness becomes clear. In Turkey, the General Directorate of Public Health within the Ministry of Health created a "Vaccine Portal", which is a platform designed to provide information on what the vaccine is, its ingredients, and side effects. Therefore, the public should be informed about where and how to find the correct and consistent information through various methods (such as SMS, press, and media).

In short, the success of vaccination policies depends on the public's attitude and demand for vaccines. In this context, the public should be informed transparently and policies that take into account vaccine hesitancy and its causes should be pursued to ensure the success of the vaccination campaign. Finally, more efforts should be made to reduce public concerns about the short and long-term side effects of the vaccine.

References

Akarsu, B., Canbay Özdemir, D., Ayhan Baser, D., Aksoy, H., Fidancı, İ., & Cankurtaran, M. (2020). While Studies on Covid-19 Vaccine Is Ongoing, the Public's Thoughts and Attitudes to the Future Covid-19 Vaccine. *The International Journal of Clinical Practice*, 75(4), 1–10. doi:10.1111/ijcp.13891

Alben, A. F. (2019). Bir Üniversite Hastanesi Sağlik Çalişanlarinin Aşi Farkindaliği Ve Aşi Reddi Konusundaki Düşünceleri. *Master Thesis*. Gaziantep University Faculty of Medicine Department of Public Health.

Ataç, Ö., & Aker, A. (2014). Aşı Karşıtlığı. *Sağlık Düşüncesi ve Tıp Kültürü Dergisi*, 30, 42–47. Retrieved from https://www.researchgate.net/publication/340594390_Asi_Karsitligi, Access date 10.04.2021

Baltacı, A. (2018). Nitel Araştırmalarda Örnekleme Yöntemleri ve Örnek Hacmi Sorunsalı Üzerine Kavramsal Bir İnceleme. *Bitlis Eren Üniversitesi Sosyal Bilimler Enstitüsü Dergisi*, 7(1), 231–274.

Basu, K. (1976). Retrospective Choice and Merit Goods. *Public Finance Analysis,* 34(2), 220–225. Retrieved from https://www.jstor.org/stable/40911199

Biasio, L. R., Bonaccorsi, G., Lorini, C., & Pecorelli, S. (2020). Assessing Covid-19 Vaccine Literacy: A Preliminary Online Survey. *Human Vaccines & Immunotherapeutics.* doi:10.1080/21645515.2020.1829315

Bozkurt, H. B. (2018). Aşı Reddine Genel Bir Bakış ve Literatürün Gözden Geçirilmesi. *Kafkas Journal of Medical Sciences,* 8(1), 71–76.

Brennan, G., & Lomasky, L. (1983). Institutional Aspects of "Merit Goods" Analysis. *Public Finance Analysis,* 41(2), 183–206.

Desmarais-Tremblay, M. (2016). The Normative Problem of Merit Goods in Perspective. *Forum for Social Economics,* 219–247. doi:https://doi.org/ 10.1080/07360932.2016.1196593

Dror, A. A., Eisenbach, N., Taiber, S., Morozov, N., Mizrachi, M., Zigron, A., ..., Sela, E. (2020). Vaccine Hesitancy: The Next Challenge in the Fight against Covid-19. *European Journal of Epidemiology.* doi:https://doi.org/10.1007/ s10654-020-00671-y

Edwards, B., Biddle, N., Gray, M., & Sollis, K. (2021). Covid-19 Vaccine Hesitancy and Resistance: Correlates in a Nationally Representative Longitudinal Survey of the Australian Population. *PLoS One,* 16(3). doi:https://doi.org/10.1371/ journal.pone.0248892

Fridman, A., Gershon, R., & Gneezy, A. (2020). Covid-19 and Vaccine Hesitancy: A Longitudinal Study. doi:https://dx.doi.org/10.2139/ssrn.3644775

Graffigna, G., Palamenghi, L., Boccia, S., & Barello, S. (2020). Relationship between Citizens' Health Engagement and Intention to Take the Covid-19 Vaccine in Italy: A Mediation Analysis. *Vaccines,* 8(576). doi:doi:10.3390/ vaccines8040576

Karlsson, L. C., Soveri, A., Lewandowsky, S., Karlsson, L., Karlsson, H., Nolvi, S., ..., Antfolk, J. (2021). Fearing the Disease or the Vaccine: The Case of Covid-19. *Personality and Individual Differences,* 172, 1–11. doi:https://doi. org/10.1016/j.paid.2020.110590

Kennedy, J. (2020). Vaccine Hesitancy: A Growing Concern. *Pediatric Drugs,* 22(51), 105–111.

Kutlu, H. H., & Altındiş, M. (2018). Aşı Karşıtlığı. *Flora,* 23(2), 47–58. doi:10.5578/flora.66355

Mendoza, R. L. (2011). Merit Goods at Fifty: Reexamining Musgrave's Theory in the Context of Health Policy. *Review of Economic and Business Studies,* 4(2), 275–284.

Murphy, J., Vallières, F., Bentall, R., Shevlin, M., McBride, O., Hartman, T., & Hyland, P. (2021). Psychological Characteristics Associated with Covid-19 Vaccine Hesitancy and Resistance in Ireland and the United Kingdom. *Nature Communications*. Retrieved from https://www.nature.com/articles/s41467-020-20226-9

Özen, F. (2020). Aile Hekimlerinin Aşı Karşıtı Ebeveynler İle İletişim Deneyimleri Üzerinden Aşı Karşıtlığının Değerlendirilmesi: Niteliksel Bir Araştırma. *Master Thesis*. Sakarya University Faculty of Medicine.

Pogue, K., Jensen, J., Stancil, C., Ferguson, D., Hughes, S., Mello, E., & Poole, B. (2020). Influences on Attitudes Regarding Potential Covid-19 Vaccination in the United States. *Vaccines*, 8(582). doi:10.3390/vaccines8040582

Robertson, E., Reeve, K., Niedzwiedz, C., Moore, J., Blake, M., Green, M., & Benzeval, M. (2021). Predictors of Covid-19 Vaccine Hesitancy in the UK Household Longitudinal Study. *Brain Behavior and Immunity*. doi:https://doi.org/10.1016/j.bbi.2021.03.008

Sallam, M., Dababseh, D., Eid, H., Al-Mahzoum, K., Al-Haidar, A., Taim, D., & Mahafzah, A. (2021). High Rates of Covid-19 Vaccine Hesitancy and Its Association with Conspiracy Beliefs: A Study in Jordan and Kuwait among Other Arab Countries. *Vaccines*, 9(1), 42. doi:https://doi.org/10.3390/vaccines9010042

Salmon, D. A., Dudley, M., Glanz, J., & Omer, S. (2015). Vaccine Hesitancy: Causes, Consequences, and a Call to Action. *Vaccine*, 33, 66–71. doi:10.1016/j.amepre.2015.06.009

Shekhar, R., Sheikh, A., Upadhyay, S., Singh, M., Kottewar, S., Mir, H., & Pal, S. (2021). Covid-19 Vaccine Acceptance among Health Care Workers in the United States. *Vaccines*, 9(119). doi:10.3390/vaccines9020119

Sherman, S. M., Smith, L., Sim, J., Amlôt, R., Cutts, M., Dasch, H., & Sevdalis, N. (2020). Covid-19 Vaccination Intention in the UK: Results from the Covid-19 Vaccination Acceptability Study (CoVAccS), a Nationally Representative Cross-sectional Survey. *Human Vaccines & Immunotherapeutics*. doi:10.1080/21645515.2020.1846397

Sonawane, K., Troisi, C., & Deshmukh, A. (2021). Covid-19 Vaccination in the UK: Addressing Vaccine Hesitancy. *The Lancet Regional Health – Europe, 1*. doi:https://doi.org/10.1016/j.lanepe.2020.100016

Wang, J., Jing, R., Lai, X., Zhang, H., Lyu, Y., Knoll, M., & Fang, H. (2020). Acceptance of Covid-19 Vaccination during the Covid-19 Pandemic in China. *Vaccines*, 8 (482). doi:10.3390/vaccines8030482

Ward, J. K., Alleaume, C., Peretti-Watel, P., & the COCONEL Group. (2020). The French Public's Attitudes to a Future Covid-19 Vaccine: The Politicization of a Public Health Issue. *Social Science & Medicine*, 265.

World Health Organization. (2021). *Ten Threats to Global Health in 2019*, Retrieved from (date of access: 10.04.2021).

Yiğit İltaş

Compulsory Vaccination Application in Turkish Legal System

Introduction

The fight against infectious diseases, which cause mass illness and even loss of lives, has almost always been the focus of studies conducted and policies followed in the field of health. Methods and techniques developed for protection against infectious diseases, on the other hand, are used as instruments in the fight against epidemics. At this point, vaccines, which are considered to be one of the most important advances made in the field of public health, have become one of the most important symbols of preventive healthcare (Türk Tabipler Birliği, 2018). Given that diseases affect not only the individual patient but the community around them (Yüksel, 2019), the protection sought by vaccination acts both at individual and social levels. A well-known fact that when vaccines are used by significant numbers of people within a given community, they can help eliminate preventable diseases (WHO, 2014). This is why governments run routine vaccination programs to vaccinate children, providing protection against many infectious diseases used to cost millions of lives a year in the past (WHO, 2020).

In this study, the relationship between preventive health services and vaccination will be explained primarily. After making explanations about the compulsory vaccination practices, it will be evaluated whether these practices are possible in the Turkish Legal System. Opinions on the subject will be included in the conclusion part.

I. Preventive Health Services and Vaccination

The WHO defines health not only as the absence of an illness or disability, but also a state of complete physical, mental and social well-being (WHO, 2006). The right to health, considered to be a fundamental right, is defined as having the highest attainable standard of physical and mental health (WHO, 2002; Zengin, 2010; Temiz, 2014). This right is protected by national and international laws. Article 25/1 of the Universal Declaration of Human Rights (1948) regulates the right to health: *"Everyone has the right to a standard of living adequate for the health and well-being of himself …."*. Similarly, Article 12/1 of the International Covenant on Economic, Social and Cultural Rights (ICESCR) provides for the right to health: *"The States Parties to the present Covenant recognize the right of everyone to the enjoyment of the highest attainable standard of physical and mental health"*. The Constitution of the Republic of Turkey, as part of national legislation, recognizes in the Article 56/1 that everyone has the right to live in a healthy and balanced environment. The Article 56/3 states that the government is responsible for ensuring that everyone leads their lives in conditions of physical and mental health.

Healthcare services, provided to protect the fundamental right to health, aim to protect, improve, and in case of an illness, restore health in a society. Preventive health services, on the other hand, constitute the first stage in the provision of healthcare services undertaken with these aims (Filiz & Kaya, 2019). Preventive health services are defined as pre-illness services that would minimize or eliminate the duration, severity, and risk of a future potential disease or infirmity, identify symptoms of illness that the patient themselves may not be aware of, making it possible to treat the illness at an early stage (T.C. Sağlık Bakanlığı, 2019).

Vaccines are the first thing that comes to mind when it comes to preventive health services (Filiz & Kaya, 2019). The concept of vaccine is defined in different ways. Vaccine is defined as a substance given to the body to prevent infections or to control illness due to a specific pathogen such as a virus, bacterium, or parasite (Cutcliffe, 2010); or as a biological substance that provides active adaptive immunity against a specific disease (Xiaoxia Dai et al., 2019). On the other hand, Article 4/f of the Regulation on the Registration of Medicinal Products for Human Use defines the concept of immunological product as *"Any agent used to produce active immunity, such as cholera vaccines, BCG, polio vaccines, smallpox vaccines; any agent used to diagnose the immunity status, such as tuberculin and tuberculin PPD, brucellin, Schick and Dick tests; any agent containing vaccines, toxins and serums used for producing passive immunity, such as diphteria antitoxin, anti-smallpox globulin, antilymphocytic globulin; any medicinal product comprising allergen products intended to alter or define a specific immunological response acquired against an allergen agent."* As per this clause, vaccines are immunological agents .

The goal in vaccination is not only to protect the vaccinated individuals, but also to control the spread of the disease in society (Dubé et al., 2015; Türk Tabipler Birliği, 2018). If a significant proportion of the population in a society has immunity against the infection, this breaks the chain of infection and social protection is achieved because the disease agent would no longer be present in the environment. (Orhon, 2020). In terms of cost and safety, vaccines are considered to be one of the most effective and important public health practices of the 20th century for protecting the health of children and adults and preventing infectious diseases (Keskin, 2020).

II. The Legal Basis of Vaccination in Turkish Legal System

The first intensive vaccination program in Turkey was the expanded immunization program initiated in 1981 against five diseases. As part of this program, a total of 18 doses of vaccine were administered against 7 diseases in 2005, and against 13 diseases in 2013. (Bozkurt, 2018; Paslı, 2021). The legal basis of vaccination activities is found in national regulations and the provisions of international treaties. This section will review the provisions in national and international regulations signed by Turkey provide the legal basis for vaccination.

A. National Regulations

The Article 17/2 of the Turkish Constitution states *"The corporeal integrity of the individual shall not be violated except under medical necessity and in cases prescribed by law.."* Article 56 of the Constitution states everyone has the right to live in a healthy and balanced environment, and the state is responsible for ensuring that everyone leads their lives in mental and physical health. The term "medical necessity" in the article is not explained, nor are there any further provisions in the Constitution regarding this term. Therefore, the legislature would need to define the concept of medical necessity. Similarly, the phrase "in cases prescribed by law" refers to the discretion of the legislature, within the boundaries set forth by the Constitution (Turhan, 2019).

Article 5 of the Regulation on Patient Rights(RPR) states the corporeal integrity and other personal rights of the individual shall not be violated without their consent except under medical necessity and in cases prescribed by law.

These provisions make it clear that the bodily integrity of an individual can only be violated with their consent (Aşıkoğlu Demirsoy, 2018; Atak, 2020). However, in case of medical necessity or cases prescribed by law, it would be possible to violate the bodily integrity of the person without their consent. Thus, in the case of people who consent to receiving a vaccine, their right to bodily integrity is not violated.

Article 24/1 of the Turkish Civil Code (TCC) states *"The person subject to assault on his/her personal rights may claim protection from the judge against the individuals who made the assault."* The Article 24/2 states *"Each assault against personal rights is considered illegal unless justified by the assent of the person whose personal right is damaged, a superior private or public interest, or authorization conferred by the laws*". Compulsory vaccination can be considered a superior public interest (Kahraman, 2016; Işık Yılmaz, 2018; Turhan, 2019). If one or more of the reasons listed in the law is present, namely a superior public or private interest, authorization by law etc., violations of personal rights are not considered illegal. Therefore, because the aim in vaccination is to protect other members of the society as well as the person being vaccinated, it can be justified by a superior public interest if not by consent.

Article 1 of the Public Health Law no. 1593 (PHL) states that general services provided by the state include improving the health conditions in the country, fighting against all diseases and other factors that are detrimental to public health, ensuring that future generations are brought up in a healthy manner, and providing public access to health and social aid.

Article 3 of the PHL states the duties of the Ministry of Health include taking measures to minimize child mortality, preventing the entry of infectious and epidemic diseases into the country and fighting against such diseases, fighting against all sorts of microbial, infectious, or epidemic diseases and other detriments to health that are responsible for large numbers of fatalities, taking all necessary measures for children and youths to lead a healthy life, and protecting children's health and bodies.

Article 57 of the PHL regulates the obligation to report upon encountering or suspecting one of the diseases mentioned in this article (cholera, smallpox...), or in case of deaths caused by one of these diseases or the suspicion thereof.

Article 72 of the PHL lists the measures to be taken upon encountering or suspecting one of the diseases mentioned in Article 57. These measures include health officials isolating and monitoring people who have or are suspected to have the disease or are known to spread the disease at their homes or in places where health services are provided, for the duration recommended by science, administering IV drips or vaccines to the infected or those exposed to the infection, and limiting movement into or out of the regions where the infectious or epidemic disease is seen until the danger is over.

Articles 88 to 94 of the PHL contains provisions regarding smallpox. Articles 88 and 89 state that everyone within the borders of Turkey have to receive the smallpox vaccine, and if the person to be vaccinated is a newborn, the vaccine is to be administered within 4 months of birth .

The PHL identifies smallpox as a dangerous disease, makes it compulsory to report upon encountering or suspecting the disease, and in Article 72, mentions the measures to be taken. Accordingly, the infected are to be isolated from other people, monitored, and administered IV drips and vaccines. When necessary, entries into and exits from the region where the disease is seen are to be banned until the disease agent disappears.

Thus, as per this Law, the only disease that requires compulsory vaccination in Turkey is the smallpox. Moreover, the doctrine states that in case of compulsory vaccination against epidemic diseases (smallpox), required by law to protect public order, the informed consent of the patient is not required (Gündüz et al., 2001; Işık Yılmaz, 2018). However, the last case of natural smallpox in the world was seen in Somalia in 1977. Two smallpox cases were seen in the UK in 1978 due to a laboratory accident. These cases were last time the disease was ever seen (Alkoy, 2003). In 1980, WHO declared smallpox was completely eradicated in the world (KLİMİK, 2003). As a result, the smallpox vaccine has not been administered in Turkey since 1980. Given that the only compulsory vaccine in Turkey, required by law, is the one against smallpox, which is considered to be completely eradicated by now, the Public Health Law is far from meeting contemporary needs.

One of the protective measures listed in Article 5/1 of the Child Protection Law (Law No. 5395) is health measures. The health measures in question refer to temporary or permanent medical care, treatment etc. Vaccination, a very important health service for the protection of the physical health of children (Argüt et al., 2016; Gülcü & Arslan, 2018) can be considered a protective and supportive measure included within the scope of the health measures stipulated by the law.

Article 2 of the Decree Law no. 181 on the Organization and Duties of the Ministry of Health lists the duties of the Ministry of Health. According to this article, duties of the Ministry include the following:

- Protecting individual and public health to ensure that everyone lives in a complete state of physical, mental, and social wellness, preparing and implementing or supervising countrywide plans and programs and taking all necessary measures to this end,
- Fighting against infectious, epidemic, and social diseases and providing preventive healthcare, treatment,
- Providing services to protect child health,
- Producing, supervising the production of, or if necessary, importing the required vaccine, serum,
- Taking health measures in land border gates, airports, and seaports against infectious and epidemic human diseases.

Article 26 of the Decree Law no. 663 on the Organization and Duties of the Ministry of Health and Its Affiliates mostly parallels the provisions of the Law no. 181. As per these provisions, the Ministry of Health can take measures in order to prevent infectious diseases and epidemics and ensure that people lead their lives in physical and mental health, and vaccination is one of these measures as it serves to protect both individual persons and the society in general.

The Ministry of Health Circular on Expanded Immunization Program states that immunization services aim to prevent infants and children, in particular, from contracting preventable diseases, and thus protect them from disabilities and death causes by these diseases. Within this framework, the main goals are to vaccinate all children, without exception.

B. International Conventions

Article 6 of the Convention on the Rights of the Child (CRC) stated that *"State parties admit that every child has the innate right to life and shall protect the survival and development of the child to the maximum level possible"*. Article 24 expressed that *"State parties admit the child's right to the enjoyment of the highest accessible standard of health, and facilities for the treatment of illness and rehabilitation of health and that they shall endeavor to secure that no child is destitute of her or his right of access to these health care benefits."* Article 24/2 declared that the state parties shall take suitable measures to reduce infant and child mortality, procure the necessary medical assistance and health care for children, and establish preventive health care (CRC, 1989).

Article 12/1 of ICESCR expressed *"States Parties to the current Covenant admit everyone's right to the enjoyment of the highest accessible standard of physical and mental health."* Article 12/2 declared that to secure the full attainment of this right, states shall take measures to curtail child mortality, for the healthy development of the child, and prevention of epidemic, endemic and other diseases (ICESCR, 1966).

Article 5 of the Convention on Human Rights and Biomedicine (ECHRBMed) imposed that suitable information shall be given to the person about the aim, essence, aftereffects, and dangers of the intervention to be made in the field of health and that an intervention in the health field may only be executed after the relevant person has given free and informed consent to it. Article 6 declared that *"a medical intervention may only be executed on a person who does not have the capability to consent, for her or his direct benefit."* Same article presented that *"where, according to law, a juvenile does not have the capability to consent to an intervention, the intervention may only be executed with the permission of her or his representative or an authority or a person or body provided for by law, but the opinion of the juvenile shall be taken into account as a more and more determining factor in proportion to her or his age and degree of maturity."* Article 26/1 expressed that *"no restraints shall be imposed on the practice of the rights and protective rule of laws contained in this Convention other than such as are ordained by law and are necessary in a democratic society .... for the protection of public health"* (ECHRBMed).

In Article 11 of European Social Charter (Revised) to which we are a party; *"parties will undertake to take suitable measures to eliminate so far as possible the causes of ill-health and to prevent so far as possible epidemic, endemic and other diseases"* to assure the effective practice of the right to health protection.

Contrarily, although there is no direct provision concerning compulsory vaccination within the context of the European Convention on Human Rights (ECHR), the European Court of Human Rights (ECtHR) recognizes the situations about mental and physical integrity of the person such as forced physical examination, alcohol-blood tests, forced medical interventions, forced feeding, and compulsory vaccination within the extent of the right to respect for private life, which is covered in Article 8 of the Convention. In the aforementioned article, it is expressed that the right to respect for private and family life may only be intervened if the intervention is expected by law and to protect health in a democratic society. In this regard, compulsory vaccination implementations as a form of medical intervention are also dealt with by the Court within the extent of Article 8 of the Convention. Considering the conventions, it is possible to express states may execute compulsory vaccination practices when necessary, to eradicate infectious diseases threatening the health of individuals and society and to prevent regional or state-level epidemics and child mortality due to these diseases (Karakul, 2016; Turhan, 2019).

III. Compulsory Vaccination Practices

The increase in the proportion of people who refuse or delay vaccination for themselves and for their children causes problems in the fight against diseases in countries that aim to minimize or eliminate the burden of preventable diseases through vaccination (Gravagna et al., 2020). Compulsory vaccination policies have been considered and even implemented in many countries in order to overcome anti-vaccination and vaccine hesitancy and fight preventable diseases in an effective manner (McIntosh et al., 2016; Bozzola et al., 2018; Gravagna et al., 2020). Compulsory vaccination refers to vaccination regulated by law and required and administered by governments, the refusal of which leads to various sanctions (Sindel, 2020). Vaccination system in which the implementation of a duty to vaccinate is eventually provided by compulsory administration of the vaccine means compulsory vaccination. It is suitable to define any vaccination system which stipulates any negative consequence as a result of rejecting carrying out a vaccination as compulsory vaccination subject to justification, as these consequences can (and are intended to) affect one's decision to get vaccinated (Krasser, 2021). It is expressed that compulsory vaccination programs will be accepted as ethically right to protect public health if there is a serious threat to public health, compulsory vaccination is found to be more advantageous compared to its alternatives in terms of cost and benefit, there is a strong belief to safety and effect of the vaccination and pressure for vaccination is reasonable and proportional (Savulescu, 2021).

The World Health Organization does not have an official policy regarding compulsory vaccination. However, the WHO stated that it was understandable for countries that have to deal with decreasing vaccination rates and raging epidemics to implement compulsory vaccination programs (Walkinshaw, 2011). Suits brought in countries that implement compulsory vaccination policies focus on the argument that such vaccination violates the personal rights and autonomy of the individuals concerned, but compulsory vaccination programs continue to be defended on various grounds. Defenders argue that a public health policy that solely relies on choice regarding vaccination would make the system vulnerable, and vaccination needs to remain a top priority despite concerns. (Glover-Thomas, 2019).

Individuals who contract an infectious disease not only become patients, they also become vectors, knowingly or unknowingly, in the spread of the disease. A frequently made argument is that unvaccinated people can infect other people and exacerbate an existing epidemic, which is in fact a form of harm inflicted on other people. In the case of epidemics and when public health is at stake, governments can use compulsory vaccination programs to protect, through collective immunity, vulnerable people who are unable to protect themselves for medical reasons (Pierik, 2018; Drew, 2019). It is argued that vaccinating everyone regardless of age would prevent disease, increase herd immunity in society, and protect health interests of everyone (Pierik, 2018; Glover-Thomas, 2019). Therefore, given that vaccination protects not only the vaccinated individuals but other members of society as well, refusing to be vaccinated without a justifiable reason would be ethically unacceptable because it would be a case of intentionally inflicting harm on others. Another argument is that vaccination creates mutual benefit, and in case of mutual benefits, complying with laws is an ethical responsibility as well (Glover-Thomas, 2019). For all those reasons, governments can limit the freedoms of individuals and require them to receive compulsory vaccination in order to prevent harm to others (Giubilini, 2020).

Parents have a duty to protect the rights of their children, and when they fail to perform this duty, the government can intervene. Parents' refusal to have their children vaccinated against preventable diseases exposes children to serious risks, including of death. Given this possibility, it is argued that governments should intervene in the process through compulsory vaccination policies and protect children. This government intervention does not remove parents' right to raise their children as they choose, but limits the right in question in the best interests of the children (Pierik, 2018). Many countries in the world have compulsory vaccination programs. For example, as of 2017, vaccination against diseases including diphtheria, tetanus, whooping cough, hepatitis B, and polio became compulsory for children in Italy (Bozzola et al., 2018). Parents who refuse to have their children vaccinated are fined and their children are not enrolled in schools (D'Ancona et al., 2019). Nearly all states in the US require children above the age of five to be vaccinated before they can be enrolled in school (Holland, 2012; Meningitis Research Foundation, 2017). Those who refuse to comply with compulsory vaccination programs face sanctions and fines including the barring of unvaccinated children from enrollment in schools, monetary fines, and loss of parental rights, etc. (Holland, 2012; Gravagna et al., 2020;). Another example is the case of Belgium, where the polio vaccine is the only compulsory vaccine since 1960s, and children must be vaccinated before they are 18 months old. Parents who refuse to comply face monetary fines and even prison sentences. Recently, a parent who refused to have their children receive the polio vaccine was fined EUR5,500 and sentenced to 5 months in prison (Stafford, 2008).

The first state in the US to impose compulsory vaccination for the general population was Massachusetts, which made smallpox vaccination compulsory in 1809. All adults were to be administered the smallpox vaccine, but children could be exempted for medical reasons. Debates about the constitutionality of compulsory vaccination began when a Henning Jacobson living in the state was fined USD5 for refusing to be vaccinated. Jacobson believed the vaccine had undesired side effects. He also argued that a compulsory vaccination law was unreasonable, arbitrary, and oppressive, violated the right of every free person to take the best care of their own bodies and health, and forcing someone who refuses to be vaccinated, for whatever reason, to comply with the law amounted to an assault on their person. The Supreme Court of the United States heard the case in 1905 and rejected all of these arguments in its decision. The Court ruled that the Constitution granted freedom to everyone living in the United States, but this freedom did not confer an absolute right to be free from all limitations, at all times and under all conditions. Therefore, the state had the right to enforce compulsory vaccination, and protecting public health could, within reasonable limits, have priority over certain individual interests (Salmon et al., 2006).

Various applications have also been presented to the ECtHR regarding compulsory vaccination. The Solomakhin v. Ukraine case is one of such cases. Sergey Dmitriyevich Solomakhin (applicant) is a Ukrainian national and died in 2010; afterwards his mother took up the case. According to him, he had an acute respiratory disease, after he was given diphtheria vaccination in the hospital his health condition worsened and that the vaccine had caused many chronic diseases. The Court emphasized that a person's private life and the body integrity cannot be considered separately and that mandatory medical practice, regardless of its magnitude, constituted an intervention with that right. The Court stated that compulsory vaccination, as an involuntary medical treatment, equates to an intervention with the right to respect for one's private life, including physical and psychological integrity of a person, as stipulated by Article 8 of the ECHR. However, it stated such intervention was provided by law and with the legitimate purpose of health protection. It was examined whether this intervention was necessary in a democratic society and stated the intervention with the applicant's physical integrity could be legitimized by public health considerations and the need to curb the spread of infectious diseases in the region. The Court ruled there had been no violation of Article 8 of the ECHR in the present case (Solomakhin v. Ukraine).

According to legal regulations of the Czech Republic, children must be immunized against nine diseases. Those who violate these regulations are fined. Unvaccinated children without any health reasons cannot enroll in kindergartens. In the Grand Chamber judgement in the case of Vavřička and Others, the ECtHR ruled there had been no violation of Article 8 of the ECHR. In the case presented to the ECtHR, the first applicant had been fined because he failed to comply with the compulsory vaccination schedule for his two children. All of other applicants had been denied admission to kindergartens for the same reason.

The Court emphasized compulsory vaccination, as a form of involuntary medical intervention, constituted an interference with physical integrity and therefore relates to the right to respect for private life protected by Article 8 of the ECHR. It states the Czech policy defends the legitimate aims of protecting the rights of others as well as health and thus, the vaccine to be administered protects both the vaccinated and the unvaccinated for medical reasons, and in this fashion depend on herd immunity to protect against serious infectious diseases. It was assessed that a wide "margin of appreciation" is due for the respondent State.

It was highlighted in all matters concerning children, their interests should be favoured at the highest level. It was stated that the purpose of vaccination should be to protect every child against serious diseases through vaccination or herd immunity. Therefore it can be said that the Czech health policy aiming to protect children, is in the best interests of children.

The Court then inspected the proportionality of the vaccine policy. It took into consideration the scope and content of vaccination, the existing exceptions from it and procedural safeguards available. It was highlighted that the fine imposed on Mr. Vavřička had not been unjust. Although it was put forward that child applicants' non-admission to kindergarten had meant the loss of an important opportunity to enrich their personalities, it was a preventive rather than a punitive measure, and had been limited in time because these children who were not accepted to kindergarten were accepted to primary school when they reached the age of mandatory education and their admission was not affected by their vaccination status.

As a result, measures had been in a reasonable relationship of proportionality to legitimate aims defended by the Czech State (to protect against diseases) through vaccination. Court ruled the impugned measures could be deemed necessary in a democratic society (Vavřička v. the Czech Republic, 2021).

IV. Compulsory Vaccination Practices in the Turkish Legal System

For a medical intervention to be accepted by the law it must be performed by a competent person, by the obligation of attention and care, by the latest data and possibilities of medical science; must be a medical necessity and made by the purpose stipulated by law and the informed consent of the patient must be obtained. Preventive vaccines are also known to be a form of medical intervention (Şenocak, 2001; Şimşek, 2014; Işık Yılmaz, 2018; Atak, 2020). There is no problem for adult patients who can perceive the reasons and results of medical intervention in terms of consent in vaccination applications. However, it is important to determine whose consent will be sought if the people to be vaccinated are children.

Both Article 24/1 of the RPR and Article 70/1 of the Law on the Practice of Medicine and Related Arts stipulated that if the patient to be treated is minor, permission will be obtained from the parent or guardian before the intervention. It is stated in Article 24/2 of RPR that the child is listened and supported to join information and decision process about his/her treatment to the extent that they understand as much as possible even when the consent of the legal representative is enough. Within the scope of that article, it is emphasized that children must be informed via simple and understandable expressions and consent of his/her must be required at this point except for the serious medical interventions and risky situations. The consent to medical intervention of the legal resspresentative is surely the only choice if the child has no power of discernment. The doctor will decide on whether the child has the power to distinguish or not by considering behaviours of the child, his/her maturity, ability to decide on his/her own health (Törenli Çakıroğlu, 2018). At this point, it is stated that the child who has power to distinguish and his/her legal representative must be informed together and both of their consent must be required (Gülen Kurt, 2020). As a matter of fact, it is also stated the final decision belongs to the child's legal representative about the medical interventions and providing them to take part in the process is a kind of right by which the child will know the process and join it rather than a consent issue. In this respect, it is pointed out that it an ethical responsibility of the doctor to make the child be a part of the process in terms of medical interventions as long as the right to know of the child is respected (Aydın, 2003). Unlike these provisions, in Article 16 of TCC stated that minors are not required to receive the consent of their legal representatives regarding the exercise of rights strictly bound to persons. Considering the fact that the person will have the right to decide on her /his own health, body integrity and life, it is stated that the subject of consent to medical intervention is not considered to be completely left to the legal representative of the minor. This opinion states the consent of the minor, who has the power to distinguish will make the medical intervention legal (Kahraman, 2016). On the other hand, some opinions seek the consent of their legal representative or think that the consent of their legal representative should be sought together in medical interventions directed at minors. However, in the presence of a situation that threatens the health and life of the minor, the medical intervention will be deemed urgent and the consent of the minor will not be sought considering the superior benefit of the intervention to be performed by the authorized physician (Şenocak, 2001; Törenli Çakıroğlu, 2018).

It is believed the consent of the child alone will be sufficient if the person to be vaccinated is a child and has the power to distinguish in terms of vaccination. If it is an epidemic disease and there is an existing vaccine to prevent this disease, it can be easily said that the medical intervention in the form of vaccination will not be unlawful, since it will be in the best interest of the child. At this point, as stated in Article 6 of the ECHRBMed, if the minor's benefit is in question, medical intervention may be made on the minor. However, in such a situation, it was stated the profits and losses that can be obtained by vaccination should be evaluated separately for each event and as a result of the evaluation, if it is believed that vaccination serves the best interests of the child, vaccination should be administered (Işık Yılmaz, 2018).

The most significant problem about medical intervetions towards the children arises when the legal representative does not consent to medical interventions to be carried out. In this case, the article in 24/4 of Regulations of Patient Rights that he fact that if the medical intervention is required, the patient under the custody and authority can be given medical attention is subject to court decision in accordance with Article 346 and 487 of Turkish Civil Code will be taken into account (Arpacı, 2009; Törenli Çakıroğlu, 2018). Within the scope that article, whether the medical attention will be given or not will be subject to court decision when the legal representative does not consent to concerning medical attention.

The evaluations of the Court of Cassation and Constitutional Court are important in terms of the Turkish Legal System concerning compulsory vaccination practices. Provincial Directorate of Family and Social Policies applied to the court with the request of giving a health measure within the scope of Article 5/1-d of Law No.5395, about the child who needs to be vaccinated, regarding the fact that the compulsory vaccinations as per the expanded immunization program determined by the Ministry of Health are not made and also avoided by the parents. The decision was appealed after the court rejected the request. In the decision of the 2nd Civil Chamber of the Court of Cassation, it was emphasized that if the legal representatives do not give their consent without any validate reasons despite being informed about vaccination, this attitude will not be subject to legal consequences. Consent will not be sought if the failure of the parents to give consent is clearly contrary to the best interests of the child. It was stated that opposing parents did not show any reason and evidence to rationalize their statements, and there was no evidence that the mentioned vaccine would be against the best interests of the child. Court stated this is one of the compulsory vaccines in terms of both the child's future individual health and public health, and the decision of the directorate should be accepted, but the refusal of the request was contrary to the procedure and the law, solely because the parents did not give their consent (Y. 2. HD, T. 4.5.2015, E. 2014/22611, K. 2015/9162).[1]

Various applications were made to the Constitutional Court regarding the issue. In a case brought before the Constitutional Court, the representative of the

---

1   For similar decisions: Y.2.HD, T. 07.05.2015, E. 2015/1170, K. 2015/9552; Y. 2.HD, T. 13.05.2015, E. 2015/637, K. 2015/10057. https://www.lexpera.com.tr/ictihat, Accessed: 10.05.2021.

applicant stated that although the applicant did not accept the vaccination of his child, a health measure was decided by the Court in this regard, that the bodily integrity of his child was violated due to the decision, according to Article 17 of the Constitution, the bodily integrity of the person will not be touched except for medical obligations and the cases written in the law, and these situations may come to the agenda if one of the diseases included in Article 57 of the PHL with reference to Article 72 is in question. He claimed that although there was no such situation in the present incident, a health measure was imposed on the applicant's child; his child was qualified as such even though she was not a child in need of protection within the extent of Law No. 5395, and stating that the applicant's bodily integrity was violated due to the measure, claimed the right to protect and develop the corporeal and moral property defined in Article 17 of the Constitution was violated.

It was stated the regulation indicating that in Article 17 of the Constitution everyone has the right to protect and improve their corporeal and spiritual existence and that the person's bodily integrity shall not be touched except under medical necessity and in cases determined by law, related to the right of the individual to realize her/himself and to make decisions regarding her/himself with the right of physical and mental integrity ensured within the extent of Article 8 of the ECHR. By this article, it was pointed out that, with exceptions, individuals have the right to reject medical intervention and to decide on their bodies. It was also highlighted it was clear that the execution of vaccines and health measures constituted an interference with the applicant's bodily integrity and the right to protect and develop his corporeal and spiritual existence. It was stated for an intervention within the scope of Article 17 of the Constitution to fulfil the requirement of legality, the intervention must have a legal basis. It was emphasized the criterion of restriction by law will express the accessibility, predictability and certainty of the it, and this will prevent arbitrariness and assure legal security.

Without any explanation regarding the type and scope of the medical intervention, the 5/1-d regulation of Law No. 5395 for the protection and treatment of the mental and physical health of the child, it was also stated it is not possible to understand this regulation as authorizing the administration of all types of vaccines to be determined by the administration, depending on a certain age period and contrary to the consent of the parents. Otherwise, it was stated the type and scope of the medical intervention to be applied would be uncertain, and the types of interventions whom people do not consent would be likely to be on the agenda. In terms of the concrete application, it was stated that the relevant provisions of Law No. 5395 do not have the predictability quality, which is one of the elements that the legal basis of the intervention subject to the application should contain. It was emphasized the interference in the sense of Article 17 of the Constitution does not meet the requirement of legality, which is one of the legitimacy elements.

Considering the types of vaccines included in the The Ministry of Health Circular, it was stated that the regulation in the Circular is not limited to the diseases listed as limited in Article 57 of PHL. In this respect, the vaccines that were ordered to be applied to the applicant did not fully meet the diseases that are limited in Article 57 of PHL. It was stated Article 72, which regulates the administration of serum or vaccine to patients or people exposed to the disease in case of the emergence or suspicion of one of the diseases listed in Article 57, cannot be accepted as the legal basis of the application subject to the appeal. It was stated that only the smallpox vaccine was stipulated as compulsory vaccination in PHL, and other vaccines were made within the scope of the circular. It was stated that there is no provision of law that can be used as a basis for general and compulsory vaccination.

The court stated the intervention subject to the appeal did not meet the requirement of legality, and such an intervention violated the right to protect and develop the corporeal and spiritual existence guaranteed in Article 17 of the Constitution (AYM Halime Sare Aysal Başvuru: 2013/1789, 2015).[2]

It can be deduced from the previous decisions of the Court of Cassation that the child can be vaccinated, even if the legal representatives of the child do not consent to vaccination, if the vaccine in question is a compulsory vaccine within the scope of the expanded immunization program determined by the Ministry of Health, suitable for the best interests of the child and necessary for public health (Akkoyunlu, 2017). But after the aforementioned decision of the Constitutional Court, the Court of Cassation changed its attitude and made decisions in line with the decisions of the Constitutional Court that the vaccines would not be made compulsory (Yargıtay 2. Hukuk Dairesi, E. 2015/24695, K. 2016/361, T. 12.1.2016 Sayılı İlamı).[3]

ECtHR and the Constitutional Court stated that the compulsory vaccine constitutes an intervention against the bodily and psychological integrity of the

---

2 For similar decisions; AYM Muhammed Ali Bayram, Application no: 2014/4077; AYM Salih Gökalp Sezer, 21.11.2017, Application No: 2014/5629; AYM Esme Fatıma Kızılsu & Rukiyye Erva Kızılsu, Appplication no: 2013/7246. https://kararlarbilgibankasi.anay asa.gov.tr/Ara?KelimeAra%5B%5D=kamu+sa%C4%9Fl%C4%B1%C4%9F%C4%B1 n%C4%B1n+korunmas%C4%B1&BasvuruNoYil=2013&BasvuruNoSayi=7246.

3 For similar decisions; Y.2.HD. T. 18.9.2017, E. 2017/3976, K. 2017/9562; Y.2.HD. T. 5.5.2016, E. 2016/6766, K. 2016/9249, T. 5.5.2016. https://www.kazanci.com.tr/.

person and this intervention should be regulated by law. Unless regulated by law, vaccination will be against human rights. If there is a legal regulation, the compulsory vaccine must protect public health and be a necessary, measured, and proportional intervention in a democratic society. It is also possible that the compulsory vaccine in the fight against an epidemic can be considered within the legitimate aim of protecting public health within the scope of the ECtHR case law (Turhan, 2019; Akbulut, 2020).

Lastly one of the points to be emphasized is the COVID-19 disease, which is currently considered one of the biggest problems in the world and is known to be highly contagious and deadly. (Çöl & Güneş, 2020; Varol & Tokuç, 2020). The development of vaccines in terms of combating this disease has become a global goal, a worldwide mobilization of vaccine production has begun, (Okyay, 2020) and vaccines produced by different countries such as Germany and China have been put on the market. (Independent Türkçe) With the vaccines produced against this disease, which is associated with high mortality rates, it is possible to say that anti-vaccine approaches have come to the agenda again (Yadigaroğlu, 2021) and people do not want to be vaccinated for different reasons. Considering the current legal regulations, it is possible to say that the only compulsory vaccine in Turkey is the smallpox and forcing someone to vaccinate will violate the person's right to protect and develop his corporeal and spiritual existence in line with the decisions of the Constitutional Court and the Court of Cassation. It cannot be mentioned that there is an authorization taken from the law in terms of vaccines other than smallpox. However, it is stated that the decision of the ECtHR on the case of Vavřička and Others v. the Czech Republic may constitute a case law in the context of compulsory vaccination policies for the Covid-19 vaccine (DW, AİHM: Zorunlu aşı demokratik toplumlarda gerekli).

Conclusion

Since vaccination provides protection not only for the vaccinated person but also at the social level, it can be said that the decision of whether or not to be vaccinated concerns not only that person, but the whole society and the cost of not being vaccinated can be billed to the whole society as the emergence of diseases. In this respect, the benefit of the society should be taken into consideration in preventing the emergence of vaccine-preventable epidemic diseases or in combating the diseases after they occur, and compulsory vaccination policies should be implemented. At this point the fact that only people can have a say over their bodies cannot be denied. However, it is believed that leaving the fate of societies in combating the disease to the will of the people with a vaccination policy on a volunteer basis is not acceptable in terms of protecting public health. On the other hand, the adoption of compulsory vaccination policies will undoubtedly limit the right of individuals to determine their future, as well as the custody rights of parents who do not want to have their children vaccinated. However, it is believed that parents do not have unlimited freedom in exercising their right of custody of their children and should lookout for the best interests of the children. Since vaccines aim to protect the health of the child, it can be said that vaccination serves the best interests of the child. The existence of a social benefit will also be mentioned, since the health of other people will also be protected through the vaccination of children.

There is a compulsory vaccination policy only against smallpox in line with the current legal regulations in the Turkish Legal System. This vaccine is no longer applied due to the eradication of the disease all over the world, and the voluntary basis is accepted for other vaccines applied in Turkey. As stated in the last decisions of the Constitutional Court and the Court of Cassation, vaccination without the consent of the person who is vaccinated violates the right to protect and improve the corporeal and spiritual existence of the person. However, regulations on a volunteer basis do not meet today's needs if new epidemics such as Covid-19 emerge, causing the death of millions of people, and vaccines play a key role in combating these epidemics. The absence of such regulations violates the benefit of society and public health, with the ever-increasing number of cases and deaths. In this respect, compulsory vaccination policies that prioritize the protection of public health should be included as a necessary, measured and proportional intervention in terms of democratic society. At this point, compulsory vaccination policies should be adopted with the new legal regulations to be made due to the belief that public interest outweighs individual autonomy. When deciding whether a vaccine is compulsory or not, decisions should be taken in line with various predetermined parameters such as the situation of the epidemic that is desired to be prevented by vaccination in the society, and the economic and social burden of it.

References

Akbulut, O. (2020). Covid-19'a karşı Türkiye'de zorunlu aşı mümkün mü? *İstanbul Politik Araştırmalar Enstitüsü*. https://www.istanpol.org/post/covid-19-a-kar%C5%9F%C4%B1-t%C3%BCrkiye-de-zorunlu-a%C5%9F%C4%B1-m%C3%BCmk%C3%BCn-m%C3%BC. Access Date 15.04.2021

Akkoyunlu, S. A. (2017). Genel sağlığın korunmasına ilişkin idari bir faaliyet olarak aşı uygulamasının kanuniliği. *Erzincan Üniversitesi Hukuk Fakültesi Dergisi, 21*(1–2), 43–73.

Alkoy, S. (2003). Olası biyolojik silah olarak yeniden gündeme gelen eski hastalık: Çiçek. *Sted, 12*(7), 246–247.

Argüt, N., Yetim, A., & Gökçay, G. (2016). Aşı kabulünü etkileyen faktörler. *Çocuk Dergisi, 16*(1), 16–24.

Arpacı, A. (2009). Özel hukuk açısından tıbbi müdahaleye rıza beyanı, buna ilişkin sorunlar ve çözüm yolları. *YÜHFD, 6*(2), 5–14.

Aşıkoğlu Demirsoy, E. (2018). Kişi dokunulmazlığı hakkı bağlamında rıza olmaksızın yapılan tıbbi müdahaleler. *Türkiye Adalet Akademisi Dergisi, 35*, 319–343.

Atak, İ. (2020). Tıbbi müdahalelerin hukuka uygunluk şartları. *TOTBİD Dergisi, 19*, 19–26.

Aydın, E. (2003). Çocuklarda aydınlatılmış onam sorunu. *Çocuk Sağlığı ve Hastalıkları Dergisi, 46*, 148–152.

Beşeri Tıbbi Ürünler Ruhsatlandırma Yönetmeliği. https://www.mevzuat.gov.tr/mevzuat?MevzuatNo=7281&MevzuatTur=7&MevzuatTertip=5. Access Date 29.06.2021

Bozkurt, H. B. (2018). Aşı reddine genel bir bakış ve literatürün gözden geçirilmesi. *Kafkas Tıp Bilimleri Dergisi, 8*(1), 71–76.

Bozzola, E., Spina, G., Russo, R., Bozzola, M., Corsello, G., & Villani, A. (2018). Mandatory vaccinations in European countries, undocumented information, false news and the impact on vaccination uptake: the position of the Italian pediatric society. *Italian journal of pediatrics, 44*(1), 1–4.

CRC. (1989). https://www.ohchr.org/en/professionalinterest/pages/crc.aspx. Access date 03.04.2021.

Cutcliffe, N. (2010). *Building on the Legacy of Vaccines in Canada: Value, Opportunities and Challenges.* BIOTECanada.

Çocuk Koruma Kanunu, https://www.mevzuat.gov.tr/MevzuatMetin/1.5.5395.pdf. Access Date 03.04.2021

Çöl, M. & Güneş, G. (2020). Covid-19 Salgınına Genel Bir Bakış. In Memikoğlu, O. & Genç, V. (Eds.), *Covid-19* (pp. 1–8). Ankara Üniversitesi Basımevi.

D'Ancona, F., D'Amario, C., Maraglino, F., Rezza, G., & Iannazzo, S. (2019). The law on compulsory vaccination in Italy: An update 2 years after the introduction. *Eurosurveillance, 24*(26);1–4.

Dai, X., Xiong, Y., Li, N., & Jian, C. (2019). Vaccine Types. In Kumar, V. (Ed.). *Vaccines the History and Future* (pp. 31–39). IntechOpen.

Drew, L. (2019). The case for mandatory vaccination. https://www.nature.com/articles/d41586-019-03642-w. Access Date 25.04.2021

Dubé, E., Vivion, M., & MacDonald, N. E. (2015). Vaccine hesitancy, vaccine refusal and the anti-vaccine movement: Influence, impact and implications. *Expert Review of Vaccines, 14*(1), 99–117.

DW. AİHM: Zorunlu aşı demokratik toplumlarda gerekli, https://www.dw.com/tr/aihm-zorunlu-a%C5%9F%C4%B1-demokratik-toplumlarda-gerekli/a-57132188. Access Date 27.04.2021

ECHRBMed. https://rm.coe.int/CoERMPublicCommonSearchServices/DisplayDCTMContent?documentId=090000168007cf98. Access Date 11.04.2021

ECtHR. (2021). Solomakhin v. Ukraine, https://hudoc.echr.coe.int/eng#{%22ap pno%22:[%2224429/03%22]}. Access Date 28.04.2021

ECtHR. (2021).Vavřička and Others v. the Czech Republic. https://echr.coe.int/Documents/Press_Q_A_Vavricka_Others_ENG.pdf. Access Date 28.04.2021

European Social Charter (Revised). https://rm.coe.int/CoERMPublicCommonSearchServices/DisplayDCTMContent?documentId=090000168007cf93 . Access Date 11.04.2021

Filiz, M., & Kaya, M. (2019). Systematic review of studies to determine factors affecting vaccine rejection/instability/contrast. *Türk Akademik Sosyal Bilimler Araştırma Dergisi, 2*(2), 1–8.

Genişletilmiş Bağışıklama Programı Genelgesi. https://www.saglik.gov.tr/TR,11137/genisletilmis-bagisiklama-programi-genelgesi-2009.html. Access Date 13.04.2021

Giubilini, A. (2020). An argument for compulsory vaccination: The taxation analogy. *Journal of Applied Philosophy, 37*(3), 446–466.

Glover-Thomas, N. (2019). The vaccination debate in the UK: Compulsory mandate versus voluntary action in the war against infection. *Journal of Medical Law and Ethics, 7*(1), 47–71.

Gravagna, K. et al. (2020). Global assessment of national mandatory vaccination policies and consequences of non-compliance. *Vaccine, 38*(49), 7865–7873.

Gülcü, S. & Arslan, S. (2018). Çocuklarda aşı uygulamaları: güncel bir gözden geçirme. *Düzce Üniversitesi Sağlık Bilimleri Enstitüsü Dergisi, 8*(1), 34–43.

Gülen Kurt, M. (2020). Tıbbi müdahalelerde aydınlatılmış onam. *TBB Dergisi, 146*, s.187–218.

Gündüz, T., Kırımlıoğlu, N., Eşiyok, B., & Erdemir, A. (2001). Aydınlatılmış onam ve çocuk hastaya ilişkin hukuki düzenlemeler, *Türkiye Klinikleri Tıp Etiği-Hukuku-Tarihi Dergisi, 9*(1), 27–34.

Halime Sare Aysal. (2015). B. No: 2013/1789, 11/11/2015 https://kararlarbilgi bankasi.anayasa.gov.tr/BB/2013/1789. Access Date 28.04.2021

Hasta Hakları Yönetmeliği. https://www.mevzuat.gov.tr/mevzuat?MevzuatNo= 4847&MevzuatTur=7&MevzuatTertip=5. Access Date 05.04.2021

Holland, M. (2012). Compulsory vaccination, the constitution, and the hepatitis B mandate for infants and young children. *Yale J. Health Pol'y L. & Ethics, 12*(1), 39–86.

ICESCR. (1966). https://www.ohchr.org/en/professionalinterest/pages/cescr. aspx. Access Date 03.04.2021

Independent Türkçe. Üren, Ç. Kovid-19 aşılarında son durum: Aşılar ne aşamada, hangi ülke hangisini tercih etti? https://www.indyturk.com/node/ 294491/sa%C4%9Flik/kovid-19-a%C5%9F%C4%B1lar%C4%B1nda-son-durum-a%C5%9F%C4%B1lar-ne-a%C5%9Famada-hangi-%C3%BClke-hangisini-tercih-etti. Access Date 27.04.2021

Işık Yılmaz, SB. (2018). Çocukluk çağı aşılarında hekimin cezai sorumluluğu. *Tıp Hukuku Dergisi, 7*(13), 91–122.

Kahraman, Z. (2016). Medeni hukuk bakımından tıbbi müdahaleye hastanın rızası. *İnönü Üniversitesi Hukuk Fakültesi Dergisi, 7*(1), 479–510.

Karakul, S. (2016). Avrupa İnsan Hakları Mahkemesi Kararlarında sağlık hakkı – I, *İstanbul Medipol Üniversitesi Hukuk Fakültesi Dergisi, 3*(2), 169–206.

Keskin, F. (2020). "Covid-19 pandemisinde aşılamanın önemi", https://www. ido.org.tr/userfiles/files/Covid_1_9Pandemisinde_asilanma.pdf. Access Date 05.05.2021

KLİMİK. (2003). https://www.klimik.org.tr/2003/03/01/klinik-mikrobiyoloji-ve-infeksiyon-hastaliklari-klimik-derneginin-cicek-ve-cicek-asisi-konusund aki-gorusleri/. Access Date 18.04.2021

Krasser, A. (2021). Compulsory vaccination in a fundamental rights perspective: Lessons from the ecthr. *ICL Journal, 15*(2), 207–233.

McIntosh, EDG., Janda, J., Ehrich, JH., Pettoello-Mantovani, M., & Somekh, E. (2016). Vaccine hesitancy and refusal. *The Journal of pediatrics, 175,* 248–249

Meningitis Research Foundation. (2017). Should vaccination be mandatory, https://www.meningitis.org/blogs/should-vaccination-be-mandatory. Access Date 20.04.2021

Okyay, P. (2020). Covid-19 Aşı Çalişmaları. In *Türk Tabipler Birliği COVID – 19 Pandemisi Altıncı Ay Değerlendirme Raporu* (pp. 228–252). TTB Yayınları.

Orhon, FŞ. (2020). Genişletilmiş bağışıklama programına her yönüyle bakış. *Osmangazi Tıp Dergisi Sosyal Pediatri Özel Sayısı,* 6–14.

Paslı, K. (2021). Aşı ve kamu sağlığına etkileri, *Küresel Hukuk Dergisi*, 4–9.

Pierik, R. (2018). Mandatory vaccination: An unqualified defence. *Journal of Applied Philosophy*, 35(2), 381–398.

Sağlık Bakanlığı ve Bağlı Kuruluşlarının Teşkilat ve Görevleri Hakkında Kanun Hükmünde Kararname. (2011).https://www.resmigazete.gov.tr/eskiler/2011/11/20111102M1–3.htm. Access Date 12.04.2021

Sağlık Bakanlığının Teşkilat ve Görevleri Hakkında Kanun Hükmünde Kararname. https://www.saglik.gov.tr/TR,10369/tarihi13121983--sayisi181--rg-tarihi14121983--rg-sayisi18251-saglik-bakanliginin-teskilat-ve-gorevleri-hakkinda-kanun-hukmunde-kararname.html. Access Date 15.04.2021

Salmon, D. A., Teret, S. P., MacIntyre, C. R., Salisbury, D., Burgess, M. A., & Halsey, N. A. (2006). Compulsory vaccination and conscientious or philosophical exemptions: Past, present, and future. *The Lancet*, 367(9508), 436–442.

Savulescu, J. (2021). Good reasons to vaccinate: Mandatory or payment for risk?. *Journal of Medical Ethics*, 47(2), 78–85.

Şenocak, Z. (2001). Küçüğün tıbbî müdahaleye rızası. *Ankara Üniversitesi Hukuk Fakültesi Dergisi*, 50(4), 65–80.

Şimşek, U. (2014). Sağlık hukukunda aydınlatılmış rıza. *Dokuz Eylül Üniversitesi Hukuk Fakültesi Dergisi*, 16, 3535–3556.

Sindel, E. (2020). Covid-19 aşısı bulunma ihtimaline göre Anayasa Mahkemesi aşı kararının değerlendirilmesi. http://avsa.org.tr/. Access Date 25.04.2021

Stafford, N. (2008). Belgian parents are sentenced to prison for not vaccinating children. *BMJ* 336(7640), 347–353.

T.C. Anayasası. https://www.mevzuat.gov.tr/MevzuatMetin/1.5.2709.pdf. Access Date 07.04.2021

T.C. Sağlık Bakanlığı, Kocaeli İl Sağlık Müdürlüğü İzmit Seka Devlet Hastanesi, Koruyucu Sağlık Hizmetleri. (2019). https://sekadh.saglik.gov.tr/TR,236309/koruyucu-saglik-hizmetleri.html. Access Date 03.04.2021

Tababet ve Şuabatı San'atlarının Tarzı İcrasına Dair Kanun. https://www.mevzuat.gov.tr/mevzuat?MevzuatNo=1219&MevzuatTur=1&MevzuatTertip=3. Access Date 03.04.2021

Temiz, Ö. (2014). Türk hukukunda bir temel hak olarak sağlık hakkı. *Ankara Üniversitesi SBF Dergisi*, 69(1), 165–188.

Törenli Çakıroğlu, M. (2018). Acil tıbbi müdahalelerde aydınlatılmış onam. *Uluslararası Sağlık Hukuku Kongresi*, 115–134.

Turhan, M. K. (2019). Idari kolluk yetkisi bağlamında zorunlu aşı uygulaması. *Hacettepe Hukuk Fakültesi Dergisi*, 9(1), 1–40.

Türk Medeni Kanunu. https://www.mevzuat.gov.tr/MevzuatMetin/1.5.4721.pdf. Access Date 09.04.2021

Türk Tabipler Birliği, Aşı Konusunda Yaşanan Tereddütler, Aşı Reddi ve Aşı Karşıtlığı Konusunda Etik Kurul Görüşü, 06.11.2018, https://www.ttb.org.tr/makale_goster.php?Guid=c21adfbc-e1c4-11e8-b159-336a7b2d6c99. Access Date 05.05.2021

Türk Tabipler Birliği. (2018). *Birinci Basamak Sağlık Çalışanları İçin Aşı Rehberi*. Türk Tabipler Birliği Yayınları.

Umumi Hıfzıssıhha Kanunu. https://www.mevzuat.gov.tr/MevzuatMetin/1.3.1593.pdf. Access Date 14.04.2021

Universal Declaration of Human Rights. (1948). https://www.un.org/en/about-us/universal-declaration-of-human-rights. (2006). 03.04.2021

Walkinshaw, E. (2011). Mandatory vaccinations: The international landscape. *CMAJ, 183*(16), E1167–E1168.

WHO. (2002). Sağlık ve İnsan Hakları üzerine 25 Soru – 25 Cevap., https://apps.who.int/iris/bitstream/handle/10665/42526/9241545690_tur.pdf;jsessionid=FE476A0555DF9EF0FF40B3243FAD1F7D?sequence=10. Access Date 29.06.2021

WHO. (2006). Constitution of the World Health Organization. *1946 in International Health Conference*, Bulletin of the World Health Organization.

WHO. (2014). Report of the sage working group on vaccine hesitancy. https://www.who.int/immunization/sage/meetings/2014/october/1_Report_WORKING_GROUP_vaccine_hesitancy_final.pdf. Access Date 20.04.2021

WHO. (2020). Chapter 6 Vaccine-Preventable Diseases and Vaccines (2019 Update). In: *International Travel and Health* (pp. 1–53). World Health Organization Publication.

Y. 2. HD. T. 12.1.2016, E. 2015/24695, K. 2016/361. https://www.kazanci.com.tr/. Access Date 20.04.2021

Y. 2. HD. T. 4.5.2015, E. 2014/22611, K. 2015/9162. https://www.kazanci.com.tr/. Access Date 20.04.2021

Yadigaroğlu, H. (2021). Covid-19 ve aşı karşıtlığı. *Protokol Dergisi, 1*, 61–70.

Yüksel, G. H., & Topuzoğlu, A. (2019). Aşı redlerinin artması ve aşı karşıtlığını etkileyen faktörler. *ESTÜDAM Halk Sağlığı Dergisi, 4*(2), 244–258.

Zengin, N. (2010). "Sağlık hakkı" ve Sağlık hizmetlerinin sunumu. Sağlıkta Performans ve Kalite Dergisi, *1*(1), 44–52.

Ezgi Aygün Eşitli

Informed Consent in Pandemic Processes within the Scope of "The Crime of Experimentation and Trial on Human Being"

Introduction

The area of practice of medicine focuses on humans. As a rule, physicians must use known medical methods on patients. But for a medical attempt to be technically acceptable as a known medical intervention, it has to be researched and tested in a systematic and controlled manner. The most important phase of these medical research is the clinical research on human subject.

Also, the physician could use alternative methods on patient being free to choose the treatment after it becomes evident that known medical intervention methods will not yield any results.

These medical necessities find out the importance of the term of "informed consent".

Because clinical research and trial on humans is closely related to a person's bodily inviolability and the right to free discretion on one's body, the right to life and the freedom to self-determination. In this framework, any arrangement on the subject must ensure respect to these rights and freedoms while avoiding hindering scientific development and well-being on patient.

When pandemics like COVID-19 first appear, the lack of a standard treatment pushes physicians to use off-label drugs. Since it is an alternative method that may cause an unlawful trial on patient, as a rule, off-label drug use requires the written consent of the patient in order to be legal.

On the other hand, especially in times of pandemic, may require quick decision making. This raises the question of whether it is possible to use off-label drugs on the patient without a duly received consent during pandemic times. Does public health precede the patient's consent according to General Public Health Law? Can we force a treatment to the patient who does not want to protect the life of the patient and prevent contagion?

As briefly explained above this article will define the terms of the reason of lawfulness, informed consent, criminal experimentation and trial, will focus on the informed consent in pandemic process, and will attempt an analysis of problemed areas.

I. Execution of the Medical Profession as a Reason of Lawfulness in Medical Intervention

Medical intervention refers to the physical and mental intervention carried out within the boundaries of medicine in accordance with the relevant professional obligations and standards for the protection of health, diagnosis and treatment of diseases, applied by persons authorized to perform the medical profession.

The scope and limits of the responsibilities of physicians arising from malpractices and the experiments and trials on humans could be regulated in a legal framework in parallel with the emergence and development of biomedicine.

On 04/04/1997, the Council of Europe published the "Convention for the Protection of Human Rights and Dignity of the Human Being with regard to the Application of Biology and Medicine: Convention on Human Rights and Biomedicine". Turkey became a party to the Convention in 2003.

According to Convention on Human Rights and Biomedicine; "Any intervention in the health field, including research, must be carried out in accordance with relevant professional obligations and standards (art. 4). An intervention in the health field may only be carried out after the person concerned has given free and informed consent to it. This person shall beforehand be given appropriate information as to the purpose and nature of the intervention as well as on its consequences and risks. The person concerned may freely withdraw consent at any time (art. 5). When because of an emergency situation the appropriate consent cannot be obtained, any medically necessary intervention may be carried out immediately for the benefit of the health of the individual concerned (art. 8) ".

Constitution of Turkey, in Article 17/2; "Except for medical necessities and circumstances stated in the Law, a person's bodily integrity cannot be violated; a person cannot be subjected to scientific or medical experimentation without his or her consent".

Article 90 of the Turkish Penal Code (TPC, no 5237), on the other hand, made criminal sanctions against illegal experiments and trials on human beings.

Medical intervention can be a standard medical intervention or an alternative medical intervention provided that it is in accordance with scientific methods.

Therefore, the priority issue that needs to be addressed reveals itself at the point of when the medical intervention can be considered lawful.

The question of what is the reason of lawfulness in medical interventions is a controversial issue in the doctrine. In our opinion, the reason that makes medical intervention lawful is the use of the right (TPC, art. 26/1). As a matter of fact, "no punishment is given to anyone who uses his/her rights". However, whether the right exists or not should be determined according to the fact that forms the basis of that right. This right may be based on the law, statute, regulation etc. related to the field.

In that case, the reason that makes medical intervention lawful is "execution of the medical profession" consisting of the objective and subjective conditions that constitute it is the reason of lawfulness. For this reason, it is possible to say that none of the conditions of existence of the execution of the medical profession alone have the power to constitute a reason of lawfulness in terms of medical interventions.

As a reason of lawfulness, the conditions of the execution of the medical profession are divided into two as objective and subjective conditions. While "authorization" and "medical necessity" show itself as objective conditions that should be sought in each concrete case; "consent", "defence of necessity in favor of a third party" or "executing the provisions of a statute" are subjective conditions that require the presence of someone according to the concrete event. In order to accept that the execution of the medical profession is a reason of lawfulness in that concrete case, the intervention must be carried out by the person authorized to perform the medical profession, it must have a medical necessity for the purpose of diagnosis, treatment or protection, and one of the subjective conditions must be present.

In order for the physician to be considered authorized to perform the medical profession in clinical research and clinical trial on the patient, as a rule, the written consent of the patient is required.

In pandemic processes, the failure to obtain the written consent of the patient, except in cases where the conditions of necessity requiring emergency intervention occur, will result in the crime of experimentation and trial on human.

II. Lawful Clinical Research, COVID-19 and Informed Consent in Pandemic Processes

A. Authorization

According to "Regulation on Clinical Researches of Medicinal and Biological Products", Clinical researches are human studies in order to reveal or verify the clinical, pharmacological or other pharmacodynamic effects of one or more investigational products, to identify adverse events or reactions, to determine absorption, distribution, metabolism and excretion, and to investigate the safety and efficacy (CRMBP, art 4/1-t).

Clinical research and clinical trial are two different processes carry out on humans. While one is a research intended for reaching scientific data on the patient or healthy volunteers, the other is aimed at treating the patient (Aygün Eşitli, 2012; Veli Özer Özbek et al., 2018; Hakeri, 2019).

Clinical researches are conducted under the chairmanship of the responsible investigator (CRMBP, art. 4/1-y) with a team appropriate to the nature of the research. Phase I clinical researches and bioavailability-bioequivalence studies are conducted by an appropriate team with sufficient training and experience in good clinical practice and a medical doctor pharmacologist who has completed his specialty or doctorate.

Responsible researcher in clinical researches conducted during pandemic periods; The physician who has completed his/her specialty or doctorate education in the field related to the research subject is responsible for the execution of the research.

B. Medical Necessity

In scientific research, the medical necessity emerges as the need for clinical research to find a standard treatment or prevention method with the diagnosis of the disease.

The process, determines that a study has the mentioned qualities and therefore is a clinical research, is the approval of the Ethics Committee and the permission of the T. C. Ministry of Health, Turkish Medicines and Medical Devices Agency (TMMDA).

As a minimum, when ethics committees form an opinion on the research application (CTMBP, art. 28/1-c):

1. Analysis of the expected benefits, harms and risks of the research,
2. Whether the research is based on scientific data and a new hypothesis,
3. In researches to be carried out for the first time on humans, the necessity that the research should be carried out primarily in a non-human experimental environment or on a sufficient number of animals,
4. Whether the scientific data obtained as a result of the experiments carried out in non-human experimental environments or animals, whether the research has reached the maturity that can be done on the human in order to reach the desired goal and whether it is necessary to do this on human,
5. Research protocol,
6. The content of the research brochure is evaluated and whether it has been duly prepared,

7. The adequacy of the written information given about the research, the method followed for obtaining volunteer consent, the justification for the research to be carried out on the disabled, children, pregnant women, puerperant women and breastfeeding women, intensive care and unconscious persons,
8. The responsibility of the responsible investigator or investigator or sponsor in cases of injury or death, including possible permanent health problems due to the research,
9. Compensation for an injury or death that could be attributed to an investigation,
10. Regulations regarding the inclusion of volunteers in research,
11. Evaluates the suitability of the research team involved in the research according to the nature of the research.

For clinical researches planned to be initiated and conducted by researchers in relation to COVID-19 disease, it is required to notify the "COVID-19 Scientific Research Evaluation Commission" before applying to the ethics committee.

This commission does not do any content control. In the evaluations made so far, 96 % of the researchers have been returned to continue their studies as planned. As a result of the evaluation of the limited number of studies other than this, it was invited to be included in the central data. There is no obstacle for researches who do not agree to be involved in multi-centre studies from carrying out the studies they want to carry out individually only with the data of their own centres. (T.C. Ministry of Health, https://bilimselarastirma.saglik. gov.tr.)

C. Informed Consent

The consent of the patient is required for any medical intervention (Alpa, 1999; Mantovani, 2000; Santosuosso, 2006; D' Avack, 2008).

The subjective condition that makes clinical researches lawful shows itself as written consent. It should be accepted that if the volunteer does not have a written consent, the researcher will not be authorized to conduct a clinical research on volunteer.

The consent should be based on adequate information on the subject, scope, process and consequences of the intervention.

According to the Turkish Penal Code (TPC, no 5237) art. 90, In order that scientific experiments based on consent on human beings do not require criminal liability;

a. The necessary permission has been obtained from the competent board or authorities regarding the experiment,
b. The experiment was carried out primarily in a non-human experiment environment or on a sufficient number of animals,
c. Scientific data obtained as a result of non-human experiments or experiments on animals, in order to reach the desired goal, Requiring that these be done on human beings as well,
d. The experiment does not leave a predictable harmful and permanent effect on human health,
e. Not applying painful methods that are incompatible with human dignity during the experiment,
f. The aim of the experiment outweighs the burden and the danger on the person's health,
g. The consent declared based on sufficient information about the nature and results of the experiment should be in writing and not dependent on any benefit.

A research that has obtained the necessary permission from the competent boards and authorities means that the execution of the medical profession has fulfilled the authorization and medical requirements of the reason of lawfulness. Otherwise, it is not possible for the relevant institutions to approve and give permission for the research. If a research that has received approval and permission although it does not meet these conditions, the permission will be valid until the investigation is stopped, so it does not only incur criminal liability for this reason in the process. In that case, what needs to be considered in terms of reason of lawfulness is when an action that we can accept as a clinical research will give rise to the crime of experimentation on human being.

The volunteer or his/her legal representative who wishes to volunteer to participate in the research is informed before starting the research by a principal investigator or a researcher who is a physician or dentist from the research team. The information should include the purpose of the research, its methodology, expected benefits, predictable risks, difficulties, unsuitable aspects in terms of the person's health and personal characteristics, and the conditions under which the research will be carried out, the conditions in which it will be continued, and the issues that it has the right to withdraw from the research at any time (CTMBP, art. 5).

The consent of the volunteer to be included in the study with his/her free will, which is not dependent on providing any benefits, is obtained and this situation is documented with a written Informed Consent Form covering the issues related to informing. Having a competent investigator would be in the form of the person in Turkey and must take place in this way.

Also, the legislation specifically regulates the participation of children from the vulnerable group, pregnant, puerperant and breastfeeding women, the disabled, intensive care and unconscious persons to the research and obtaining written consent (CTMBP, art. 6–9).

Although it is thought that during pandemic periods, informed consent can be obtained electronically or by the researcher participating in the information process by telephone or video conference method,[1] there are no regulations that allow these methods in Turkey.

At least one person from the research team is assigned so that the volunteer can obtain information about his/her health and the progress of the research at any time and contact for this purpose.

The volunteer may withdraw from the trial at any time, with or without justification, of his own consent, and hence no loss of his current rights may be incurred during subsequent medical follow-up and treatment.

In the doctrine, some authors state that in pandemics it is possible to obtain "deferred consent" under certain conditions. The deferred-consent procedure has been developed for two types of emergency-care settings: clear-cut cases in which patients are incapable of providing informed consent, such as seizures, sepsis, shock and severe traumatic brain injuries; and a "gray area" of emergency-care situations in which the ability of patients or their representatives to provide voluntary informed consent and to understand the

---

1   According to FDA Guidance; FDA regulations generally require that the informed consent of a trial participant (in this case, a hospitalized patient) be documented by the use of a written consent document that typically includes the elements of informed consent, as described in 21 CFR 50.25, and that has been approved by the IRB and signed and dated by the trial participant or their legally authorized representative at the time of consent (21 CFR 50.27(a)). When feasible, we recommend a traditional method of obtaining and documenting informed consent using a signed paper copy of the consent form, or use of electronic informed consent. If neither of these approaches are possible, the following procedures would be considered to satisfy FDA's informed consent documentation requirement.

Method 1: A photograph of the signed informed consent document can be transmitted to the trial staff

Method 2: A witness can attest to the signature, but a photograph of the signed informed consent document cannot be transmitted (FDA Guidance on Conduct of Clinical Trials of Medical Products during the COVID-19 Pandemic, March 2020/ Updated on January 27, 2021, 15–16).

information may be diminished, such as in the case of respiratory distress, depression or acute myocardial infarction. Consent for continuation of trial enrollment and data collection is obtained only when the patient is capable of providing informed consent or the representative is available, which renders the consent "deferred".[2] (Rieke van der Graaf et al., 2020) However, there is no regulation in the Turkish legal system that approves deferred consent in clinical researches, and the consent given subsequently to the research is not considered a valid consent.

III. Crime of Experimentation on Human Being in Turkey

According to TPC, art. 90, "Anyone performing a unlawful scientific experiment on a human being shall be sentenced to prison for one to three years".[3]

The crime of experimentation on human being is a crime that can be committed by direct intent (Aygün Eşitli, 2012; Zeki Hafızoğulları&Özen, 2013). In the event that the victim is injured or dies due to this crime, the perpetrator will be held responsible for the crime of probable intentional killing/injury due to the indifference to the result of that death or injury, as well as the crime of experimentation on human being.

---

2   Several documents legislate the right for those carrying out the trial to use deferred consent, but by and large they have in common the following:
     • The research participant suffers from an emergency condition that needs immediate treatment;
     • This condition renders the participant incapable of giving informed consent;
     • An attempt has been made to obtain informed consent from the participant's legal representative;
     • The study cannot be conducted in a population that has not developed the condition under study;
     • Informed consent to remain in the study is obtained from the participant or the legal representative as soon as possible;
     • The treatment under investigation is considered to be potentially beneficial for the participant;
     • The research participant has not objected in advance to research participation;
     • The research cannot be conducted without the option of deferred consent;
     • The risks of receiving the intervention are minimal, at least in comparison with the standard treatment of the research participant; and
     • The research ethics committee has approved the deferred-consent procedure (Van der Graaf, 2020; Jones, Gupta, & Zimba, 2021).
3   For detailed information, see also Aygün Eşitli, 2012; Hafızoğulları & Özen, 2013; Bayındır, 2018; Aygörmez Uğurlubay, 2015; Güner, 2015.

There is probable intent (Aygün Eşitli, 2012) when the individual conducts an act while foreseeing that the elements in the legal definition of an offence may occur. Although the perpetrator who committed the criminal experimentation did not want to kill or injure directly, he remained indifferent to the realization of these results.

IV. Lawful Clinical Trial on Patient, COVID-19 and Informed Consent in Pandemic Processes

A. Authorization

According to TPC, art. 90/4, A person can perform a treatment-oriented trial on a sick person in conformity with consensual scientific methods administered to the person after it becomes evident that known medical intervention methods will not yield any results does not give rise to criminal liability. The treatment must be administered by a specialized physician in a hospital environment.

Until the diagnosis of COVID-19 is finalized, it is obligatory for the patients who apply to health institutions to be admitted and treated by Ministry of Health hospitals, State and Foundation University hospitals and all private health institutions (https://hasta.saglik.gov.tr/Eklenti/36907/0/pandemi-hastaneleri pdf.pdf).

Hospitals with at least two of the infectious diseases and clinical microbiology, chest diseases and internal medicine specialists and a 3rd level adult intensive care bed are accepted as Pandemic Hospitals.

During the pandemic, Infectious Diseases and Clinical Microbiology, Internal Diseases or Chest Diseases Specialist can be met by assigning from another hospital.

Pandemic Hospital; It is defined as the hospital where the treatment process of cases diagnosed with COVID-19 (test positive) has been performed.

In places where pandemic hospitals are insufficient, hospitals with a second level adult intensive care unit should also be organized to serve as pandemic hospitals.

The chief physician/responsible manager of the pandemic hospital is fully authorized to use the clinical beds, intensive care units, operating room and assign personnel, without disrupting its normal functioning.

Since patients diagnosed with COVID-19 use off-label drugs, the treatment should be performed in the hospital environment by a specialist physician within the above-mentioned criteria. Because off-label drug use is considered as an unconventional treatment and the conditions of a legal trial must be available.

On the other hand, in accordance with Articles 64, 69 and 72 of the General Public Health Law,[4] it is possible to take a test sample from the patient or from the person suspected of being sick, in order to keep the epidemic under control within the scope of the fulfilment of the provisions of the Law and based on the authority given by the Law.

Besides, the delivery of drugs to COVID-positive cases who are treated at their homes due to epidemic and actual impossibilities and remote patient follow-up are legal in accordance with the General Public Health Law. Because a person who fulfils the provision of the law is not punished (TPC, art. 24/1).

However, the law will not protect the abuse of the right. Therefore, before off-label medication is given, an evaluation should be made in accordance with the algorithm and guidelines. It should be progressed under the control and supervision of the physician in terms of diagnosis, treatment and follow-up. In the event that the healthcare professional deliberately or negligently exceeds the limit in the authority granted by the law, he will be liable. If the fact that caused the limit to be exceeded is given by the competent authority and the fulfilment of which is obligatory due to the duty, If there is an excessive order, the person who executes

---

4   Art. 64 – If any disease other than those mentioned in Article 57 invades or if such a danger arises, declare that the disease or any form of disease must be notified all over the country or in a part of the country and to implement all or some of the measures included in this law against that disease. Ministry is authorized.

Art. 69 – In the event of an infectious and epidemic disease, healthcare professionals are obliged to take the necessary measures immediately and all administrative authorities to assist in the implementation of these measures.

Art. 72 – If one of the diseases mentioned in Article 57 emerges or is suspected, the following measures are applied:

1. Those who are sick or suspected to be sick and those who have spread the disease by scientific analysis shall be kept in isolation and observation by healthcare professionals at their homes or in places with sanitary and scientific conditions for a period of time.

2. Serum or vaccine implementation to patients or those exposed to the disease.

3. Disinfection of persons, belongings, clothes, laundry and buildings and other things that appear to be contaminated.

4. Culling of infected insects and animals.

5. The examination of the people traveling within the country where necessary and the disinfection of their belongings.

6. Prohibition of consumption of foodstuffs that cause contamination and spread of the disease.

7. Quarantine and evacuation of places where infectious and epidemic diseases occur until the danger is over.

the order is not responsible, but the person who gave the order is responsible. If the subject of the order constitutes a crime, both the one who gives the order and the one who fulfils it will be responsible for the result.

B. Medical Necessity

The essential element that distinguishes clinical trial from clinical research is that the intervention is aimed at treating the patient, not the disease.

As a result of clinical or laboratory examinations, when it is determined that known conventional treatment methods will not benefit the patient and the beneficial effects are understood by having sufficient experience on experimental animals before and the conditions of the patient's consent are present, another treatment method can be applied instead of the known classical treatment methods. In addition, in order to be able to apply a method other than the known classical treatment method, it is likely that it will be beneficial to the patient and that this treatment will not give more unfavourable results than the conventional treatment methods.

A medical treatment and intervention procedure that has not been experienced before can only be done if it is absolutely predicted that it will not harm and save the patient.

Since there is no classical treatment method in COVID-19 disease, the drugs and treatments used must meet the conditions of a legal trial.

When it is understood that the application of known medical intervention methods will not give results, in accordance with the TPC the treatment for the purpose of the scientific methods based on the consent of the person does not require criminal liability.

Following the guidelines and treatment algorithms recommended by the Ministry of Health for the use of off-label drugs indicates that the scientific method is used, which is one of the conditions of the legal trial. Testing this drug in a hospital setting by a specialist physician upon written consent should be considered lawful.

As long as a scientific method in accordance with international medical standards can be accepted, based on the principle that there is a patient, not a disease, and the physician is free to choose the treatment to be applied, off-label drug use and treatment techniques should be accepted in accordance with the law in the presence of other conditions, apart from the treatment algorithms and guidelines of the Ministry.

In accordance with the Ministry of Health TMMDA Treatment Approaches and Scientific Research Circular in COVID-19 Patients; "First of all, it is important to follow the guidelines and algorithms published by the Ministry and updated periodically, in terms of the clinical course of the patients. It is known that some sources prepared by different professional associations and also guides followed by some countries are used from time to time. In this case, again, it is important that the guidelines prepared by the Scientific Committee and published by the Ministry constitute the basis for the patient approach in the clinic in order to ensure standardization".

C. Informed Consent

According to TPC, art. 90/4, The consent given in a lawful clinical trial must be in writing and must be based on sufficient information about the nature and results of the trial.

As a rule, written consent should be obtained[5] when trying off-label drugs[6] and other alternative scientific methods in pandemic processes.

According to WHO; "It can be ethically appropriate to offer individual patients experimental interventions on an emergency basis outside clinical trials, provided that no proven effective treatment exists; it is not possible to initiate clinical studies immediately; the patient or his or her legal representative has given informed consent; and the emergency use of the intervention is monitored, and the results are documented and shared in a timely manner with the wider medical and scientific community" (WHO, 2020).

It is essential that consent is obtained by giving information about;

a. Possible causes of the disease and how it will progress,
b. The nature of the trial, by whom, where, how and how it will be done and its estimated duration,
c. It is understood that known medical intervention methods will not give results,
d. Other diagnosis and treatment options and the benefits and risks of these options and their possible effects on the patient's health,
e. Possible complications of the trial,
f. Possible benefits and risks that may arise in case of rejection,
g. Important characteristics of the drugs to be used,
h. Lifestyle recommendations that are critical for the patient's health,

---

5   See also TMMDA Off-label Drug Use Guidelines, 08 February 2019.
6   According to WHO, the use of licensed medicines for indications that have not been approved by a national medicines regulatory authority is considered "off-label" use (World Health Organization, 31 March 2020).

1. How to get medical help on the same subject when necessary.

On the other hand, if the conditions of the medical necessity exist, the necessary urgent medical intervention can be made without written consent, even if the patient refuses the treatment. Because, although the right to refuse treatment stems from the fact that the person has the power of disposition over his body, it is not unlimited and can be limited by law provided that the essence of the right is not eliminated.

Pursuant to Article 25/2 of the TPC regulating the defence of necessity in favour of a third party within the scope of the obligation; The perpetrator is not punished for acts committed against someone else's right, with the obligation to save someone else from a serious and certain danger that is not caused deliberately and which cannot be protected by any other means, and on the condition that there is a proportion between the gravity of the danger and the subject and the means used.

In emergency situations where the patient's consent cannot be obtained, there is a life-threatening and unconscious state or in the presence of a situation that causes the patient to lose an organ or become unable to perform its function, there is the defence of medical necessity in favour of a third party (Patient Right Regulation, art. 24/7). In such a case, medical intervention to the patient does not depend on consent. In addition, when the need arises to expand the procedure performed during medical intervention to the patient, if there is a medical necessity that may cause the patient to lose an organ or become unable to perform its function if the intervention is not extended, medical intervention can be extended without seeking consent (Patient Right Regulation, art. 31/4).

Another important issue in pandemics is whether an off-label drug can be applied to the patient without written consent or against the written consent of the patient, even if the conditions of medical necessity do not occur.

The Turkish General Public Health Law (art. 72) makes it possible to administer serum and vaccines to patients and those exposed to the disease in case of epidemic diseases.

Serum; It can be defined as the remaining fluid part of the blood plasma following coagulation and is injected into the body to create passive immunity against the disease.

Vaccine; on the other hand, is a product that is obtained from bacteria and viruses whose disease-causing ability has been eliminated or consists of mRNAs produced artificially in the laboratory and injected into the body to create immunity against the disease.

However, serum and vaccine can be applied against consent in cases of epidemic diseases if a standard treatment or protection method with the qualifications and conditions determined by the Ministry of Health is accepted. Otherwise, the conditions of the legal trial should be sought and it is not possible to apply it against written consent unless there is a medical necessity.

Since the law does not explicitly authorize the practices that are not accepted within the scope of serum and vaccine application and the use of off-label drugs, it is not possible to try on the patient without the written consent of the patient. The provisions regarding the medical necessity in favour of the third party are reserved.

V. Crime of Clinical Trial on Patient in Turkey

According to TPC, art. 90/4, "A person performing a treatment-oriented trial on a sick person without the person's consent shall be sentenced to imprisonment for up to one year".

In the event that the victim is injured or dies as a result of committing crime of clinical trial, the provisions regarding the crime of probable intentional injury (TPC, art. 86,87) or the crime of probable intentional killing (TPC, art. 81, 82) are applied (Aygün Eşitli, 2012; Hafızoğulları & Özen, 2013).

VI. Medical Malpractice in Legal Clinical Research and Trial

Even if a clinical research or clinical trial is legal, the physician is obliged to make an intervention in accordance with the medical attention and care standarts. The physician who causes damage by acting carelessly and cautiously will have a negligent liability. Medical malpractice is considered as medical malpractice when a medical professional acts carelessly and without precaution, and differs from complications in this respect (Ersoy, 2004).

The crime of killing by negligence in article 85 of the TPC, and the offense of injuring by negligence is regulated in article 89. Negligence can be simple or conscious negligence.

The punishment to be given for the crime committed by negligence is determined according to the fault of the perpetrator.

In crimes committed by more than one person with negligence, everyone is responsible for their own fault. The punishment of each perpetrator is determined separately according to his/her fault.

Conclusion

Clinical research and clinical trials performed by an authorized physician in the pandemic processes in the presence of the informed written consent of the patient within the medical requirements are considered lawful and do not create any legal liability, provided that the obligation of professional attention and care is followed. Otherwise, the principal researcher and the research team may be held responsible for the crime of experimentation on human being, in the extent of their causal contributions.

Before starting the research, the volunteer or his legal representative who wants to participate in the research carried out for the prevention, diagnosis and treatment of the disease causing the pandemic in pandemic processes; must be informed by a principal investigator or a physician from research team, and his/her written consent must be obtained.

On the other hand, if certain conditions exist it is also possible to use alternative treatment methods on a patient not included in a clinical research. The fact that it takes time to find treatment in diseases that cause pandemics may require alternative treatment options on the patient and the use of off-label drugs in this context. However, the alternative treatment to be applied must have a scientific basis and the patient must give informed written consent to this treatment. Emergency medical interventions in the event of the conditions of medical necessity in favour of a third party constitute an exception to the rule of obtaining informed written consent.

In the COVID-19 pandemic, it should be considered by physicians that the implementation of off-label drugs to patients without the written consent of the patient may constitute a crime of clinical trial. As with the vaccine consent forms, care should be taken to obtain informed written consent in the treatment of COVID-19.

References

Alpa, G. (1999). La responsabilità medica, *Responsabilità civile e previdenza, 02*.

Aygörmez Uğurlubay, G. A. (2015). İnsan Üzerinde Deney ve Deneme Suçuna İlişkin Bazı Tespitler, *İÜHFD, 1*, 165–206.

Aygün Eşitli, E. (2012). İnsan Üzerinde Deney ve Deneme Suçları. *Yetkin Yayınevi*.

Bayındır, S. (2018). İnsan Üzerinde Deney ve Deneme Suçları. *MÜHFD, 1(24)*, 77–121.

D' Avack, L. (2008). Sul consenso informato all' atto medico. *Diritto famiglia, 02,* 759–789.

Ersoy, Y. (2004). Tıbbi Hatanın Hukuki ve Cezai Sonuçları. *TBBD,* 53, 161–189.

Güner, U. (2015). İnsan Üzerinde Deney Suçu. *CHD, 29(10),* 319–344.

Hafızoğulları, Z. & Özen, M. (2013). Türk Ceza Hukuku Özel Hükümler Kişilere Karşı Suçlar. *US-A Yayınevi.*

Hakeri, H. (2019). Tıp Hukuku (17. baskı). *Seçkin Yayınevi.* https://bilimselarasti rma.saglik.gov.t, Access Date 23.05.2021.

https://hasta.saglik.gov.tr/Eklenti/36907/0/pandemi-hastaneleripdf.pdf, Access Date 06.06.2021.

Jones, X. M., Gupta, L. & Zimba, O. (2021) Informed Consent for Scholarly Articles during the COVID-19 Pandemic. *Journal of Korean Medical Science,* 36(3), doi: 10.3346/jkms.2021.36.e31.

Mantovani, F. (2000). Il consenso informato: Pratiche consensuali. *Rivista italiana di medicina legale, 01,* 9–26.

Özbek, V. Ö., Doğan, K., Bacaksız, P. & Tepe, İ. (2018), Türk Ceza Hukuku Özel Hükümler (13. baskı). *Seçkin Yayınevi.*

Santosuosso, A. (2006). Consenso informato. *A cura di Gilberto Colbellini, Pino Donghi e Armando Masserenti, BIbliOETİCA,* 36–41.

World Health Organization. (2020). Off-label use of medicines for Covid-19, Scientific brief, 31 March 2020, https//apps.who.int/iris/handle/10665/331 640, Access date 26.06.2021.

Van der Graaf, R., Hoogerwerf, M. A. & C. de Vries, M. (2020) The ethics of deferred consent in times of pandemics. *Nature Medicine, 26,* 1328–1330.

Part V Reflections of Covid-19 in Law and Economics

Eda Yeşil Balıkçıoğlu

H. Hakan Yılmaz

The Effect of Health Programs and Expenditures on Credit Ratings under Pandemic Era

Introduction

The main motivation of this study is to understand the responses of credit rating agencies to health policies in pandemic conditions. In this period when public expenditures are expanding and financial risks are widespread due to the fiscal measures, the study has been tried to be developed on how credit institutions will handle COVID-19 and the change in health expenditures.

Health expenditures have become the second largest expenditure area in many countries following social protection expenditures, especially in developed economies. With the ageing of the population and the development of health technologies, this structure would be expected to continue increasingly. Early in the COVID-19 pandemic, it was not clear how healthcare utilization and spending would change. Although one might expect health costs to increase during a pandemic, there were other factors driving spending and utilization down.

Although it has been observed by differentiating between countries, health expenditures have increased with the additional measures taken in this period. The public expenditure structure and financing of this increase with supplementary budgets have also come to the fore as a matter of discussion.

Expanding in financial markets and opening to international financial flows, enlargement in world trade and credit volume and heavy increases in debt ratio caused to come out new financial instruments after 1980s. Along with the openness in national economies, and change in financial markets cause to be discussed the questions such as what the government's role should be, how the government should intervene in financial markets, how the financial developments affect countries and how the changes in financial markets result in financial crises. By those discussions, the importance of credit scores and credit rating agencies began to increase in forming and practicing macro financial policies. Economic crises encountered by developing countries after 2008 in global financial crisis environment faced by USA and Euro zone, causes and effects of those crises and defects of main parties especially in perceiving structural problems in the system, also credit rating agencies' calculation methods and approaches begin to be criticized (Balıkçıoğlu and Yılmaz, 2019: 6).

According to this situation our model implies the determinants of credit ratings especially public health expenditures for selected countries. We aim to study to determine credit ratings predictions by countries using ordered probit models for the period of 2000–2020.

I. Public Health Programs and Expenditures under COVID-19 Era

The intervention of state or in general terms the public sector in health sector is explained mainly by two arguments in theory. The first argument is the market failure that diverts the market from Pareto efficiency. The imperfect competition among the producers, imperfect information among the consumers and the externalities are main factors to justify the existence of the government. The second argument supporting the state intervention is the income inequality. Everyone has the right to have access to a minimum level of health services. The countries adopting this approach frequently face with a problem that is the economic efficiency of the alternative methods used to provide minimum level of health services to everyone (Stiglitz, 1988:288; Yilmaz, 2006).

In theory research expenditures are also deemed as public goods. The inventions and novelties are somewhat under patent protection, but some others may not enjoy this protection. On the other hand, any patented invention is somewhat protected but the level of protection is under debate. The increase of prices of such drugs or vaccination may be as a result of the decrease in such benefits. This issue is more significant since the world suffers from new contagious diseases. Very recently the contagious Covid19 and SARS outbreak originated in Asian countries are striking examples. It is not rational to expect from the market to successfully complete such researches in the due time against such instantaneous contagious diseases.

The health services should be separately evaluated due to its nature comparing other public goods and services. In general, the preventive health services covered under the scope of useful goods and services are considered as one of the main liabilities of the public authority. Similarly, it is generally accepted that the priority of the public sector in expenditures is to be the preventive health services instead of curative services. The main argument is related to the scope of the health insurance undertaken by the public sector, efficiency of the alternative service methods and the medical treatment health services rendered by the public sector (Yılmaz, 2016).

Public health is defined as "the art and science of preventing disease, prolonging life and promoting health through the organized efforts of society" (Acheson, 1988). Public health programs are important to sustain the health and well-being of communities. As a public good, it focuses on the whole population rather than individuals, and is consumed collectively. It affects a wide range of people. Mainly public health functions are preventative to support that citizens' health situation become better for a more effective and economic health system. Good health is accepted as a human right and the existence of advanced and targeted public health policies is a key factor towards closing the inequality gap between people regardless of genders, ethnicities, ages, and socio-economic background. Main functions of public health start from healthy daily activities including sports, good nutrition, prevention of diseases and awareness of health risks. This can be done with a broad spectrum from educational programs, campaigns, to influencing government policies.

The public sector renders health services through the institutions of central government or local institutions. This factor does not bring an end to the general debate; on the contrary, it brings out another debate on the level three, which is defined as the efficient use of resources.

Considering government budget constraint, government expenditures are supposed to be financed by increasing taxes, changing the composition of expenditures or raising public debt. However, a shift in the composition of government expenditures, especially a decrease in investment expenditures or health and education expenditures in sectoral base is in question, could lead to a slowdown and has an effect on factor productivity (Iyidogan et al., 2017). The fiscal pressure of public health expenditures resulting from mainly ageing and technology which is a major component of government expenditures carries a great importance for the public policies and programs.

The economic contraction and unemployment experienced with the pandemic highlighted public fiscal policies in 2020. Together with the measures taken against the crisis, the increase in public expenditures and the slowdown in tax revenues have brought the approach to public policy to a different point in the global crisis environment.

The ongoing coronavirus (COVID-19) outbreak has put governments across the OECD under considerable pressure to deliver emergency support to the healthcare sector, households and several sectors of the economy, whose activity was temporarily frozen (OECD, 2020a).

The COVID-19 pandemic has important consequences for both GDP and health spending growth in 2020. While there remains much uncertainty at the time of writing, it is clear that GDP will substantially contract in all EU member states, even under the most optimistic scenarios. For health spending, further increases can be expected – at least in some countries. As a result, another hike in the health spending to GDP ratio is likely in 2020 (OECD, 2020b).

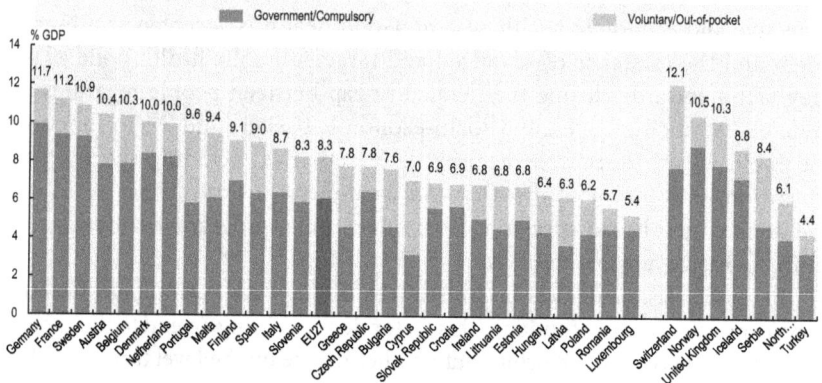

Fig. 1: Health expenditures in OECD Countries (% of GDP), 2019

Source: OECD Health Statistics 2020; Eurostat Database; WHO Global Health Expenditure Database.

Especially after the 2008 global crisis, health expenditures, which continued to increase above the growth in general, caused an additional increase in health expenditures due to the measures taken in a period of discussions about the effectiveness of public policies.

Figure 1 shows the additional healthcare expenditures in response to the Covid 19 pandemic period. UK is the country with the highest increase in health expenditures as above the line measure with 7.5 % as a share of GDP. Following that USA and Canada's health expenditures are also high. On the contrary, Turkey, Chine, India, Argentina and Italy have not increased health expenditures much in this period. When we look at the health expenditures among the measures implemented, we see that Britain, Saudi Arabia and Mexico stand out. Considering that the total fiscal measures of the last two countries are low, the UK and Canada are distinctly countries where health measures are heavily followed (Figure 2).

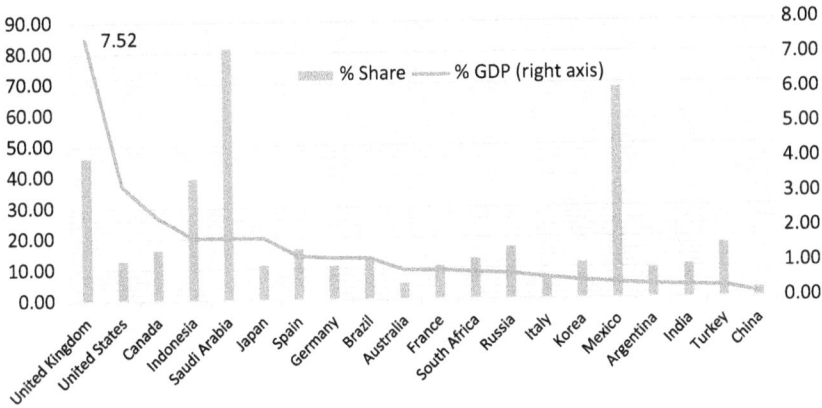

Fig. 2: Health Expenditure Measures of G20 Countries in Response to COVID19 (2020–2021)

Source: IMF, Country Fiscal Measures in Response to the Covid 19 pandemic, April 2021.

In the following graph, the size of the measures implemented by G20 countries during the COVID19 process is given under two main groups (above the line fiscal measures and financial-liquidity measures). The size and scope of the financial measures implemented by countries against the pandemic significantly vary even in G20 group This differentiation seems to depend on the ability of countries to adapt their economic programs rapidly during the pandemic period and financial resilience (Figure 3).

In terms of the size of additional public expenditure and tax measures, Turkey is among the countries with the lowest public expenditure and income measures, together with Mexico, among the G20 countries. USA and UK stand out as the principles with the highest financial measures under above the line items.

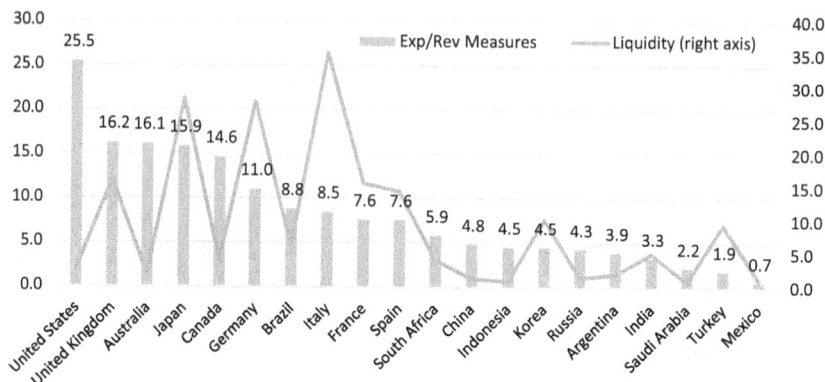

Fig. 3: Above the Line Measures (Public Exp./Rev.) and Liquidity Support (% of GDP) in Response to COVID19 (2020–2021)

Source: IMF, Country Fiscal Measures in Response to the Covid 19 pandemic, April 2021.

II. Theoretical Discussions on the Effect of Health Expenditures on Credit Ratings under COVID-19

Credit rating agencies consider information from economic, social, political behaviours to assess the country's willingness to repay its current and future debt obligations (Bissoondoyal-Bheenick, 2005). And after that all countries have been faced with Covid-19 which has become pandemic. It has originated from China at the beginning of the year 2020. The virus has hit advanced and emerging countries alike, and governments around the world are scrambling for funds to prevent a breakdown of their health infrastructure and economy. The enforced shutdown around the world is helping to contain the spread, but at substantial economic costs.

The literature on credit ratings Cantor and Packer (1996), Afonso (2002) and Canuto et al. (2004) indicated that, growth, per capita income, inflation, foreign debt, economic development level and default history of the country are the most prominent factors in determining the credit ratings. In studies of Mulder and Perrelli (2001) and Mora (2006) crises are up to the serious factors those are assumed to affect credit ratings, Bissoondoyal-Bheenick et al. (2005) studies showed that technologic development is one of the important factors of credit ratings determinants. Emara (2012) argued that strengthening the financial structure and inflation are the main factors in determining the credit ratings.

Josip (2014) analyses 46 European countries by using discriminant analyses and the paper implied that GDP per capita, inflation and international reserves are affecting credit ratings. Kabaday and Çelik (2015), Reusens and Croux (2017) applied probit models to find the determinants of credit ratings and implied that growth, inflation, unemployment, current account are the significant factors. Athari et al. (2021) analysed 1990Q1-2018Q4 period for Balkan countries and they find there is a relation between economic risks and sovereign credit ratings. And added these literature Tab. 1 emphasizes the credit rating literature by term of Covid 19.

Tab. 1. Credit Ratings Literature about Covid 19 pandemics

Authors	Model/Period/Countries	Results
Benmelech and Tzur-Ilan (2020)	Multivariate panel regression 35 advanced, 50 emerging and developing countries	In the pandemic process low income countries has poor credit rates, high interest rates but high income countries low interest rate and credit rates decreasing slowly
Tran et al. (2021)	Ordered probit model, 30 January-16 August 2020 period, IMF regions	Economic Outlook, government responses to the health crises and pandemic itself determine the intensity of rating actions.
Kartal (2020)	Multivariate Adaptive Regression Splines (MARS) method, December 2019- June 2020 period, Turkey	The importance of deaths number from Covid-19 pandemic, decreasing credit ratings in Turkey.
Balajee et al. (2020)	cross-section panel data analysis, Oxford Government response tracker (OXCERT) data, 22 countries	Economic stringency and rating determine fiscal stimulus
Jinjarak et.al. (2020)	Dynamic factor model, January 2014-June 2019 and March 2020	Covid 19 shifted resources to health expenditures
Augustin et al. (2021)	30 developed countries, cross-section panel data analysis, January 2020-October 2020	Fiscal capacity and spread of virüs effected credit ratings

III. Data and Methodology

In this study, S&P and Fitch and Moody's credit ratings for 12 countries between 2000–2020 (USA, Canada, Japan, England, Germany, France, Italy, Ireland, Spain, Portugal, Greece and Turkey) are examined by ordered probit models. In these models growth, unemployment, inflation, current deficit, public revenue, public expenditures, budget deficit, primary deficit, public health expenditures and ratio of public debt to GDP are used to analyse effect of sovereign credit ratings. Data has been taken from IMF World Economic Outlook Database. An ordered probit model in which the dependent variable is a sovereign rating in order to set up a model investigating the sovereign credit ratings by international credit rating agencies for Covid 19 pandemic period. Due to this, it has been analysed public health expenditures are effective in the ratings given to countries by international credit rating agencies

Ordered probit model is the most appropriate model for credit ratings. Because of the discrete, ordinal nature of the dependent variable in the estimation The central idea is that there is a latent continuous metric underlying the ordinal responses observed by the analyst. The ordered probit model is shown,

$$Y_{it} = X_{it}\,\beta + yZ_{it} + \varepsilon_{it} \tag{1}$$

where Y_{it} is an unobservable latent variable that measures the credit rates of a country in period t. X_{it} is a vector of time varying explanatory variables and is a vector of unknown parameters. Zit contains time invariant regressors that are generally dummy variables and ε_{it} is a random disturbance term. If the distribution of ε_{it} is chosen to be normal, then ultimately this produces an ordered probit model.

Y_{it} determinants show,

$$Y_{it} \rightarrow \quad Y_{it} < \tau 1 \; ise \; 1 = \text{investment grade} \tag{2}$$
$$\tau 1 \leq Y_{it} < \tau 2 \; ise \; 2 = \text{low credit risk} \tag{3}$$
$$\tau 2 \leq Y_{it} < \tau 3 \; ise \; 3 = \text{high credit risk} \tag{4}$$

In order to estimate the probit model, repeating and non-repeating observations should be distinguished from each other. For this purpose, likelihood method is the method that is most widely benefited. This method generally indicates the error in the model when an independent variable is added to the analysis. Log likelihood value has values in the range of 0 – 1. This ratio shows the probability of estimation of dependent variables by independent variables. Therefore, significance of undetermined variance in the dependent variable is indicated with -2log L. -2 LogL statistics in probit analysis resembles sum of error squares in regression analysis. Hence, if likelihood ratio is 1, -2 LogL statistics is equal to zero. As a result, a smaller – 2 LogL statistics always indicates a better model (Almendros et al., 2011: 5).

We could detect the influence of financial ratios on credit ratings by calculating the marginal effects of the explanatory variables on the probability of ratings (Yang and Raehsler, 2005). In this study, marginal effects are also measured in order to show the relative effects of independent variables on dependent variables which are explained in Tab. 2. Marginal effects regarding each independent variable are obtained by making use of sample averages of dependent variables. This situation is presented in the equation below (Akay and Oskonbaeva, 2018: 433).

$$Pr(Y_{it}=j_1, Y_{it}=j_2, \ldots Y_{it}=IX_i, v_i) \tag{5}$$

$$\pi^{ti}_{t=1} ¥ (\eta_j - \beta' \times_{it} - \Omega v_i) - ¥ (\eta_{j-1} - \beta' \times_{it} - \Omega v_i) \tag{6}$$

Tab. 2: Variable Definitions

VARIABLES	DEFINITIONS
Dependent Variables	
S&P Credit Ratings	Ysp= 1=Investment grade, 2=Low credit risk, 3=High Credit Risk
Moody's Credit Ratings	Ym= 1=Investment grade, 2=Low credit risk, 3=High Credit Risk
Fitch Credit Ratings	Yf= 1=Investment grade, 2=Low credit risk, 3=High Credit Risk
Independent Variables	
Growth	X_1= GDP Growth
Unemp	X_2= Unemployment
İnf	X_3= Consumer price index(end of period)/GDP
Curbal	X_4= Current account balance
Pubrev	X5= Public revenue/GDP
Pubexp	X6= Public expenditure/GDP
Budbal	X7= Budget balance/GDP
Primbal	X8= Primary balance/GDP
Pubhealth	X9= Public health expenditures/GDP
Pubdebt	X10= Public debt/GDP
Dummy	X11= 2020 pandemic period

The model is,

$$Ysp,m,f=\beta_1 X_1+ \beta_2 X_2+ \beta_3 X_3+ \beta_4 X_4+ \beta_5 X_5+ \beta_6 X_6+ \beta_7 X_7+ \beta_8 X_8+ \beta_9 X_9+ \quad (7)$$
$$\beta_{10}X_{10}+ \beta_{11}X_{11}+\varepsilon_i$$

Tab. 3 indicated S&P ordered probit results. Growth, unemployment, current account balance, public health and public debt are the significant determinant on S&P credit ratings. And following these results, column 3,4 and 5 implies the predicted probability of S&P's changing the credit ratings according to the marginal effects of variables assumed statistically significant. Coefficients show the direction of relation between dependent and independent variables. According to the analysis, one unit increase in growth, increase the probability of changing S&P's rating for investment grade, decrease the probability of changing S&P's rating for high and low credit risk. One unit increase of unemployment decreases the probability of S&P changing the credit rating by 0,0246 units for investment grade but on the other hand increasing low and high credit risk predictions. For current account balance and public debt the same as unemployment. And decreasing in health expenditures increasing the investment grade but on the other hand decreasing low and high credit risk. The differences of direction means the different rating scales and structures of countries. In the countries that their credit rates are in the investment rate grade adversely effect of growth, health expenditures.

Tab. 3: S&P Ordered Probit Results

Variables	OProbit(S&P) Coefficients	Dy/dx(predict= 1)	Dy/dx(predict= 2)	Dy/dx(predict= 3)
Growth	-0.1370** (-2.46)	0.0165**	-0.0145**	-0.0019**
Unemp	0.2045*** (5.63)	-0.0246	0.0217	0.0029
İnf	-0.0084 (-0.24)	0.0010	-0.0008	-0.0001
Curbal	0.0909** (2.56)	-0.0109**	0.0096**	0.0012**
Pubrev	-0.0682 (-0.74)	0.0082	-0.0007	-0.0009
Pubexp	0.020 (0.24)	-0.0025	0.0022	0.0002
Budbal	-0.0220 (-0.25)	0.0022	-0.0023	-0.0003
Primbal	0.0267 (0.53)	-0.0032	0.0028	0.0003
Pubhealth	-1.0700*** (-5.09)	0.1290***	-0.1137***	-0.0152***
Pubdebt	0.0210*** (-4.48)	-0.0025***	0.0022***	0.0003***
Dummy	-0.8786 (0.167)	0.0105	-0.0934	-0.125
Threshold 1	-4.1729	-		
Threshold 2	0.1915	-		
Loglikelihood	-59.8275	-		
LR chi2(11)	214.81	-		
N	252	-		

Note: Paranthesis show z statistics, *** $p<0.01$, ** $p<0.05$, *$p<0.1$

Tab. 4 clearly shows that, growth, unemployment, current account balance, public health expenditures, public debts and Covid 19 period are main characters of credit ratings to determine all of credit ratings scenarios. And resembling the S&P rating Moody's ratings are changed by countries credit ratings. But in Moody's ratings Covid 19 period is significant to change the credit ratings. Growth, public health expenditures and Covid 19 period increase the countries credit rates to investment grade but decrease the low and high credit risks. Contrarily, other dependent variables that are unemployment, current account balance and primary balance and public debts decrease the investment grade, increase prediction of 2 and 3.

Tab. 4: Moody's Ordered Probit Results

Variables	OProbit(Moody's)			
	Coefficients	Dy/dx(predict= 1)	Dy/dx(predict= 2)	Dy/dx(predict= 3)
Growth	-0.02189*** (-3.80)	0.0245	-0.0212	-0.0032
Unemp	0.0868** (2.51)	-0.0097**	0.0084**	0.0013**
İnf	-0.0014 (-0.04)	-0.0001	0.0002	0.0001
Curbal	0.1804*** (4.90)	-0.0202***	0.0175***	0.0027***
Pubrev	-0.0224 (-0.23)	0.0025	-0.0021	-0.0003
Pubexp	-0.0526 (-0.53)	0.0059	-0.0051	-0.0007
Budbal	0.0226 (0.25)	-0.0025	0.0022	0.0003
Primbal	-0.1902* (-2.01)	0.0213	-0.0184	-0.0002
Pubhealth	-1.5554*** (-6.62)	0.1744***	-0.1511***	-0.0232***
Pubdebt	0.03618*** (5.30)	-0.0004***	0.0034***	0.0005***
Dummy	-2.4268*** (-3.54)	0.2721***	-0.2358***	-0.0363***
Threshold1	-9.0246	-	-	-
Threshold2	-4.1824	-	-	-
Loglikelihood	-57.6809	-	-	-
LR chi2(11)	255.17	-	-	-
N	252	-	-	-

Note: Paranthesis show z statistics, *** p<0.01, ** p<0.05, *p<0.1

In Tab. 5, Fitch ordered probit results are shown. GDP growth, unemployment, current account balance, public health expenditures and public debts are main determinants of Fitch's credit ratings. In the prediction 1 means investment grade, increase the probability of changing the credit rating increases GDP growth and public health expenditures and decreases unemployment, current account balance, public debt. In the prediction 2 and 3, means high and low credit risk ratings, the probability of changing the credit rating increases unemployment, current account balance and public debt, decrease growth and public health expenditure.

Tab. 5: Fitch Ordered Probit Results

Variables	OProbit(Fitch)			
	Coefficients	Dy/dx(predict= 1)	Dy/dx(predict= 2)	Dy/dx(predict= 3)
Growth	-0.1235*	0.0013*	-0.0120*	-0.0015*
	(-2.20)			
Unemp	0.1950***	-0.0215***	0.0019***	0.0024***
	(5.23)			
İnf	0.0020	-0.0002	0.0002	0.0001
	(0.06)			
Curbal	0.1146***	-0.0126***	0.0112***	0.0014**
	(2.91)			
Pubrev	-0.0039	0.0043	-0.0038	-0.0005
	(-0.30)			
Pubexp	0.0320	-0.0003	0.0031	0.0004
	(0.33)			
Budbal	0.0020	-0.0002	0.0002	0.0002
	(0.02)			
Primbal	-0.0184	0.0020	-0.0017	-0.0002
	(-0.20)			
Pubhealth	-1.2364***	0.1366***	-0.1208***	-0.0015***
	(-1.24)			
Pubdebt	0.0220***	-0.0024***	0.0021***	0.0002***
	(3.95)			
Dummy	-0.7663	0.0847	-0.074	-0.0097
	(-1.17)			
Threshold1	-3.5748	-	-	-
Threshold2	0.0954	-	-	-
Loglikelihood	-54.9732	-	-	-
LR chi2(11)	222.20	-	-	-
N	252	-	-	-

Note: Paranthesis shows z statistics, *** p<0.01, ** p<0.05, *p<0.1

As a result of the ordered probit model GDP growth, unemployment, current account balance, public health expenditures and public debt are common determinants of credit ratings for three agencies. Primary budget balance and Covid 19 are also found significant in Moody's (Tab. 6).

Tab. 6: Summary table of significant results

Credit Rating Agencies (Significant Results)	S&P	Moody's	Fitch
Determinants	Growth	Growth	Growth
	Unemployment	Unemployment	Unemployment
	Current account balance	Current account balance	Current account balance
	Public health exp.	Public health exp.	Public health exp.
	Public debt	Public debt	Public debt
		Primary balance	
		Covid 19 period	

Conclusion

The coronavirus pandemic provides researchers with a unique opportunity to shed new light on a sovereign's resilience to external shocks. According to our analysis, growth, unemployment, current account balance, public health expenditures and public debts are the main determinants of sovereign credit ratings. In generally, Moody's predictions consist of primary budget balance and Covid 19 period. Fitch and S&P's predictions have not shown the Covid 19 period yet.

The impact of public health expenditures has been evaluated within the scope of this study, among other parameters. The result shows that public health expenditures have different effect comparing the effect of public expenditures and this differentiation varies according to the credit grade levels of the countries categorized their credit scoring level.

To the point public health expenditures and credit ratings are important factors to this pandemic era. Our analyses also supported these theories. But the pandemic time is not ever yet. So our analyses give us limited result about effect of pandemic.

We consider that we will enter a period in which the results of the fiscal policies implemented in the following period and the programs aimed at correcting the fiscal balances after the pandemic will have an impact on credit evaluation of the credit rating agencies. The new world normal that has been changing after the pandemic, we think that credit rating agencies should reconsider medium and long-term public policies by taking into account the differences of countries and the effects of non-financial consequences of policies.

References

Afonso. A. (2002). Understanding the Determinants of Government Debt Ratings: Evidence for the Two Leading Agencies, Department of Economics and Research Center on the Portuguese Economy (CISEP), Lisbon.

Akay, E. Ç. & Oskonbaeva, Z. (2018). Panel Sıralı Probit Modelinin Kredi Derecelendirilmesine Uygulanması, International Conference on Eurosian Economies, Tashkent/Uzbekistan.

Augustin, P., Sokolovski, V., Subrahmamyam, M, G. & Tomio, D. (2021). In Sickness and in Debt: The COVID-19 Impact on Sovereign Credit Risk, https://ssrn.com/abstract=3613432, Access date 10.05.2021.

Athari, S.A, Kondoz, M. & Kirikkaleli, D. (2021). Dependency between sovereign creditratingsand economic risk: Insight from Balkan countries, *Journal of Ecomics and Business*, available online 27 January 2021. 0148-6195/© 2021 Elsevier Inc.

Balajee, A., Tomar., S. & Udupa, G. (2020). Covid 19, Fiscal Stimulus and Credit Ratings, Electronic copy available at: https://ssrn.com/abstract=3577115

Balıkçıoğlu E. & Yılmaz, H. H. (2019). How Fiscal Policies Effect Credit Ratings: Probit Analysis of Three Main Credit Rating Agencies Sovereign Credit Notes, Transylvanian Review of Administrative Sciences, No. 56, E/ 2019, pp. 5–22.

Benmelech, E. & Tzur-Ilan, N. (2020). "The Determinants of Fiscal and Monetary Policies during the Covid 19 Crises", NBER Working Paper Series, No. 27461, http://www.nber.org/papers/w27461.

Bissondoyal-Bheenick, E., Brooks, R. & Yip, A. Y. N. (2005). Determinants of Sovereign Ratings: A Comparison of Case-Based Reasoning and Ordered Probit Approaches, Working Paper, Department of Econometrics and Business Statistics.

Cantor, R. & Packer, F. (1996). Determinants and Impact of Sovereign Credit Ratings, Economic Policy Review, Federal Reserve Bank of New York, Kasım, pp. 37–53.

Canuto, O, Santos, P., F., P. & Porto, P. C. (2004). Macroeconomics and Sovereign Risk Ratings, www.worldbank.org.

Emara, N. (2012). Inflation Volatility, Financial Institutions, and Sovereign Debt Rating, *Journal of Development and Economic Policies*, 14(1), 1–44.

Jinjarak, Y., Ahmed, R., Nair-Desai, S., Xin, W. & Aizenman, J. (2020). Pandemic Shocks and Fiscal-Monetary Policies in The Eurozone, Covid!9 Dominance during January-June 2020, NBER Working Paper Series, No. 27451.

Josip, V. (2014). Determinants of Sovereign Credit Ratings and Credit Rating Agencies Fault, *Sarajevo Business and Economics Review*, 33, 55–71.

Kabaday, B. & Çelik, A. A. (2015). Determinants of Sovereign Ratings in Emerging Countries: A Qualitative, Dependent Variable Panel Data Analysis. *International Journal of Economics and Financial Issues*, 5(3), 656–662.

Kartal, M, T. (2020). The Behavior of Sovereign Credit Default Swaps (CDS) Spread: Evidence from Turkey with the Effect of Covid-19 Pandemic. *Quantitive Finance and Economics*, 4/3, 489–502.

Mora, N. (2006). Sovereign Credit Ratings: Guilty Beyond Reasonable Doubt. *Journal of Banking & Finance*, 30, 2041–2062.

Mulder, C. & Perrelli, R., A. (2001). Foreign Currency Credit ratings for Emerging Market Economics, IMF Working Paper, No. 01/ 191.

OECD (2020a). Government Financial Management and Reporting in Times of Crisis, https://www.oecd-ilibrary.org/social-issues-migration-health/government-financial-management-and-reporting-in-times-of-crisis_3f87c7d8-en, Access date 15.05.2021.

OECD Health Statistics (2020b). Eurostat Database; WHO Global Health Expenditure Database.

Reusens, C. & Croux, C., (2017). Sovereign Credit Rating Determinants: A Comparison Before and After the European Debt Crisis. *Journal of Banking and Finance*, 77, 108–121.

Tran, Y., Vu, H., Klusak, P., Kramer, M. & Hoang, T., (2021). Leading from Behind: Sovereign Credit Ratings during COVID-19 Pandemic. https://ssrn.com/abstract=3809701.

Yılmaz, H. H. (2016). Quality Problem in Fiscal Adjustment of Stabilization Programs Implemented in Turkey after 2000, Ph.D. Thesis.

Çetin Arslan

Eylül Erdem

The Evaluation of the Measures Taken Within the Scope of the Covid-19 Pandemic in Turkey in Terms of Misdemeanor and Criminal Law

Introduction

On March 11, 2020, Covid-19 disease was declared as a pandemic by the World Health Organization (WHO, 2020).

Due to the dynamic nature and widespread global effects of the Covid-19 pandemic, the implications of the issue on various disciplines such as health, economics, politics, and law are widely explored. However, of course, at this stage, there is no summative study in terms of the final results of the problem as the subject is still current. The effects of the Covid-19 pandemic on the discipline of criminal law are also discussed and examined by academic circles at various academic events. It is understood that the studies carried out in this context are generally focused on determining the relationship between the Covid-19 pandemic and the current criminal law regulations, evaluating and improving the effectiveness of criminal law methods in the fight against the epidemic. In our study, the resources that can be accessed via the Internet and dealing with the relationship between the Covid-19 pandemic and criminal law were used mostly.

In this study, with the research made with the formal-logical method, the legal framework of the measures taken within the scope of combating the Covid-19 epidemic in Turkey and the consequences of non-compliance with these measures in terms of misdemeanor law and criminal law will be examined. In this context, in the first part of the study, it will be revealed that the measures taken within the scope of combating the Covid-19 epidemic in Turkey have no legal basis. The application of the Supreme Court on the subject will be explained later. Finally, the consequences of not complying with the measures taken in terms of combating the Covid-19 epidemic will be evaluated in terms of criminal law and misdemeanor law provisions, which we consider as a sub-discipline of criminal law.

I. The Legal Framework of the Measures Taken in the Scope of Combatıng against the Covıd-19 in Turkey

The aims of the Turkish Penal Code are explained in the first article of the Code. Accordingly, one of the aims of the Code is to protect public health. Again, in the first article of the misdemeanor law, which is a part of the criminal law legislation, it is stated that one of the purposes of the Code is to protect general health.

It goes without saying that public health is at great risk during the COVID-19 pandemic. In this case, it is necessary to take some measures in order to reduce the risks posed by the epidemic. These measures prohibit citizens from engaging in behaviours that endanger public health during the epidemic process. Undoubtedly, in order for these behaviours to be subject to criminal law sanctions, they must first be regulated by law. As a matter of fact, article 7 of the European Convention on Human Rights ("ECHR"), article 38 of the Constitution of the Republic of Turkey ("CS") and article 2 of the TPC clearly adopt the principle of "lawfulness in crime and punishment". In this case, an act that is not explicitly regulated as a crime in the law cannot be considered a crime, no matter how harmful the consequences are for public health. It should be noted that the principle of legality, which is universally accepted with regard to criminal law, is also valid in terms of misdemeanors (Akbulut, 2021: 6–34). As a matter of fact, although the content of the framework provision determined by the law in terms of scope and conditions regarding which acts constitute misdemeanor, unlike the criminal law, can be filled with the general and regulatory actions of the administration, the type, duration and amount of the sanctions against misdemeanor can only be determined by law (ML art. 4/2).

Based on this, in order to determine whether criminal law sanctions can be applied in case of violation of the measures taken within the extent of combating the epidemic, it is necessary to determine the legal framework of the measures applied first.

Since the beginning of the pandemic in Turkey, the measures to be taken regarding the regulation of daily life within the scope of combating the epidemic are primarily recommended by the Coronavirus Science Board. The Board was established as an advisory board on 10 January 2020 under the Ministry of Health (2021).

In the President's Cabinet consisting of the President, vice-presidents and ministers, the recommendations of the Board are discussed and the measures to be implemented within the scope of combating the epidemic are decided. After the decisions taken by the Cabinet are announced to the public by the President through the press, the Ministry of Interior sends a circular announcing these decisions to the governorships of 81 provinces in the country. Provincial Public

Health Assemblies, established under the governorship of each province, take and implement measures in line with the circular of the Ministry of Internal Affairs. The issue of how the measures within the scope of combating the epidemic were taken was expressed in this way in the Ministry of Internal Affairs Circular dated 01.06.2021. When the circulars published by the Ministry of Internal Affairs are examined, it is seen that the expression of *taking the decisions of the Provincial/ District Public Health Assemblies immediately, pursuant to Articles 27 and 72 of the General Public Health Law*.[1] In that respect, all the measures taken within the scope of combating the pandemic in Turkey are decided by the Provincial Health Assemblies in line with the circulars of the Ministry of Internal Affairs. These decisions are mostly announced by publishing on the governorships' websites. When the aforementioned decisions are considered, it is understood that the contents of the decisions mostly consist of enumerating the measures specified in the Ministry of Internal Affairs' Circular. However, it appears that the majority of the decisions published on the governorships' official websites do not include the signatures of the members of the Assembly, and it is not stated whether the decision was taken unanimously or by majority of votes.[2] Briefly, it is understood that the decisions of the Assembly, which are the source of the measures to be implemented on a provincial basis, are presented to the public without the formal elements. When the relevant decisions are reviewed, it is seen that the sanctions to be applied against the people who do not comply with the injunction orders are also mentioned in the last part of the decisions. Accordingly, in accordance with Article 282 of the Public Health Law, Article 32 of the Misdemeanor Law No. 5236, Article 66 of the Provincial Administration Law, or the offense regulated in Article 195 of the Turkish Penal Code No. 5237, for those who do not comply with the measures in the decisions appears to be punishable.[3] It should be noted that the mentioned articles are the common articles mentioned in the Assembly resolutions, and at least one of the provisions listed in each resolution is requested to be implemented. Although, there are also decisions in which the implementation of more than one or all of the aforementioned articles is stated.[4]

---

1 See as an e.g. https://www.icisleri.gov.tr/81-il-valiligine-kademeli-normallesme-tedbirleri-genelgesi-gonderildi

2 See for e.g. http://www.ankara.gov.tr/kurumlar/ankara.gov.tr/Ankara2021/UHK-kararlari/UHK2021_31.pdf

3 See for e.g. http://www.istanbul.gov.tr/kurumlar/istanbul.gov.tr/il_Hifzissihha_Meclis_Karari_No_47.pdf

4 See for e.g. http://www.tunceli.gov.tr/tunceli-valiligi-il-umumi-hifzissihha-kurulunun-02032021-tarihli-ve-11-sayili-karari

As can be seen, there is no unity of practice in Turkey regarding which sanctions will be applied in case of violation of the measures taken within the scope of combating the epidemic.

It should be noted that almost all of the measures taken regarding the pandemic have restrictive attributes towards fundamental rights and freedoms. Within this framework, the measures taken within the scope of combating the epidemic such as; The obligation to wear a mask, the curfew and quarantine obligations, the limitation of intercity travel, the abolition of flights to certain countries, the prohibition of travelling abroad for public employees,of worship in worship places, of all kinds of meetings and activities stopping all kinds of scientific and artistic activities, postponement of judicial hearings, suspension of enforcement proceedings, suspending face-to-face education, prohibiting certain businesses from operating and stopping health workers from taking a leave, prohibiting the termination of employment contracts and application of unpaid leave without seeking consent, all of these had resulted in the restriction of personal immunity (CS art. 17), personal freedom (CS art. 19), the freedom of travel (CS art. 23), the freedom of religion and belief (CS art. 24), the freedom of science and arts (CS art. 27), the right to organize meetings (CS art. 34), the right to legal remedies (CS art. 36),the right to education and training (CS art. 42) and the liberty of labour (CS art. 49) (Gözler, 2020).

Of course, there is no doubt that these measures are mandatory in terms of combating the epidemic. So much so that in a situation where public health and personal fundamental rights and freedoms compete, the right that should be prioritized will be the right to public health. However, it is imperative that the measures that seriously interfere with fundamental rights and freedoms should be taken with legal methods. Because in case of non-compliance with these measures, the possibility of imposing sanctions on individuals depends on the compliance of the measure with the law. Even though a measure taken within the context of the epidemic serves a legitimate purpose in terms of content, it cannot be applicable in a state of law unless it is taken by lawful methods. When all these issues are evaluated together, it is understood that the measures taken for combating the COVID-19 disease in Turkey do not have a legal framework. Because, as mentioned above, many measures taken for combating the epidemic restrict fundamental rights and freedoms. In Article 13 of the Constitution; It is stated that *"fundamental rights and freedoms can only be limited by law, depending on the reasons specified in the relevant articles of the Constitution, without touching their essence"*. However, *"these restrictions cannot be contrary to the word and spirit of the Constitution, the requirements of the democratic social order and the secular Republic, and the principle of proportionality."*

As can be seen, it is clearly unconstitutional to limit fundamental rights and freedoms with measures that are not primarily prescribed by law, in other words, they do not derive their source from the law (Aslan, 2020; Gözler, 2020). However, in Article 15 of the Constitution; It is envisaged that restrictive measures regarding fundamental rights and freedoms may be taken in cases of war, mobilization and emergency. In such cases, the obligation to limit the fundamental rights and freedoms by law is no longer required, so in extraordinary cases, fundamental rights and freedoms can be limited with regulation, for example, with a presidential decree. (CS art. 119/6) (Şirin, 2020). However, since a state of emergency has not been declared in Turkey due to the COVID-19 outbreak, this article cannot be applied (Aslan, 2020; Gözler, 2020). In this case, the measures envisaging restrictions on fundamental rights and freedoms must be prescribed by law.

As mentioned above; In Turkey, regarding the measures to be taken about the pandemic, a de facto implementation has developed as follows; The measures which were decided in the Presidential Cabinet and shared by the President through the press are issued in a circular of the Ministry of Internal Affairs and taken and implemented by Provincial Public Health Assemblies. However, this de facto practice is not in accordance with the law since, as mentioned above, all measures that result in the restriction of fundamental rights and freedoms must be prescribed by law. However, there is no legal source of the measures taken in Turkey. There is no legal provision for the measures to be decided by the Presidential Cabinet and announced to the public by the President through the press. First of all, the Presidential Cabinet is not a constitutional organ (Gözler, 2021a). In this case, the council gathered under the name of the Presidential Cabinet has neither advisory nor decision-making power. It is also not legally binding for the President to share the measures taken by this committee, with the public through the press. As a matter of fact, since the Presidential Cabinet is not a council with a legal basis, in other words, since it takes its source only from practice, it is out of question for the measures decided by this board to be published in the Official Gazette. Additionally, the announcement of the Cabinet decisions under the name of a circular by the Ministry of Internal Affairs to the governorships of 81 provinces is also not binding on the citizens. Because circulars are internal letters sent to relevant places and relevant persons for purposes such as guiding the implementation of laws, by-laws and regulations, illuminating any issue, drawing attention to a situation. In this case, circulars do not bind citizens, but institutions (Gözler, 2021b). In line with the circulars issued by the Ministry of Interior, it is also illegal for Provincial Public Health Assemblies to take and implement decisions restricting fundamental rights and freedoms. Because, as mentioned, measures restricting fundamental rights and freedoms can only be enacted by law, not by the decisions of the Assembly established under the Governorship.

II. Practice of the Supreme Court

As mentioned above, there are two types of sanctions in terms of violation of the measures taken by the Provincial Public Health Assemblies regarding the pandemic; either an administrative fine pursuant to Provincial Administration Law art. 66, Misdemeanors Law, art. 32, Public Health Law, art. 282, or imprisonment pursuant to TPC art. 195. In this context, in the decisions of the Assembly, administrative sanction in the context of misdemeanor law or criminal liability within the framework of the crime regulated in TPC art. 195 is foreseen for those who do not comply with the measures. On the other hand, in terms of persons who do not comply with the measures, no decision has been found yet that has passed the Supreme Court's control within the scope of TPC art. 195. Therefore, the explanations regarding the current Supreme Court practice under this title are limited to the decisions subject to administrative sanctions.

In Turkish law, the Supreme Court, as a rule, is the Supreme Court responsible for reviewing appeals. However, first of all, it should be noted that it is not possible for disputes regarding administrative sanction decisions to come before the Court of Cassation within the framework of ordinary legal remedies.

The provisions of the Misdemeanor Law regarding the remedy against administrative sanction decisions are in the nature of public act unless there is a contrary provision in other laws. (ML md. 3/1). In this case, unless there is a contrary provision in the relevant law, an application can be made to the criminal court of peace against the administrative fine and the administrative sanction decision regarding the transfer of the property to public ownership, within 15 days at the latest from the notification or annotation of the decision. If the application is not made within this period, the administrative sanction decision becomes final. (ML md.27/1). In terms of the decisions to be made by the criminal court of peace upon the application, an appeal can be made in accordance with the provisions of the Criminal Procedure Code No. 5271 ("CPC"), (ML. art. 29). The decisions of the appeal authority are final (CPC md.271/4). As can be seen, it is not possible to appeal against decisions subject to administrative sanctions through ordinary legal remedies. These decisions become final in the courts of first instance. On the other hand, decisions subject to administrative sanction can be reviewed by the Supreme Court through extraordinary legal remedies through reversing for the benefit of the law (CPC art. 309).

Below, the events that were the subject of three different decisions brought before the Court of Cassation with the method described above will be explained.

In the case subject to the first decision (19th Criminal Chamber, 09.11.2020, 4354/14250); An administrative fine of 392.00 TL was imposed on the person who went out without a mask, in accordance with Article 32 of the Misdemeanor Law.[5]

In the cases subject to the second and third decisions (19. Criminal Chamber, 14.12.2020, 5699/19579-19. Criminal Chamber, 14.12.2020, 5700/19580); An administrative fine of 900.00 TL has been imposed on persons who wear masks in accordance with the standards, without covering their mouth and nose, in accordance with Article 282 of the Public Health Law No. 1593.

The objections made by the culpables for the annulment of the decisions were examined by the Bolu Criminal Court of Peace, which is the first instance court. In all three applications, for similar reasons and in summary; According to the 13th and 19th articles of the Constitution, the freedom of the person cannot be restricted without a court decision, the General Hygiene Law No. 1593 does not include the obligation to wear a mask, a person who has to be outside 12 hours a day should change 3–4 masks a day, and this has a certain financial burden. It has decided to accept the objections on the grounds that the Constitution states that the Republic of Turkey is a social state, that the state must meet this financial burden, but there is no such practice, and therefore people cannot be obliged to wear masks. Decisions became final without appeal or appeal.

The Ministry of Justice, which ruled that the aforementioned provisions were unlawful, sent a notice to the Office of the Chief Public Prosecutor of the Court of Cassation to apply for reversing in accordance with CMK art. 309. In the notice, it was requested that the judgement be reversed on the grounds that there is no scientific basis for the assessment that *the obligation to wear masks in the judgment of the judge imposes financial burden on individuals.*

As a result of the examination, the Supreme Court made a joint assessment of all three decisions as follows;

Pursuant to Article 27 of the General Public Health Law No. 1593, the measures listed in Article 72 of the Law within the scope of combating epidemic disease can be taken by the Provincial Public Health Assemblies, the obligation to wear a mask is not among these measures, but the measures that the Assembly can take are not limited to those listed in this article. Law No. 5442

---

5   See. Decisions of Bolu Criminal Judgeship of Peace dated 29.06.2020 and numbered 2020/1604, dated dated 06/07/2020 and numbered 2020/1914, 07/07/2020 and numbered 2020/1915, dated 06/07/2020 and numbered 2020/1914

on Provincial Administration, which regulates that the Governors will execute the decisions of the assembly in Article 28 of the Law, that the Governors must duly announce to the people living throughout the province that the decisions of the Assembly are complied with, and that in case of failure, Article 32 of the Misdemeanors Law No. 66/1 of Article 32 of the Misdemeanor Law No. 5326 is regulated for those who do not comply with the orders issued by the governors based on the authority given by the laws. He evaluated that the misdemeanor of violating the order regulated in Article 32 would occur, and that there would be no misdemeanor without a duly made announcement. Again, it was stated that the authority to decide on administrative fines within the scope of the Law belongs to the Governor, that the administrative sanction cannot be applied by law enforcement officers, and the decision was reversed in terms of the afore-mentioned issues. On the other hand, the Court of Cassation has also made it a reason to overturn the issue that the Law No. 1593 cannot be applied in the second and third case decisions. The decisions of the 19th Penal Chamber of the Court of Cassation were appealed by the Office of the Chief Public Prosecutor of the Court of Cassation in accordance with CPC art. 308.[6] In the aforementioned objections, it is stated that the examinations to be made within the scope of CPC art. 309 should be limited to the request, that it is unlawful for the Chamber to make the grounds for reversing the issues other than the ones requested to be reversed, and in terms of the ex officio determined reasons for the reversal, the Ministry of Justice is informed to apply for the reversal for the benefit of the law. It was also stated that in the cases in dispute, the Sanitary Law No. 1593 should be applied, not the Article 32 of the Law on Misdemeanors, that there is no obli-gation to announce in this context and that it is possible to apply the penalties by the law enforcement.

The 19th Penal Chamber of the Court of Cassation, with its decisions dated 25.01.2021 and numbered 627/465, 628/466, 267/464, accepted the objections of the Chief Public Prosecutor of the Court of Cassation and abolished the annul-ment decisions and accepted that action should be taken pursuant to Article 282 of the Public Health Law. However, when the aforementioned Supreme Court decisions are examined, it is understood that the decisions subject to the change of opinion do not contain sufficient justification, and it is sufficient to refer to the reasons in the appeal of the Office of the Chief Public Prosecutor of the Court of

---

6   See. Appeals of the Chief Public Prosecutor's Office of the Supreme Court of Appeals dated 31.12.2020 and numbered KD-2020/75964, dated 12.01.2021 and numbered KD-2020/91873, dated 12.01.2021 and numbered KD-2020/92275

Cassation. It should be noted that this situation is contrary to Article 141 of the Constitution, which includes the provision that all decisions of all courts shall be written with justification. Because, although Supreme Audit courts can make judgements in reference to first instance court judgements containing sufficient justification, even this situation is criticized in the doctrine. In addition, considering that the extraordinary legal remedies damage the reliability of the final judgement, we believe that it is not correct for the legal precedent change to be the source of a uniform application throughout the country to be unjustified.

III. Our Evaluation in Terms of Misdemeanor Law

As can be seen after these general explanations, it is controversial whether administrative sanctions can be applied to individuals in case of violation of the measures taken within the framework of the COVID-19 epidemic, and if so, under which law it will be applied. As mentioned above, while the Court of Cassation was of the opinion that administrative sanctions could be applied in line with the misdemeanor of the violation of the order regulated in ML art. 32, it decided that article 282 of the Law No. 1593 would be applied by amending its legal precedent in a short time. In the following, it will be evaluated whether both faults will occur in terms of their elements.

A. Misdemeanor of Opposing the Order (Ml Art. 32)

The misdemeanor of violation of the order was regulated in Article 32 of the ML. The said arrangement is as follows:

Article 32 –

1. *An administrative fine of one hundred Turkish liras shall be imposed on a person who violates the lawful order given by the competent authorities due to judicial proceedings or for the purpose of protecting public security, public order or general health. This penalty is decided by the authority that issued the order.*
2. *This article can only be applied in cases where there is an explicit provision in the relevant law.*

In the second paragraph of the misdemeanor, it is stated that this article can only be applied in cases where there is a clear provision in the relevant law. In this case, it is not possible for the perpetrator to be punished for misconduct, unless the relevant law clearly states that this article will be applied.

The material subject of the misdemeanor is the orders given by the competent authorities in accordance with the law due to *judicial proceedings or for the protection of public security, public order or general health.*

In regards to the orders that do not meet the aforementioned conditions, it cannot be said that the misdemeanor is formed in terms of the material subject.

The fact that the order is given by the competent authority means that there is no usurpation of function, usurpation of authority or infringement of authority. In other words, if the authority giving the order is not legally authorized to give this order, even if the order is appropriate in terms of purpose and content, no misdemeanor will occur.

The order must have been given for the purposes specified in the law. In this case, not every order given by the competent authorities, but orders aimed at protecting certain legal values constitute the material subject of the crime.

The lawfulness of the order means that it complies with the entire legal order. In this case, there is no fault for anyone who does not fulfil an unlawful order in terms of authority, form, reason, subject, purpose or other aspects.

It should be noted that although it is stated in the justification of the article that the order constituting the subject of the misdemeanor must have also been announced by the competent authority, the justification is not included in the text of the law. On the other hand, it is a requirement of the principle of certainty that the wrongful order be known and understood by the addressees.

The criminal act is to act in violation of the lawful order given by the competent authority. A certain behaviour may be ordered by the authority to "do" or "not do" in a certain way. In this context, misdemeanor can be committed with an executive action or negligence (ML art. 7). Such that, a misdemeanor will be committed with an executive act in the case of performing a behaviour prohibited by the competent authority, and with a negligent act in case of not performing a behaviour ordered by the competent authority. For example, neglecting to wear a mask means to act contrary to the order by negligence while to act against the curfew means to act against the order by execution.

As a result of these general statements, we are of the opinion that in case of violation of the measures taken by the Provincial Health Assemblies, a misconduct will not occur. Because, although it is foreseen to impose administrative sanctions in line with the misconduct in terms of acts regulated in various articles of the Law (see: art. 287, 291, 299, 301), acting contrary to the decisions of the Provincial Hygiene Council is not considered within the scope of these articles. For the explained reason, since there is no direct reference to ML art. 32 within the scope of Law No. 1593, the article does not have the ability to apply primarily for this reason (ML md.32/2).

On the other hand, it should be emphasized that, as seen in practice and the Supreme Court decision, the Provincial Administration Law No. 5442

(5442 S.K.), it is not possible to apply the misdemeanor of violating the order. In practice, it is understood that the following articles of the aforementioned Law are based on the administrative fines imposed within the scope of ML art. 32.

5442 S.K. art. 9-ç ;*"Governors can issue general orders and announce them in order to use the authority given by the law, Presidential decree and other legislation and to fulfill the duties imposed by them."*

5442 S.K. art. 11-c; *"Providing peace and security, inviolability of the person, security in terms of disposition, public welfare and preventive law enforcement authority within the borders of the province are among the duties and duties of the governor. To ensure these, the governor takes the necessary decisions and measures. The provisions of Article 66 shall apply to those who do not comply with the decisions and measures taken and announced in this regard."*

5442 S.K. art. 66;*"…Those who oppose the implementation and execution of the decisions and measures promulgated or promulgated pursuant to the authority given by the laws by the provincial general assembly or administrative boards or the highest civil authorities, or those who show difficulties or do not comply with the provisions of Article 32 of the Misdemeanor Law, by the local civilian authority. punished accordingly …"*

In this framework, the governor's authority to issue general orders is regulated in Article 9 of the Law, the governor's authority to take decisions and measures to ensure public well-being is regulated in Article 11, and the sanctions to be imposed on those who do not comply with the measures taken within the framework of the provincial general administration are regulated in Article 66.

As can be seen, it is clearly stated in Article 66 of the Law that ML art. 32 will be applied (ML art. 32/2). However, this article may be applied to persons who do not comply with the decisions taken by the provincial general assembly, provincial administrative boards or the highest civilian authority. However, all of the measures to be implemented on a provincial basis during the COVID-19 epidemic were taken by the Provincial Public Health Assemblies. Although the Governor presides over this Assembly and although the Assembly is in charge of executing its decisions, it is not possible to evaluate the Assembly's decisions, which are in the nature of a collective action, as a general order or decision of the governor, which is a simple-willed action. In this context, we do not agree with the view of the Court of Cassation that ML art. 32 can be applied for those who do not comply with these decisions, if the decisions of the Assembly are duly announced by the Governor. Because the mere announcement of the decisions of the Assembly cannot be considered as a "general order" as stipulated in Article 9 of the Law No. 5442. Again, the announcement of the decisions of the Assembly cannot be considered in accordance with the law within the scope of

Article 11. Because the powers given to the Governor within the scope of Article 11 should not be interpreted broadly to allow taking measures restricting fundamental rights and freedoms (Akbulut, 2021; Şirin, 2020). Otherwise, it will be clearly contrary to Article 13 of the Constitution.

B. Misdemeanor of Objection to Public Health Law (Phl Art. 282)

The Public Health Law No. 1593, which started with the provisions of combating infectious and epidemic diseases, entered into force on 6.05.1930. In the context of our work, the provisions on combating epidemics are regulated in the 57th and following articles of the Law, and acting in violation of these measures is subject to an administrative fine as a misdemeanor. The relevant article of the law is as follows:

Article 282 – (amended: 23/1/2008-5728/48 art.)

Those who act contrary to the prohibitions written in this law or do not comply with the obligations, are punished with an administrative fine from two hundred and fifty Turkish liras to one thousand Turkish liras, unless their acts also constitute a crime. Misdemeanor is typical in terms of measures regulated under Law No. 1593.

In this context, the material subject of the misdemeanor consists of the measures regulated in the Law No. 1593. Measures regulated in connection with our working subject within the scope of the Law are counted as a limitation in Article 72 of the Law, and it is stated that these measures can be applied in terms of diseases listed as a limitation in Article 57 of the Law.

However, in article 64 of the Law, it is stipulated that in the event of an epidemic disease other than those listed in article 57, the Ministry of Health will declare the disease as an epidemic and be authorized to implement all or some of the measures regulated in the Law.

In such a case, in case of an epidemic disease other than those listed in Article 57, the measures implemented by the Ministry of Health will also constitute the material subject of the misdemeanor. In this context, the COVID-19 disease can be considered within the scope of Article 64 of the Law. However, it should be noted that the measures taken within the scope of the COVID-19 disease have been taken by the Provincial Health Councils, not the Ministry of Health, since the beginning of the epidemic, in accordance with Article 64. The act that gives rise to misdemeanor is to act contrary to the prohibitions written in the law numbered 1593 or not to comply with the obligations. In this context, misdemeanor can be committed by executive action or by negligence. The measures that can be taken within the scope of combating the epidemic are regulated in Article 72 of the Law. In this context, acting contrary to these measures will constitute the act of misdemeanor. The measures regulated in the aforementioned article are as follows:

- Keeping people who are sick or suspected of being ill under quarantine in their homes or health institutions,
- Administration of serum or vaccine to those who are sick or exposed to the disease,
- Disinfecting people, things, buildings and other things that carry germs,
- Extermination of disease-producing vermin and animal,
- Inspection of travellers at certain points and disinfecting their belongings,
- Prohibition of consumption of foodstuffs that cause disease,
- Evacuation of public places where the epidemic has started until the danger has passed.

Within the framework of all these explanations, it is understood that if the measures decided by the Public Health Council are violated, the misdemeanor regulated in Article 282 of the Law will not occur. Because although the orders given by the Provincial Public Health Council within the scope of combating the COVID-19 epidemic have the purpose of protecting general health, these Assemblies do not have the authority to give orders restricting fundamental rights and freedoms. Because measures restricting fundamental rights and freedoms cannot be considered lawful unless they are taken in accordance with the procedures in Articles 13 or 15 of the Constitution. As a matter of fact, the measures that the Assembly may decide within the scope of combating the epidemic are listed in Article 72 of the Law.

When the measures in the article are examined, it is understood that almost none of the restrictions applied in Turkey are within the scope of the article. Because the measures regulated in the Law No. 1930 foresee appropriate measures to combat the epidemic diseases of that period. In this context, we are of the opinion that the Court of Cassation's opinion that the Assembly may order other measures, such as the obligation to wear a mask, apart from the measures listed in Article 72, is contrary to the prohibition of comparison.

IV. Our Evaluation in Terms of Criminal Law

As mentioned above, in the decisions of the Provincial Health Council, it is stated that legal action will be taken against persons who do not comply with the measures taken within the scope of combating epidemics, within the scope of the crime of violating the measures regarding infectious diseases regulated in Article 195 of the TPC. The said arrangement is as follows:

Article 195- (1) A person who does not comply with the measures taken by the competent authorities to quarantine the place where a person who has caught or died from one of the contagious diseases is located, is sentenced to imprisonment from two months to one year.

The legal interest protected by crime is the protection of public health. The act element of the crime consists of not complying with the measures taken by the competent authorities to quarantine the place where the person who has caught one of the infectious diseases or died from these diseases is located. In this context, for the crime to occur;

- Must be a person who has contracted or died from one of the infectious diseases,
- The place where this person is located must be quarantined by the competent authorities,
- The measures taken by the competent authorities regarding quarantine should not be followed (Arslan & Azizağaoğlu, 2004).

What should be understood from the quarantine within the scope of the article is the protection measures taken in the form of isolating "the place where a person who has caught one of the contagious diseases or died from these diseases is located".

As can be seen, TPC art. 195 is a type of crime with a very limited area of application. Indeed, although the title of the article is "crime of violating the measures regarding communicable diseases", the actual element of the crime is a violation of the measures that can only be applied to the quarantined regions. For this reason, when there is a violation of the measures taken within the framework of the COVID-19 epidemic in Turkey, it is clear that this crime will not occur due to its elements (in a similar direction, Kahraman, 2020). In addition, crime can only come up in terms of measures given by the competent authorities (Bayzit, 2020). As explained above, Provincial Health Assemblies do not have the authority to take measures restricting fundamental rights and freedoms, so the provision cannot be applied in this aspect.

Conclusion

Each country has produced different legal remedies in terms of combating the COVID-19 epidemic, which affects the whole world. In this context, some countries have managed the legal process within the scope of the state of emergency, some have made arrangements in their existing laws, and some have enacted new laws to meet the needs brought by the epidemic (Evran Topuzkanamış,

2020). It should be noted with regret that Turkey did not resort to any of these methods and preferred to carry out the process with the current regulations. However, the current regulations in our law do not allow taking measures that result in restriction of fundamental rights and freedoms within the scope of combating the epidemic. For this reason, in Turkey, regarding the measures to be taken about the pandemic, a de facto implementation has developed as follows; The measures which were decided in the Presidential Cabinet and shared by the President through the press are issued in a circular of the Ministry of Internal Affairs and taken and implemented by Provincial Public Health Assemblies. This practice is unconstitutional.

The illegality of the measures taken within the scope of combating the epidemic makes it impossible to apply the law of misdemeanor and criminal law sanctions in case of violation of these measures. This situation, of course, constitutes a weakness within the scope of the fight against the epidemic. First of all, there is no unity of practice regarding the scope of the law under which administrative sanctions will be applied to those who violate the measures. The approach of the Court of Cassation, which is expected to provide a unity of jurisprudence on the subject, is criticizable. Because, the Court of Cassation first predicted that administrative sanctions would be applied in accordance with ML art. 32 for those who violated the measures, and then decided that Article 282 of the Law No. 1593 would be applied. It is not appropriate that the Supreme Court's case-law change is unjustified. Moreover, there is no possibility of administrative sanctions under both laws for those who violate the measures.

The Turkish Penal Code, which came into force in 2005, gives its first test in terms of protecting public health during the epidemic. In the decisions of the Provincial Health Council, it is stated that Article 195 of the TPC should be applied for those who do not comply with the measures. However, the relevant provision has a very limited scope of application and there is no application area in terms of the measures taken in Turkey.

In accordance with the crime policy followed, if criminal law sanctions are deemed necessary within the scope of combating the epidemic, it is clear that there is a need for revision in the legal regulations. However, in our opinion, the truer thing in this case would be to prepare a new law in accordance with the experiences gained during the epidemic and the emerging needs and to include criminal law sanctions in this law. Unfortunately, while it is possible to amend the relevant law and to prepare a new law that meets the needs of the period, it is not understandable to try to expand the provisions of the 1930 Public Health Law by analogy.

References

Akbulut, B. (2021). Kabahatler Hukukunda Kanunilik İlkesi ve Covid-19 Nedeniyle Alınan Tedbirlere Aykırılık. Ceza Hukuku ve Kriminoloji Dergisi, 1–57. https://doi.org/10.26650/JPLC2020-837085

Arslan, Ç., & Azizağaoğlu, B. (2004). *Yeni Türk Ceza Kanunu Şerhi*. Ankara: Asil Yayın, Dağıtım Ltd. Şti.

Aslan, V. (2020). COVID-19 Salgını Sebebiyle Uygulanan Sokağa Çıkma Kısıtlamalarının 1982 Anayasası'na Uygunluğu . İstanbul Hukuk Mecmuası, 78(2), 809–835. DOI: 10.26650/mecmua.2020.78.2.0018

Bayzit, T. (2020). Bulaşıcı Hastalıklara İlişkin Tedbirlere Aykırı Davranma Suçu (TCK m. 195). Lexpera Blog. https://blog.lexpera.com.tr/bulasici-hastalikl ara-iliskin-tedbirlere-aykiri-davranma-sucu-tck-m-195/.

Evran, Topuzkanamış, Ş. (2020). Olağanüstü Zamanlarda Anayasa Hukuku. Lexpera Blog. https://blog.lexpera.com.tr/olaganustu-zamanlarda-anayasa-hukuku/.

Gözler, K. (2020, Temmuz 6). Korona Virüs Salgınıyla Mücadele İçin Alınan Tedbirler Hukuka Uygun mu? (2). www.anayasa.gen.tr/korona-2.htm

Gözler, K. (2021a, Mayıs 14). Genelge Devleti: Hukukta Şeklin Önemi Üzerine. www.anayasa.gen.tr/genelge-devleti.htm

Gözler, K. (2021b, Mayıs 16). "Cumhurbaşkanlığı Kabinesi: Var mı Böyle Bir Şey?" https://www.anayasa.gen.tr/cb-kabinesi.htm

Kahraman, R. (2020). The Crime of Violating the Measures Related to Infectious Diseases (TCC Art 195). *Istanbul Law Review*, 78(2), 737–767. https://doi. org/10.26650/mecmua.2020.78.2.0016

Şirin, M. C. (2020). Fransa'da Covıd-19 ile Mücadele Kapsamında Ulusal Düzeyde Alınan Kolluk Tedbirlerinin Hukuki Rejimi: İlk İzlenimler. İstanbul Üniversitesi Hukuk Fakültesi Mecmuası, 78(2). 1009–1046. https://dergipark. org.tr/tr/pub/ihm/issue/57316/812472

www.who.int

www.wikipedia.com.tr

www.icisleri.gov.tr

www.ankara.gov.tr

www.istanbul.gov.tr

www.tunceli.gov

Ayşe Nil Tosun

Oytun Canyaş

Necati Nurcalı

A Comparative Analysis of Taxation Practices during the COVID-19 Pandemic in Turkey and Selected OECD Countries

Introduction

COVID-19 first appeared in a group of patients in the city of Wuhan, China, in December 2019, causing respiratory symptoms. On March 11, 2020, the World Health Organization declared COVID-19 a global pandemic. As it spreads rapidly globally, the pandemic has damaged many economic units at all scales. Consumption and investment spending are falling while the production chain network is suffering. The pandemic has brought unprecedented challenges to the lives of many people worldwide. Unemployment, and therefore poverty, has increased, with small-scale enterprises particularly at risk of collapse. States have had to rapidly take many steps to support their citizens and businesses during these difficult times to mitigate the impact of these sudden and profound shocks on individual households, businesses, and the wider economy. However, without state economic support, full or partial lockdowns to overcome the pandemic will clearly be catastrophic for businesses and their employees because of the need to cover fixed costs while they remain closed. To overcome such problems, states have offered various solutions, such as direct financial aid programs for the people facing these challenges. These programs usually include financial aid for citizens, employers, and the working class, such as new unemployment benefits for all households with an income below a certain level, individuals who lost their jobs, unemployed students and recent graduates, self-employed citizens suffering from reduced demand as a result of lockdown measures, employer subsidies so that businesses do not lay off workers, and subsidies for companies at risk of bankruptcy due to liquidity problems.

The COVID-19 pandemic has created many new issues that need research, such as the economic losses caused by the recession due to the pandemic (Carletti et al., 2020:534; Chernick et al., 2020:699), the pandemic's specific impact on different sectors (Munavar et al., 2021:1), the measures needed to protect small and medium-sized enterprises (Lu et al., 2020:323; McGeever et al., 2020:1; Tian, 2020:75), and the short-term and long-term measures to be taken during the pandemic (Collier et al., 2020:794; Devereux et al., 2020:225). Thus, the subject is wide-ranging and current. Taxation policies implemented to respond to the COVID-19 pandemic can be added to this list. The pandemic has halted many economic sectors, which has created a panic. However, taxation policies can provide effective, albeit short-term solutions. States have also turned to taxation policies to combat the effects of the pandemic by introducing various tax measures to the extent of their financial organization and financial means.

The extraordinary situation caused by the COVID-19 pandemic has required many changes in taxation policies. The new normal has changed consumption habits and the composition of direct tax revenue. For example, remote working has reduced tax revenue from sales of goods and services like gas, travel tickets, and clothing. To compensate for tax losses due to the pandemic (Clemens &Veuger, 2020:619; Coffey et al., 2020:14–15), governments have proposed various new taxes, such as a minimum tax on the total profits of international companies and a COVID-19 income tax (Karnon, 2020:335; Laffitte et al., 2020:1). While fighting the pandemic, states have had to waive some normal taxes, so additional revenue is needed to solve the liquidity problems of both households and business sectors.

The main purpose of this study is to comparatively investigate how taxation policies have been used in Turkey and various other countries to overcome the pandemic with minimum economic damage, to identify differences, and to identify the effective policies. The study is limited to corporate tax, income tax, and social security legislation, VAT, and other consumption taxes since tax legislation is very comprehensive and varies significantly between countries. This study firstly addresses Turkish Tax Law regulations due to the COVID-19 pandemic before comparing them to those in selected countries. Their regulations are analysed based on information in the OECD's report, Tax Policy Reform 2021 (Special edition on Tax Policy during the COVID-19 Pandemic). The OECD collected data in 66 countries for 2020 and early 2021 from a survey (the OECD Tax Policy Reform Questionnaire).

I. Evaluation of New Regulations in Turkish Tax Law due to the Covid-19 Pandemic

According to the first paragraph of Article 73 of the Turkish Constitution,[1] taxation power in Turkish Law is exercised to "finance public expenditure". That

---

1   Article 73/1 of the Constitution: "Everyone is under the obligation to pay taxes according to their financial resources, in order to meet public expenditures."

is, taxation power is used for fiscal purposes (Turhan, 1987: 38; Akdoğan, 2009:121). However, both doctrine (Turhan, 1987, 39–45; Akdoğan, 2009:123) and jurisprudence indicates that the concept of public expenditure should not be interpreted narrowly (Çağan, 1980:172; Öncel et al., 2019:61). Rather, taxation power can be used as a tool to achieve non-fiscal goals to fulfil the duties entrusted to the State by the Constitution (Çağan, 1980: 145; Göker, 2011: 15–16). Thus, taxation power can be exercised for various purposes: to ensure that private enterprises operate in accordance with national economic requirements and social objectives, and in conditions of security and stability, as stipulated in Article 48/2 of the Constitution; to ensure they take necessary measures to raise workers' living standards; to protect workers to improve labour conditions; to promote labour; and to create suitable economic conditions to minimize unemployment, as stipulated in Article 49 of the Constitution. More examples can be provided here.[2]

It is also not unconstitutional for the state to make regulations that change tax laws, such as exceptions, discounts, exemptions, rates, or formal duties, to perform these duties. That is, the State can exercise its taxation power for extra-fiscal purposes. As Constitutional Court Decision E:1967/41, K: 1969/57 puts it:

> The execution of the social and economic development plan is among the duties entrusted to the state pursuant to Articles 41 and 129 of the Constitution, in other words, the public works stipulated by the Constitution. Giving loans to the private sector that will help with these works, to a certain extent, does not mean that state expenses that are covered by taxes are spent for purposes other than public works, and the law principle authorizing such expenditure cannot be contrary to Article 61 of the Constitution.

Here, the Constitutional Court considers State regulations in tax laws to fulfil its constitutional duties as norms established to "meet public expenditure", as stipulated in Article 73/1 of the Constitution. Hence, it did not consider them unconstitutional.

The negative impact of the COVID-19 pandemic on the economic life of taxpayers in all countries, including Turkey, has reduced their ability to pay taxes and fulfil their formal tax obligations. Accordingly, certain material and formal tax duties in Turkey have been deferred since the pandemic began while certain taxpayer groups affected by the pandemic have been supported. Furthermore, the State exercised its taxation power to fulfil its constitutional duties, just like

---

2   The taxation power can also be exercised, for example, to protect the family, as stipulated in Article 41, or ensure the right to education and training, as stipulated in Article 42.

its duty to ensure that private enterprises operate in accordance with national economic requirements and social objectives, as stipulated in Article 48/2 of the Constitution.

This study therefore first identifies the new measures and incentives introduced under the Turkish Tax Law due to the pandemic to compare these with OECD countries. To make a full comparison, this part is not confined to measures and incentives regarding taxes due to financial obligations but also includes social security payments. These are described as "similar financial obligations" in Article 73/3 of the Constitution. This is because social security payments, which are financial obligations, are also included as "similar financial obligations" in Article 73/3 of the Constitution. Thus, they fall within the scope of tax law in a broad sense.

A. Corporate Tax

In Turkey, income is taxed in two ways: income tax and corporate tax, with no separate business tax. Upon the examination of the regulations made in corporate tax to reduce or postpone tax dues due to the Pandemic; it is safe to say that firstly, there was facilitation in filing tax returns and tax payment deadlines. Pursuant to Article 14/1-3 of the Corporate Tax Law, annual corporate tax returns should be filed with the tax office of the taxpayer by the evening of April 25th, following the month in which the accounting period closed. Pursuant to the first paragraph of Article 21 of the same law, it should be paid by April 30th. During the pandemic, one of the government's first measures was to extend the deadline for filing of corporate tax returns for the 2019 accounting period and payment of taxes accrued on these returns to end of day April 30, 2020, and end of day Monday, June 1, 2020, respectively. Similarly, the deadlines for filing income and corporate provisional tax returns for the first provisional tax period of 2021 (January-February-March) and payment of the taxes accrued on these returns were extended from end of day May 17, 2021 until end of day Monday, May 31, 2021.

In addition, the government introduced provisions to reduce the burden of tax and secondary public receivables on taxpayers. Under Law No. 7256 on the Restructuring of Certain Receivables and the Making Amendments on Certain Laws, which entered into force on November 16, 2020[3] the government stopped collecting certain public receivables. For example, pursuant to Article 2/1-a of

---

3   The enactment date of the provisions of Law No. 7256 are provided in Article 45 of the same law.

Law No. 7256, auxiliary public receivables, such as late interest rates and delay penalties, and all tax penalties based on the principle tax debt and late interest, including those whose original was paid before the effective date of this law, were waived, provided that the amount calculated based on the Domestic Price Index at the publication date of the law was paid instead of all the unpaid portion of the taxes that had accrued but was not yet paid or whose payment deadline had not yet expired, and auxiliary receivables, such as late interest and delay penalties.

It should be noted that not all the new corporate tax regulations during the pandemic favoured taxpayers. In order to finance increased public spending due to the pandemic, the government increased the corporate tax rate in both 2021 and 2022. Specifically, having been 20 %, pursuant to Provisional Article 13 added to the Corporate Tax Law No. 5520, it increased to 25 % for corporate earnings for the 2021 taxation period and 23 % for the 2022 taxation period. However, the general communiqué of May 25, 2021, announced a 2-point discount for businesses offered to the public at a rate of at least 20 % in order for them to be traded for the first time on the Borsa Istanbul Equity Market.

B. Income Tax and Social Security Legislation

The government also introduced facilitating measures for certain taxpayer groups regarding income tax and social security payments (premiums, deductions, etc.), which are duty-like financial obligations. The tax administration's approach here contrasted with that for corporate tax. More specifically, it declared a force majeure event, as provided for in the Tax Procedure Law, for taxpayers adversely affected by the pandemic (and for social security payments). Accordingly, instead of adjusting tax return filing and payment periods for these taxes, it simply deferred the tax duties.

Here, we should first consider the power of the Tax Administration to declare a force majeure event in order to explain the new regulations. The Turkish Tax Law defines "force majeure" in Article 13 and other articles of the Tax Procedure Law No. 213 (TPL). According to the TPL, once force majeure is accepted, the statute of limitations and other periods for the taxpayer (and those responsible) do not apply, and no tax penalty can be imposed due to failure to fulfil tax obligations during this period (TPL Articles 15 and 373). The COVID-19 pandemic can be considered a force majeure for various reasons stipulated in Article 13. It can also be considered under Article 12, which defines force majeure as taxpayers and those responsible being exposed to "disasters such as fire, earthquake, and flooding that will prevent the fulfillment of their tax duties" or failure to fulfil the tax obligations due to "compulsory absences that occur beyond the will of the person".

The Ministry of Finance exercised this power with the General Communiqué on Tax Procedure Law No. 518,[4] which entered into force on 24/3/2020. It declared a force majeure event for taxpayers obliged to pay income tax on their commercial, agricultural, or professional income who were directly affected by the pandemic, and for taxpayers operating in sectors that temporarily suspended their activities due to measures taken by the Ministry of Interior.[5] According to the communiqué,[6] the force majeure provisions, covering 1 April 2020 to 30 June 2020 inclusive, applied to the following three groups: first, tax payers required to pay income tax on commercial, agricultural, or professional revenue; second, tax payers directly affected by the COVID-19 pandemic and whose main area of activity related to retail, including shopping centres, health services, furniture manufacturing, iron, steel, and metal industry, mining and quarries, building construction services, industrial kitchen manufacturing, automotive manufacturing and trade, and automotive parts and accessories manufacturing, logistics and transportation services, including car rental and storage services, artistic services, such cinema and theaters, publication activities of books, newspapers, magazines, and similar printed materials, including printing services, accommodation activities, including tour operators and travel agencies, food and drinks services, including restaurants and coffee houses, textile and garment manufacturing, and trade, event, and organization services, including public relations; third, tax payers whose main area of activity was in workplaces temporarily been closed due to measures adopted by the Ministry for Internal Affairs. In this contex the filing date for withholding tax returns and duties related to e-books was delayed from 27/04/2020 to 27/07/2020 while the payment date for taxes accrued on the basis of these tax returns was deferred until 27/10/2020.[7] The payment periods for taxes accrued on the basis of the tax returns that should have been filed by May and June, were extended until 27/11/2020 and 28/12/2020, respectively.

With the Tax Procedure Law General Communiqué No. 524, the Ministry of Finance then declared a force majeure, as allowed in TPL Article 15 for the second time during the pandemic. This applied to taxpayers operating in sectors having workplaces that had to temporarily suspend or stop their

---

4   See Duplicate Official Gazette No:31078 dated 24/03/2020.
5   Article 2 of the TPL General Communiqué No. 518.
6   Article 3/1 of the TPL General Communiqué No. 518.
7   Article 4/1-a. of the Communiqué No. 518.

activities due to measures taken by the Ministry of Interior, from 01.12.2020 until whenever it would be appropriate to resume their activities.[8] The new regulation postponed until the end of day on the 26th day of the month following the ending of the force majeure by the Ministry withholding tax returns to be filed (including withholding and tax premium returns) and duties to be fulfilled regarding e-books within the force majeure period. Likewise, the payment periods of the taxes accrued based on these tax returns were deferred.

The Income Tax Law was also changed by reducing tax withholding rates for leasing certain properties/rights. Pursuant to Article 1 of the Presidential Decree No. 2813, dated 31/7/2020, the rates were reduced from 20 % to 10 %. Presidential Decree No. 3319, dated 23.12.2020, extended the new withholding tax rate until 31/05/2021.

The Ministry of Finance's force majeure declaration also affected social security legislation. Pursuant to Article 91/3 of Law No. 5510, with the decision of the Board of Directors of the Social Security Institution, No. 2020/188, dated 26/03/2020, the deadlines for payment of insurance premiums for March, April, and May 2020 for taxpayers within the scope of TPL General Communiqué No. 518 and insured under Article 4/1-a and Article 4/1-b of Law No 5510 were extended until 2/11/2020, 30/11/2020, and 31/12/2020, respectively.[9]

As with corporate taxation, for periods up to and including 31/08/2020, the government introduced new regulations to reduce the burden on taxes and secondary public receivables on taxpayers (related tax fines, late interest, and late

---

8   See Article 2 of the Communiqué No. 524.
9   Certain measures were also taken regarding Turkish Labor Law. The first concerned the short-term work allowance, stipulated in Annex Article 2 of the Unemployment Insurance Law No. 4447. This defines short-term work as work in a workplace (maximum three months) in case the weekly working hours in the workplace are significantly reduced or the business temporarily suspends its operations in full or in part due to general economic, sectoral, or regional crisis or compelling reasons. For short-term work, a short-term work allowance is paid from the Unemployment Insurance Fund under certain conditions. This study does not cover the short-term work allowance as it is not considered a financial obligation within the scope of tax law.
    The second new labor law regulation prohibited termination of employment/service contracts. The prohibition on termination was last extended from 17.05.2021 until 30.06.2021 in accordance with Presidential Decree No. 3930, dated 30.4.2021. This study does not investigate the prohibition of termination since it is not part of tax law.

fees for tax returns due to be filed until that date) under Law No. 7256 on the Restructuring of Certain Receivables and the Making Amendments on Certain Laws, which entered into force on November 16, 2020[10] the government stopped collecting certain public receivables. Given that the reductions from this regulation are the same as those for the corporate tax, they are not repeated here.

Likewise, regarding those covered by Article 2/11 of Law No. 7256, the new regulation waived the collection of all auxiliary receivables, such as the delay penalties and late fees applied to these receivables. This law mostly provided a partial deduction on the interest and fees of receivables covered.

Finally, grant and rental support provided by Presidential Decree No. 3323, dated 23/12/2020, should also be mentioned since this is directly related to certain income taxpayers and the spending of tax revenues in accordance with the social state principle, albeit not related to financial obligations. The grant and rent support was later extended for one more month by Presidential Decree No. 3929, dated 30.04.2021.

C. Measures Taken for Value-Added Tax and Other Consumption Taxes

Turkey's tax system includes many consumption taxes, such as Value–Added Tax (VAT), excise duty, customs duty, special communication tax, stamp duty, BSMV (banking and insurance transaction tax), entertainment tax, and advertisement tax. Some of these taxes were reduced to support sectors affected by the pandemic, particularly tourism.

For example, VAT on domestic plane tickets was reduced from 18 % to 1 % between 1/4/2020 and 30/6/2020.[11] VAT on overnight services was also reduced to 1 % on 1/6/2021[12] while implementation of the new accommodation tax was postponed until 1/2/2021.[13] Under Article 34 of the Expenses Tax Law No. 6802,[14] the accommodation tax is supposed to be collected at 2 %[15] on overnight

---

10 The enactment date of the provisions of Law No. 7256 are provided in Article 45 of the same law.

11 Presidential Decree No. 2278 (https://www.resmigazete.gov.tr/eskiler/2020/03/20200 322-1.pdf, 20.5.2021)

12 Presidential Decree No. 3931, dated 30/4/2021

13 See Article 51 of Law No. 7226 Making Amendments to Certain Laws.

14 It was created to be effective as of 1/4/2020 as per the provisions of Article 9 and others of Law no. 7194.

15 Article 42 of Law No. 7194 stipulates that the accommodation tax should be applied at 1 % until 30/12/2020.

services in accommodation facilities, such as hotels, motels, holiday villages, hostels, apart-hotels, guest houses, camping sites, chalets, highland houses, and all other services offered there (foods, beverages, activities, entertainment, use of swimming pools, gyms, thermal baths, etc.) sold with this service. This tax was clearly created to reduce the state's budget deficit due to Turkey's economic crisis. However, its implementation was postponed to protect the tourism sector from the effects of the pandemic.

Given that the entertainment sector has also been heavily affected by the pandemic, the government mostly reduced its VAT rate to 1 %. This includes the services provided at cafes, tea houses, tea shops, cafeterias, patisseries, fast food restaurants, take-out restaurants, and other food service businesses, such as diners, diners selling alcohol, kebab restaurants, and similar places (except for alcoholic beverages). However, casinos, open-air casinos, bars, dance halls, discotheques, night clubs, taverns, pubs, cocktail lounges, and similar places were not included.

The entertainment tax was also reduced,[16] which is another consumption tax,[17] levied on local or foreign film screenings, theaters, operas, ballets, sports competitions, horse races, concerts, circuses, amusement parks, joint bets, and entertainment venues that do not require tickets. The entertainment tax for domestic and foreign film screenings was reduced from 10 % to 0 % until 31/5/2021.

VAT was also reduced from 18 % to 8 % until 31/12/2020 for workplace rental services, passenger transportation services, congress, conference, seminar, concert, fair, and amusement park entrance fees, organization services for weddings, balls and cocktail halls, services provided in barbershops and hairdressing and beauty salons, tailoring, clothing, and home textile products, repair services for shoes and leather goods, dry cleaning, laundry, ironing services, carpet and rug cleaning services, maintenance and repair services of appliances like bicycles, motorcycles, and household electrical appliances, maintenance and repair of consumer electronics (TVs, radios, CDs, etc.), maintenance and repair of domestic heating products like water heaters, maintenance and repair of garden equipment, maintenance and repair of furniture and flooring, maintenance and repair of computers, communication tools and equipment, and watches, maintenance and repair of musical instruments, locksmith and key duplication services,

---

16 For the entertainment tax, see Municipal Revenues Law Article 17 and others.
17 For the entertainment tax, see Municipal Revenues Law Article 17 and others.

porter services, oiling, washing, cleaning, polishing services for motor vehicles, housing maintenance, repair, painting and cleaning services, ornamental plants and flower deliveries.[18] These changes aimed to reduce the tax burden on low or middle-income taxpayer groups affected by the pandemic. With the same Presidential Decree, VAT was reduced from 18 % to 1 % for certain food and beverage services, which are among the sectors most affected by the pandemic, until 31/12/2020. VAT reductions in the delivery of goods and services in question were extended until 31/5/2021 with Presidential Decree No. 3318, dated 23.12.2020. Finally, VAT rate was reduced for certain deliveries in the healthcare sector. For example, VAT for COVID-19 vaccine delivery was reduced to 1 %.[19]

On the other hand, Communiqué No. 32, Amending the Value Added Tax General Communiqué, published in the Official Gazette No. 31121, dated May 8, 2020, announced measures to accelerate VAT returns for a few taxpayers with high tax compliance, subject to certain criteria.

As with income tax, corporate tax, and social security payments, the government postponed the tax return filing and payment periods for VAT. Specifically, the deadline for filing and payment of the February tax returns, originally 26.3.2020, was extended until 24.4.2020. Pursuant to TPL General Communiqué No. 518, mentioned above, the filing period for the April, May, and June VAT returns was extended until 27/7/2020 while the payment deadlines for the accrued taxes based on these were extended until 27/10/2020, 27/11/2020, and 28/12/2020, respectively. Furthermore, TLP Circular No. 126 deferred the imposition of VAT withholding on invoices issued to taxpayers considered within the scope of force majeure between 1.4.2020 and 30.6.2020.[20]

With Presidential Decree No. 2301, dated 26.03.2020, the 25 % Excise Duty levied on cola sodas was increased to 35 % while the proportional tax on certain cigars and cigarettes was increased from 40 % to 80 %. However, there was a partial tax discount for pipe tobacco and chopped smoking tobacco.

Finally, the regulation introduced for certain public receivables under Law No. 7256, which was mentioned in the section on income and corporate tax, also applies to VAT and customs taxes. Therefore, auxiliary public receivables, such as late interest and delay penalties, and all tax penalties imposed based on the

---

18 See Provisional Article 6 added to the Decree on the Determination of Value Added Tax Rates to be Applied to Goods and Services, which was implemented with the Council of Ministers Decision No. 2007/13033, dated 24/12/2007 and Presidential Decree No. 2812, dated 31/7/2020.

19 Presidential Decree No.3318, dated 23/12/2020

20 https://www.gib.gov.tr/node/143122/pdf, 20.5.2021

principle tax debt and late interest, including those whose original is paid before the effective date of this law, were waived, with certain conditions (Law No. 7256 art. 2/1-a; art. 2/2-a).

II. Comparison of Tax Measures Taken in Other Countries During the Pandemic Period

In 2021, the OECD published its report, Tax Policy Reforms 2021: Special Edition on Tax Policy during the COVID-19 Pandemic, which describes the tax measures that countries have taken against the pandemic. It provides information on tax regulations and broader fiscal measures since the start of the outbreak. Based on this information, this section comparatively evaluates tax policies in various countries as well as Turkey. The report classifies the measures in general before providing country examples for each measure.

In the first half of 2020, many countries took urgent measures to provide relief for businesses and households against large-scale lockdowns. Once these large-scale lockdowns ended, they took further measures to stimulate the economy and solve the state's financing problem. Table 1 presents these tax measures, as categorized in the report.

Tab. 1: Typology of tax measures introduced in response to the COVID-19 crisis

	Relief	Recovery-Oriented Stimulus	Tax Increases
Objectives of policies	Cushion the economic and social impacts of virus containment policies	Stimulate aggregate demand and investment	Finance part of the government's response to the crisis
Main types of tax measures	Tax deferrals Tax filing extensions Accelerated tax refunds Loss-carry back provisions Temporary tax waivers Temporary tax reductions	Tax incentives for investment Reduced corporate or other business taxes Tax incentives for employment Temporary VAT reductions Lower property transaction taxes	Increases in top personal income tax rates Health excise tax increases Environmental tax increases Property tax increases Business tax increases

Source: OECD (2021), Tax Policy Reforms 2021: Special Edition on Tax Policy during the COVID-19 Pandemic, OECD Publishing, Paris (Tab. 2.1); 2021 OECD Tax Policy Reform Questionnaire

As seen in Tab. 1, States intervened early in the crisis and tried to offset the sudden devastating effects of the pandemic on national economies. Following these initial interventions, states' increasing need for resources to fight the pandemic required different measures to increase government revenue. The measures required to restore the economy after the pandemic are also a subject of discussion. However, their implementation requires time since policies aimed at stimulating the economy during a pandemic will be ineffective given restrictions on economic activity and may even cause the virus to spread further in an environment where social distance must be maintained.

Different countries have different tax classification systems. Here, we will use the classification in the OECD report and examine practices in Turkey using this classification to facilitate the comparison. We will examine the tax types under the general headings of corporate tax and other business taxes, personal income taxes and social security contributions, value added tax and other consumption taxes.

A. Measures Taken Regarding Corporate Tax and Other Business Taxes

Countries took two kinds of measures regarding corporate tax and other business taxes. The first type aimed to protect those institutions required to pay these taxes but in danger of insolvency. The measures included deferring tax prepayments, accelerating tax refunds, developing retroactive loss reduction practices, reducing tax rates, or waiving taxes. Corporate tax and income tax payments for commercial enterprises generally use a prepayment system. Many countries, such as Chili, Greece, Indonesia, Luxembourg, Mauritius, Slovenia, and Uruguay, suspended prepayment during the pandemic while others, such as Portugal and Chile, reduced the amount of prepayments from medium and small-sized enterprises. Finally, prepayment systems may require taxpayers to pay more tax than necessary during the year, so the state then has to reimburse them. However, because this takes time, some countries, such as Israel and Portugal, reimbursed the prepayments while others, such as Barbados, Seychelles, Trinidad and Tobago, and the United States, expedited the reimbursement payments.

Other countries preferred the second type of measure, namely more taxpayer-oriented policies, and largely opted out of collecting all corporate or business-related income taxes from those sectors most affected by the pandemic. For example, Singapore provided a 25 % corporate tax refund for 2019. Other countries focused support on small and medium-sized enterprises. For example, Korea reduced income tax by 60 % for qualified small and medium-sized enterprises and by 30 % for some medium-sized enterprises. Another measure was to deduct damages suffered by taxpayers retrospectively or prospectively. Each country had different policies on this issue before the pandemic. For example, some countries do not recognize a long period for loss-carry back provisions, such as England, Japan, and Germany. However, they extended this period for companies suffering losses during the pandemic. Many countries, including China, Portugal, Peru, the Slovak Republic, and Uruguay, changed the prospective deductibility of these losses, mostly by binding them to temporary periods.

On the other hand, because states needed more revenues to fight the pandemic, some governments increased the corporate and other business taxes for those sectors that they considered had not been badly affected by the pandemic, especially high-income taxpayers. For example, the UK increased its corporate tax rate for 2023 from 19 % to 25 % for businesses with an income above GBP 250,000. Finally, many countries, such as Australia, China, Finland, Germany, Indonesia, Italy, and Mauritius, increased incentives for research and development activities, and intellectual property rights in 2020 (OECD 2021).

This comparison of regulations in various countries raises several interesting points (see Tab. 2). First, in Turkey, the government postponed corporate tax returns and corporate tax temporary returns filing deadlines but did not introduce any regulations to accelerate state reimbursements of taxpayers. Second, while some corporate tax receivables were waived in Turkey, these waivers are mostly related to public receivables, such as delay interests, late fees, or tax penalties that taxpayers have to pay in relation to corporate taxes. Third, unlike in many other countries, Turkey introduced no new regulations in favour of the taxpayer regarding loss deductions, although taxpayers in Turkey can deduct their losses from their profits for the next 5 years, unlike in other countries. Fourth, Turkey's flat-rate corporate tax rate was increased from 20 % to 25 % for 2021 and 23 % for 2022. However, for companies traded on the Borsa Istanbul equity market for the first time, the government provided a 2-point discount on their corporate tax rate. Finally, incentives for research and development activities in Turkey were extended until 2028.

Tab. 2: Cross-Country Comparison of Corporate and Other Business Taxes

Corporate and Other Business Taxes	Examples in other Countries	Practice in Turkey
Deferment of temporary taxes	Chili, Greece, Indonesia, Luxembourg, Mauritius, Slovenia, Uruguay	Yes
Accelerating the refund or deduction of provisional taxes	Israel, Portugal	No
Tax Waivers and discounts	Singapore, Korea	Only deductions related to delay interest, late fees, and tax penalties
Increasing the possibility of retroactive deduction of losses	England, Japan, Germany	No
Increasing the possibility of prospective deduction of losses	China, Portugal, Peru, Slovakia	Already possible for 5 years in the current situation
Increase in corporate tax rate	England	In general, there has been an increase in the corporate tax but there is a conditional discount for companies traded on the stock market for the first time.
Discounts at various withholding rates	Thailand	Yes
Increase in incentives granted to research and development activities and intellectual property rights	Australia, China, Finland, Germany, Indonesia, Italy, Mauritius	Extended until 2028

B. Personal Income Taxes and Social Security Contributions

Many countries have taken measures during the pandemic regarding income tax and social security contributions to relieve employees and households. For example, some have extended the deadlines for filing tax returns and delaying the payment of taxes due (e.g., Israel, Italy, Spain, Sweden, Italy, Poland, Russia, and Slovenia). Other countries have increased tax rates on high-income earners (e.g., Korea, New Zealand, and Spain); increased the standard tax allowance (e.g., Canada, Germany, and the United Kingdom); increased the general tax credit (e.g., Czech Republic, Finland, and Italy); developed policies targeting low-income individuals and families with children (e.g., Germany, Canada, and Nigeria); provided tax exemptions for the elderly (e.g., Sweden, Canada, Thailand); introduced tax exemptions for students and educators (e.g., Lithuania, Netherlands, and the USA); or increased incentives for philanthropic donations (e.g., China, Croatia, France, Iceland, Indonesia, Nigeria, South Africa, and the USA) (OECD, 2021).

In Turkey, the government only introduced measures for income tax and social security contribution payments for those considered to be in difficulties due to the pandemic, and for certain taxpayer groups (Tab. 3). The government extended deadlines for social security contributions and filing tax returns and deferred payment deadlines of taxes due for those taxpayers whose activities were temporarily suspended due to anti-pandemic measures. It also partially waived receivables, such as delay interest, late fees, or tax penalties related to these payments. However, no changes were made to the standard tax allowance or policies regarding families with children, the elderly, and students. In line with the principle of the social state, registered taxpayers operating in sectors affected by the pandemic and meeting certain criteria received direct support and rental assistance. Tax withholding rates for renting certain properties and rights were reduced and state receivables were deferred.

Tab. 3: Personal Income Taxes and Social Security Contributions

Personal Income Taxes and Social Security Contributions	Examples in Other Countries	Practice in Turkey
Postponing the filing of tax returns/postponing tax payment deadlines	Israel, Italy, Spain, Sweden, Italy, Poland, Russia, Slovenia	Only for Specific Taxpayer Groups Affected by the Pandemic
Increasing standard income tax discounts	Canada, Germany, United Kingdom	No
Increasing tax credits	Czech Republic, Finland, Italy	No
Tax exemptions for low-income families and families with children	Germany, Canada, Nigeria	No
Tax exemptions for the elderly	Sweden, Canada, Thailand	No
Tax exemptions for students	Lithuania, Netherlands, USA	No
Increasing tax rates for high-income earners	Korea, New Zealand, and Spain	No
Increasing philanthropic donation incentives	China, Croatia, France, Iceland, Indonesia, Nigeria, South Africa, USA	No new regulation was introduced. Pursuant to Article 89/10 of the current Income Tax Law, all donations made to the aid campaign initiated by the President can be deducted from the income tax base.
Discounts at various withholding rates	Thailand	Yes

C. Measures Taken Regarding VAT and Other Consumption Taxes

The primary purpose of measures taken for VAT and other consumption taxes during the pandemic was to alleviate liquidity pressure on businesses and encourage consumption. Many countries, including Canada, Chile, and Finland, took measures to facilitate VAT refunds while 40 % of countries in the OECD study extended the deadlines for filing VAT returns and a few countries temporarily reduced their VAT rates. For example, Germany reduced its standard VAT rate from 19 % to 16 % for 6 months, and Ireland from 23 % to 21 %. More than half of countries reduced VAT rates for healthcare products to zero whereas they increased excise duties on harmful goods, such as cigarettes and alcohol. Only a few countries (e.g., Paraguay) reduced excise duties on healthcare-related goods, such as alcohol products used for cleaning. Customs duties on healthcare-related products were generally reduced in almost three-fifths of the countries in the study (OECD 2021).

Generally, VAT is a significant financial burden for taxpayers in Turkey. However, during the pandemic, the deadlines for filling VAT returns and paying the taxes deferred to the government also accelerated and facilitated VAT refunds for a few taxpayers meeting certain tax-compliant criteria. VAT rates were also significantly reduced in many sectors. As mentioned above, VAT rates were reduced from 18 % to 1 % in domestic air transportation, overnight services in the tourism sector, and the entertainment sector. In certain other sectors, such as passenger transportation, hairdressing, tailoring, various maintenance and repair, and various similar services, the VAT rate was temporarily reduced from 18 % to 8 %. In the healthcare sector, the VAT rate for delivery of COVID-19 vaccines was reduced to 1 %.

Tab. 4: *VAT and Other Consumption Taxes*

VAT and Other Consumption Taxes	Examples in Other Countries	Practice in Turkey
Facilitating VAT returns	Canada, Chili, Finland	Yes (for a limited number of taxpayers)
Extending VAT returns filing deadlines	40 % of countries in the OECD study	Yes
Temporary reduction in VAT rates	Germany, Ireland	Yes
Zeroing VAT products on medical products	In more than half of the countries	Yes
Increasing excise duty on goods harmful to health	Majority of the countries	Yes
Decreasing or zeroing customs duties on healthcare products	3/5 of countries in the study; all European Union countries	Yes
Discount or deferral of certain consumption taxes	Hungary (tourism tax)	Yes (e.g., accommodation tax, entertainment tax)

Discussion and Conclusion

The first part of this study investigated selected tax policies implemented during the Covid 19 pandemic in Turkey. The second part compared these practices with other OECD countries. Because each country has its own very comprehensive and unique tax legislation, this study was limited to corporate tax and other business taxes, income tax and social security legislation, VAT, and other consumption taxes. Various countries' tax policies were examined, based on the OECD's report, Tax Policy Reform 2021 (Special edition on Tax Policy during the COVID-19 Pandemic). Comparing their practices with those in Turkey during the pandemic revealed the following differences.

First, regarding corporate tax and other business taxes, Turkey alone did not refund or deduct temporary taxes, and did not provide any opportunity to deduct losses retrospectively. Clearly, such practices require a cash flow from the state to the taxpayers. Like many other countries, Turkey implemented practices like deferring taxes and waiving certain public receivables, such as delay interest and late fees. Turkey also increased the corporate tax rate. These regulations indicate that Turkey avoided practices that would create cash needs; instead, the government waived taxes and similar incomes that it should have been receiving from taxpayers.

Second, Turkey did not introduce regulations regarding standard tax allowances, there were no new regulations for taxes paid by students, the elderly, or families with children. Beyond that, Turkey differentiated between taxpayers who had suffered or not due to the pandemic and introduced supportive measures, for the former, regarding filing tax returns and deferment. This may have caused problems between these two groups in terms of the principle of equality in taxation. The state's classification of those who were or were not economically affected by the pandemic was based on criteria that sometimes resulted in support being given for those who did not really need it and vice versa.

Third, Turkey, like other countries, reduced VAT rates on many goods and services, and accelerated VAT refunds for a limited number of taxpayers with high tax compliance, subject to certain criteria. As in many countries, the Turkish government also raised excise duty on unhealthy products, such as cola soda, cigarettes, and cigars, to increase state revenue.

Fourth, the Turkish government introduced other measures to protect the cash flows of individuals, including tax deferrals, lower tax rates, waiving of certain auxiliary public receivables, such as delay interest. However, it did not apply some of the methods used by other countries that require direct cash flow to taxpayers, such as refunds on prepaid taxes. But although it is not directly related to tax practices, the state has also provided direct monetary or rental support to some groups that it thinks are affected by the pandemic. Apart from these, Turkey's government took the necessary measures to avoid penal sanctions on those taxpayers who could not fulfil their tax obligations due to lockdowns.

Overall, this comparative analysis of practices in Turkey shows that the state distinguished between taxpayers in implementing measures discussed in this paper, and provided tax facilities based on specific criteria (e.g., difficulties due to the pandemic or taxpayers with high tax compliance before the pandemic). However, while these practices have benefits, they may contradict the principle of equality in taxation due to implementation problems. Future studies should therefore investigate how much of pandemic-related tax benefits in Turkey were actually received by those who really needed them, and how many people were unable to benefit from tax benefits despite being affected by the pandemic.

In this study, the tax systems of countries other than Turkey were not separately examined. The OECD report was the only source used and thus demonstrates a limitation of the study.

References

Akdoğan, A., (2009). Kamu Maliyesi, Gazi Kitabevi, 13. Baskı, Ankara.

Clemens, J. & Veuger, S., (2020). Implications of the COVID-19 Pandemic for State Government Tax Revenues, *National Tax Journal*, 73(3), pp. 619–644.

Coffey, C., Doorley, K., O'Toole, C. & Roantree, B. (2020). The Effect of the COVID-19 Pandemic on Consumption and Indirect Tax in Ireland. *Budget Perspectives. No. 2021/3, ESRI Series*, Available online: https://www.esri.ie/sys tem/files/publications/BP202103.pdf (accessed on 1 October 2020).

Collier, R., Pirlot, A. & Vella, J. (2020). Tax Policy and the COVID-19 Crisis. *Intertax* 48(8), 794–804

Çağan, N. (1980). Türk Anayasası Açısından Vergilendirme Yetkisi, *Anayasa Yargısı Dergisi*, C:1, 1980, s.171–183.

Carletti E., Oliviero T., Pagano M., Pelizzon L. & Subrahmanyam M. G. (2020). The COVID-19 Shock and Equity Shortfall: Firm-Level Evidence from Italy. *The Review of Corporate Finance Studies*, 9(3), pp. 534–568, https://doi. org/10.1093/rcfs/cfaa014

Chernick H., Copeland D., & Reschovsky A. (2020). The Fiscal Effects of the Covid-19 Pandemic on Cities: An Initial Assessment. *National Tax Journal*, September 73(3), 699–732

Devereux, M. O., Güçeri, I., Simmler, M., & Tam, E. H. F. (2020). Discretionary Fiscal Responses to the Covid-19 Pandemic, *Oxford Review of Economic Policy*, 36 (Suppl 1), 225–241

Göker, C. (2011). Yönlendirici Vergilendirme, *Marmara Üniversitesi Hukuk Fakültesi Hukuk Araştırmaları Dergisi*, 17 (3–4). Retrieved from https://dergip ark.org.tr/tr/pub/maruhad/issue/316/1493, pp. 11–30

Karnon, J. (2020). The case for a temporary COVID-19 income tax levy now, during the crisis, *Applied Health Economics Health Policy*, 18, 335–337.

Laffitte, S, Martin, J., Parenti, M., Souillard, B., & Toubal, F. (2020). International Corporate Taxation after Covid-19: Minimum Taxation as the New Normal, in CEPII Policy Brief no:30, 1–6 http://www.cepii.fr/PDF_PUB/pb/2020/pb2 020-30.pdf (accessed date: 1 May 2020.

Lu, Y., Wu, J., Peng, J., & Lu, L. (2020). The Perceived Impact of the Covid-19 Epidemic: Evidence from a Sample of 4807 SMEs in Sichuan Province, China. *Environmental Hazards*, 19(4), 323–340. doi: 10.1080/ 17477891.2020.1763902.

McGeever, N., McQuinn, J., & Myers, S. (2020). SME liquidity needs during the COVID-19 shock, Financial Stability Notes 2/FS/20, Central Bank of Ireland. pp. 1–12

Munawar, H. S., Khan, S. I., Qadir, Z., Kouzani, A. Z., & Mahmud, M. A. P. (2021). Insight into the Impact of COVID-19 on Australian Transportation Sector: An Economic and Community-Based Perspective, *Sustainability*, 13(3), 1276, 1–24. https://doi.org/10.3390/su13031276

OECD (2021), Tax Policy Reforms 2021: Special Edition on Tax Policy during the COVID-19 Pandemic, OECD Publishing, Paris. https://doi.org/10.1787/ 427d2616-en (accessed date: 22 April 2021)

Öncel, M., Kumrulu, A., Çağan, N. & Göker, C. (2019). *Vergi Hukuku*, Turhan Kitabevi, 28. Baskı, Ankara.

Tian, W. (2020). How China Managed the COVID-19 Pandemic, *Asian Economic Papers*, 20(1), 75–101. DOI: 10.1162/asep_a_00800

Turhan, S. (1987). *Vergi Teorisi ve Politikası*, Der Yayınları, Istanbul.

Fatma Didem Sevgili Gencay

The Continuity Principle of Public Service and the Working Conditions of Physicians in Turkey (Before and During the Covid-19 Pandemic)[1]

Introduction

The concept of public service designates a mission to satisfy the public interest and is fulfilled by the administration or by a private law person acting under the authority and supervision of the administration.

In Turkish administrative law (as in the French administrative law on which it was modelled) there are several key principles of public service such as continuity, adaptability, equality, neutrality, secularity, and the provision of said services without charge. The continuity principle requires the service to be delivered continuously, reliably, and without interruptions unless otherwise dictated by a regulation currently in force. In order to maintain continuity of a service, certain provisions have been made in the legislation, such as the prohibition of strikes for all civil servants. Based on this principle, certain regulations were already in force regarding physicians before the COVID-19 pandemic even started, such as residing near their place of work, and the fulfilment of obligatory service. With the start of the pandemic, additional restrictions in the form of annual leave suspension and a ban on resignations have also been imposed on healthcare workers.

Considering the extraordinary conditions of the pandemic, such restrictions may appear reasonable, but they should never be at the expense of the physicians' basic human rights, such as the right to free choice of employment, the right to decent work, and the right to rest. In this instance, the necessities of a pandemic prevented the rights of healthcare workers from being protected. In addition to these, I will demonstrate that the administration has no authority to impose such restrictions. Furthermore, as healthcare workers are at a greater risk of infection

---

1 This manuscript is an extended version of the oral communication presented at the Colloquium of General Public Law Professionals organized by the Turkish Society of General Theory of State on April 9–11, 2021.

due to increased exposure time to COVID-19, the administration has an added responsibility towards them.

I. The Principles of Public Service and Their Effects on Public Officials

The most basic duty of the state, and the very reason for its existence, is to provide services to the public. The state is granted privileges of public power to fulfil such services (Karahanoğulları, 2004). A public service can briefly be defined as an activity for the benefit of the public determined by political bodies and carried out by public or private entities under the supervision and control of the administration (Günday, 2011; Gözübüyük & Tan, 2019). In other words, public service is an activity of public utility carried out directly or indirectly by the administration (Atay, 2018).

A. The Principles of Public Service

In Turkish administrative law, it is recognized that public services are subject to certain common rules of such paramount importance that they are called public service principles. These principles are continuity, adaptability, equality, and gratuity.

Starting from the end and working our way back, it can be seen that today there are few services where the principle of gratuity is in existence, i.e. provided without receiving money for their use (Günday, 2011). Currently, education is the only public service being provided free of charge in Turkey as per Article 42 of the Turkish Constitution, which states that "primary education is compulsory for all citizens of both sexes and is free of charge in state schools." Of course, one could argue that education, like all other public services, is already paid for by the public through taxes. (Karahanoğulları, 2004).

The principle of equality implies that all individuals are to be treated equally when they enter and benefit from a public service (Günday, 2011). Everyone should have equal access to public services. Who will benefit from a public service and under which conditions are determined in advance by objectively drafted regulations and all those who are included in this parameter can make use of it under the same conditions (Yıldırım et al., 2018). Unequal treatment is possible in cases of positive discrimination or for those people with special circumstances. The principles of neutrality and secularity are related to equality. Neutrality requires equal treatment regardless of political opinion and secularity requires equal treatment regardless of religious beliefs.

According to the principle of adaptability (or adaptation), public services should adapt to the changing needs of society and in line with technological improvements (Günday, 2011). The administration has the privileges of public power to take necessary measures to adapt the services to the public interest, including abrogation of a service if there is no further need for it. The adaptation of the national education system from in-person to online classes during the pandemic by the Ministry of Education is a prime example of adaptability.

Lastly, the principle of continuity implies that a public service activity must be fulfilled continuously and regularly for as long and as frequently as the need for the service continues (Giritli, Bilgen & Akgüner, 2006; Günday, 2011; Kalabalık, 2014). Depending on the nature of the service, the principle of continuity may require the service to be provided without interruption, as in the case of firefighters, security forces, or other emergency services. For other services, such as education, regulations may prescribe not to carry it out at certain times of the day, week, month, or year (Atay, 2018). In other words, although the principle of continuity may require uninterrupted service in some areas, it usually highlights the regularity of an operation (Karahanoğulları, 2004).

B. Effects of the Continuity Principle on Public Officials

The effects of the continuity principle are felt by the administration, private individuals who have a contract with the administration for executing a public service, and by public officials.

A rule that immediately comes to mind as an example of the effects of this principle on civil servants is Article 94 of the Civil Servants Act (Law No. 657), which stipulates that if a civil servant resigns, he may not leave his position until another civil servant arrives to take over his duties (Giritli, Bilgen & Akgüner, 2006; Günday, 2011; Gözler, 2019).

According to Article 26 of the same law, "It is forbidden for civil servants to retract collectively from the civil service or refuse to perform their duties to deliberately disrupt the public service or to take measures and actions that will cause a slowdown or disruption of public services and activities".

Another effect of the principle of continuity on civil servants is the prohibition of strikes. Under Act No. 657, civil servants are prohibited from striking (Art. 27). The principal goal of this ban is to ensure that the continuity of public services is not disrupted in case of a strike (Giritli, Bilgen & Akgüner, 2006; Yıldırım et al, 2018; Atay, 2018; Gözler, 2019; Ulusoy, 2020).

Civil servants in France can enjoy the right to go on strike, while Turkish administrative law inspired by French administrative law does not recognize this right for its civil servants. The ways in which the French Constitution and the Turkish Constitution regulate the right to strike differ considerably; while in France, the right to strike is granted to every working person, in Turkey, this right is recognized for "workers" only.

In fact, paragraph seven of the preamble of the French Constitution of 1946, which is considered a part of the Constitution of 1958 currently in force, states that "The right to strike is exercised within the framework of the laws that regulate it." So, whereas the French Constitution does not stipulate a specific beneficiary, the Turkish Constitution states categorically that "workers have the right to strike." To clarify this point, the Turkish legal system does not consider civil servants "workers" as they do not work under contract and are not subject to the Labour Law. Rather, the administration appoints civil servants and the Civil Servants Act regulates their working conditions, which are non-negotiable.

The provision in Law No. 657 prohibiting strikes for public officials was ruled by the Constitutional Court as being constitutionally sound, since the Constitution does not directly grant public officials and civil servants the right to strike. This conclusion was reached after further consideration that the interdiction of strikes imposed on public officials was for the purpose of ensuring the continuity of public services without disruption (CC, 23.06.1970, E.1970/11, K.1970/36; for a review of this ruling: Ulusoy, 2020).

II. The Principle of Continuity in Public Healthcare Services

Although all public services are essential, healthcare services stand somewhat apart. The purpose of the public healthcare service is to meet the medical needs of individuals in society, thereby ensuring their right to health and medical care, with particular emphasis on equal and continuous access to this service on a national scale.

Due to the importance of healthcare as a public service, special regulations concerning physicians were already in effect prior to the advent of COVID-19. Undoubtedly, the most prominent of these regulations is obligatory service, which highlights the difference between physicians and other public service employees. According to Additional Article 3 of the Basic Law on Healthcare Services, "... those who have completed their studies at home or abroad and gained the title of physician or specialist physician following completion of their physician, specialist physician and subspecialty training, are required to complete a separate government service for each title (...)."

This law requiring obligatory medical service was brought before the Constitutional Court, but the Court did not qualify this as forced labour, since physicians who are subject to this ruling have the status of contractual personnel and are employed by the state for their services. The Court reiterated that the state instituted the obligation of "state service" on physicians "because everyone has the right to live in a healthy and balanced environment and the right to demand equal access to healthcare services in all regions of the country" and concluded by citing Article 18 of the Constitution, which states that "physical and intellectual work, which is a civic duty required by those fields provided to meet the needs of the country, is not considered forced labour" (CC, 13.03.2006, E.2006/21, K.2006/38).

Contrary to the prohibition of forced labour, the Court did not consider the fact that physicians do not receive their diplomas from the Ministry of Health until after they have completed their obligatory service, thereby being prevented from practicing their profession. The court also concluded that, considering the purpose of this service, the separate obligatory services imposed for each specialty and subspecialty could not be considered impractical, unnecessary or disproportionate to the desired purpose. The final ruling of the Court upheld the regulation as a civic duty that is proportionate and therefore consistent with the Constitution.

In 2016, a physician, Meltem Sukan, began her obligatory medical service following the completion of her specialist training but applied for a change of position due to health and family related problems. The administration rejected this request, despite the issuance of a 14-month medical report citing a diagnosis of major depression. Finally, the applicant resigned and requested her medical diplomas and a certificate of specialization. The administration did not respond to her request and at the end of 60 days their silence constituted a formal rejection under Turkish law. She filed for an appeal in the administrative courts, and this was also rejected. Finally, she made an individual application to the Constitutional Court in which she argued that, despite having received specialist training, she could not even work as a general practitioner or practice her profession under any circumstance, and that this was a violation of "the prohibition of forced labour, freedom of work and contract, the principle of protection of the family and the principle of legal security." The Constitutional Court did not find any of the applicant's claims to be warranted. (CC, 21.04.2016, Meltem Sukan Decision).

In a statement about the individual application of the physician, the Constitutional Court concluded that "it was not possible (to) qualify the work under the said obligation as forced labour, since physicians subject to the public service obligation are remunerated for their services". This interpretation is consistent with its decision about the law requiring obligatory medical service discussed above. Meltem Sukan case was an individual application, and as such the Court should have considered the circumstances of the event. Furthermore, although it was later recalled that "for there to be forced labour, the person must be employed under threat of penalty and without personal consent" (CC, 14.02.2013, E.2011/150, K.213/30), this condition was not considered when the verdict was given. In this instance it is unquestionably clear that the physician in question had not given consent.

The European Court of Human Rights (ECHR) states that "for there to be forced or compulsory labour, for the purposes of Article 4 § 2 (Art. 4-2) of the European Convention, two cumulative conditions have to be satisfied: not only must the labour be performed against the person's will, but either the obligation to carry it out must be "unjust" or "oppressive" or its performance must constitute "an avoidable hardship". In other words, it must be "needlessly distressing" or "somewhat harassing"" (Van De Mussele v. Belgium).

The ECHR rules that the "threat of penalty" should not be perceived as a criminal sanction, so failure to deliver the diplomas and certificates of specialization to any physicians who fail to fulfil their civil service obligations can be perceived as a penalty. Indeed, whether the work in question is carried out under threat of penalty and against the will of the person is examined by the ECHR, and any obstruction to the practice of a profession is considered to be a threat of penalty. The knowledge of the future obligation of forced labour at the time of entry into the profession and the conscious request of the individual in question to enter into the profession should not be considered sufficient grounds for the obligatory service to be deemed acceptable. The service should also not impose an unreasonable and disproportionate burden considering the advantages of the profession for the person under obligation (Van der Mussele v. Belgium). In Turkey, physicians in training are fully aware of the impending "state service" but its execution often generates problems like in the case for Meltem Sukan. In addition, as a separate obligatory service is required for each specialty and subspecialty training received, the duration can be quite lengthy. However, the obligatory medical service was not considered forced labour by the Constitutional Court in either of the abovementioned cases and it was concluded that this obligation was proportionate and constitutionally could not be claimed to be inadequate, unnecessary or disproportionate to the purpose.

In determining whether work or service falls under the scope of forced labour, the ECHR indicates that the conformance of conditions of the concrete event with the principal purposes of Article 4 of the convention should be examined. For example, in an appeal concerning the obligatory medical service for physicians, the ECHR examined whether the obligation in question was within the scope of the existing normal professional activities, whether people under the obligation were remunerated for the services they provided, whether these services fell within the framework of professional or civil solidarity, and lastly whether the burden imposed on the physician was proportionate or not (Steindel v. Germany). However, the case in question here was not regarding obligatory service in Turkey. Specifically, the application was filed by an ophthalmologist alleging that the legal obligation to take part in an emergency room program organized by a public institution was contrary to his human rights. The ECHR declared the claim to be ill-founded, noting that this obligation was "founded on a concept of professional and civil solidarity and aimed at avoiding emergencies" (Steindel v. Germany). Moreover, 6 days of service imposed on the applicant in a three-month interval was not disproportionate and therefore could not be considered "forced or compulsory labour". The obligatory service in this case also carries a much lighter burden than the obligatory medical service practice in Turkey which takes years of full-time work.

III. Healthcare Professionals during the Pandemic

A. Restrictions Imposed on Healthcare Professionals

During the COVID-19 pandemic, physicians were treated differently from other civil servants by the Turkish administration on many fronts. Flexible working conditions, such as remote working and rotational shifts, were envisaged for public officials working in other fields (Circular of the President n.2020/4) while more intensive working conditions were introduced for healthcare professionals. It must not be overlooked that the reason for this difference lay in the extraordinary circumstances brought about by the pandemic that represented a major threat to public health. One of the first measures taken, which was announced by the General Directorate of Healthcare Services of the Ministry of Health (2020a) in a circular dated March 27, 2020, was a three-month ban on all healthcare personnel in both the public and private sectors from taking leave or resigning. The ban was later lifted with the circular of June 7, 2020 (2020b), then put back into effect with the circular of October 27, 2020 (2020c).

The Ministry of Health prohibited healthcare professionals from taking leave, transferring to other institutions, or resigning from their positions, except in some exceptional cases (2020c). Restrictions on the retirement and annual leave rights of healthcare workers were lifted by the Ministry with the circular issued on January 19, 2021 (2021a), but the ban on resignation was upheld with a new circular dated March 3, 2021, stating that the resignations of healthcare workers would not be accepted regardless of the reasons (2021b).

It could be argued that these measures were necessary to ensure the uninterrupted provision of healthcare services during what were undoubtedly extraordinary circumstances. Nevertheless, a case could be made that as an alternative to placing restrictions, the administration could have used positive reinforcement methods to encourage physicians who are already bound by their Hippocratic oath to remain at their posts and carry out their duties. As it stands, the legality of these prohibitions, just like the other COVID-19 measures taken in Turkey, are questionable.

With regard to the restrictions placed on retirement, neither the Social Insurance and General Health Law No. 5510 nor the Pension Fund Law No. 5434 make allowances for the placement of conditions on or the postponement of retirement. Once all the eligibility requirements for retirement have been met, any efforts to deny that right to someone is tantamount to "forced labour".

As for the prohibition of resignation, the right to enter the public service is stated in Article 70 of the Turkish Constitution, but there are no stipulations requiring an employee to remain in that position for a specific length of time. Therefore, just as entering the civil service is a right, so should leaving it be considered a right (Şahin, 2019). It is stated in Article 20 of the Civil Servants' Act No. 657 that civil servants may withdraw from the civil service according to the principles set out in the law. Under Article 94 of the Act, a request to withdraw from public service may be made to the institution of affiliation in writing after which the employment will continue (to ensure continuity of service) until the appointment of a replacement or acceptance of the request. In case the appointed replacement does not come within 1 month or if a replacement is not appointed, the officer may quit the service after informing his or her superior. So, in any case the civil servant cannot be forced to continue his/her work more than a month except during state of emergency. In short, withdrawal from the civil service is not a request conditional on approval, but a right exercised by the civil servant. In fact, the Council of State concedes that resignation is an entirely legal act of the public officer's will and not one that is dependent on the acceptance of the administration (CS, 5th Ch., E.1991/2002, K.1993/999).

It is also recognized in the Act that a civil servant who does not come to work for 10 consecutive days without an excuse is deemed to have withdrawn from the civil service without the requirement of a written petition. No disciplinary measures are proposed in the legislation in such an event, which can be construed as a reflection of the prohibition of forced labour stipulated in Article 18 of the Constitution. Şahin (2019) argues that by giving the civil servant the opportunity to terminate the existing employment with immediate effect, the legislation recognizes the right of an employee to leave the service without any notice if they so choose. However, this is not to say that this route will not carry any consequences: by quitting without giving any notice, the civil servant has not complied with the principle of the continuity of service, so whereas the reinstatement period for any returning employee who has made a formal request for withdrawal is 6 months, it is 1 year for the employee who has left without notice.

During a state of emergency, regulations also see some changes. Firstly, during the state of emergency, civil servants are not permitted to resign from their positions unless their withdrawal request is accepted or until "their replacement has arrived to take over from them" (Art. 96 Law no. 657). So, the civil servant can be forced to fulfil his/her service until the end of the state of emergency.

Secondly, Article 8 of the State of Emergency Law grants the government the authority to oblige healthcare workers to continue working, which is not possible during "ordinary" times. Likewise, the said article provides that "The terms of the Weekly Holiday Act, the National and General Holidays Act and the Lunch Break Act may not be implemented in part or in whole", essentially permitting the government to restrict the rights of all healthcare personnel. Furthermore, Article 9 subclause (d) permits the government to limit or suspend the annual leave of personnel in charge of providing services as it deems appropriate.

Article 18 of the Constitution allows for these limitations and obligations by saying that "work required of an individual while serving a sentence or under detention provided that the form and conditions of such labour are prescribed by law; services required from citizens during a state of emergency; and physical or intellectual work necessitated by the needs of the country as a civic obligation" do not constitute forced labour. Article 4 § 3 (c) of the ECHR also exempts "any service exacted in case of an emergency or calamity threatening the life or well-being of the community" from forced or compulsory labour.

If the government in Turkey had declared a state of emergency, the restrictions imposed in healthcare workers would have been within the confines of the law. But no such declaration was made. Regrettably, the government decided to manage the pandemic with everyday regulations, resulting in the illegality of many of the restrictions placed and measures taken in the name of weathering the pandemic (Gözler, 2020; Sevgili, 2020).

B. Problems Faced by Healthcare Professionals during the Pandemic

In a statement entitled "Covid-19: the rights and obligations of physicians (healthcare professionals), the responsibilities of the Ministry of Health and employers" issued by the Turkish Medical Association (TMA) on April 3, 2020 (TMA. 2020), it was announced that in the early stages of the COVID-19 pandemic many institutions were unprepared and experienced problems in the form of sub-standard working conditions and lack of personal protective equipment. In all such instances, the administration has an obligation to protect its employees, and to provide a safe work environment by providing, for example, protective clothing where necessary. This requirement is addressed already in Article 27 of the Regulation on the Control of Medical Waste and Article 36 of the Regulation on Municipality Firefighters, so failure to provide protective equipment and clothing, as was the case in the early days of COVID-19, may result in the government being held liable for fault.

Additionally, the TMA specifically highlights that healthcare workers were not provided with details regarding the changes to their working conditions or with the necessary training by their institutions, thereby not permitting healthcare workers to make essential arrangements or protect themselves: a deficiency that the administration could again be held responsible for.

Another cause for concern for the TMA was the failure to provide guidance and training materials for the diagnosis and treatment of COVID-19. Such oversights result in a lower standard of care for which the administration would normally be held responsible, but the scientific uncertainty experienced globally during the first months of the pandemic lessens their accountability in this instance. There are nevertheless some examples of mismanagement such as the removal of hydroxychloroquine from the COVID-19 treatment protocol by the Ministry of Health on May 2021 – a considerable time after the WHO and TMA warnings were made – making the administration liable if any patients suffer long term side effects as a result of this treatment.

Furthermore, no alternative triage arrangements to respond to the COVID-19 pandemic were made; rather than increasing the number of employees, the government simply forced healthcare employees to work even if they were sick. The oppressive environment made it impossible for the employees to report their claims to the government and ultimately physicians were required to work 24-hour shifts drawn up by the hospital authorities.

It is clear that a conflict exists between the principle of the continuity of public service and a physician's right to rest, right to work in humanitarian conditions, and right to health. Professional ethics are also a factor: just as a firefighter must intervene in a fire despite the danger, so too must a physician care for a patient regardless of the personal health risks involved. However, the TMA argues that obliging physicians to fulfil their duties despite a risk to their health and their lives is unreasonable. In this respect, the healthcare workers' demands that all precautionary measures are taken to ensure their own protection is completely justified.

The list of concerns published by the TMA are likely to result in the administration being found liable for fault. Of course, it is also necessary to check whether the government resolved any of the problems cited, some of which including the risks posed by the physical condition of the hospitals. Indeed, in its one-year report the TMA calls attention to the high rate of illness among healthcare workers, especially those who work in hospitals that do not have operable windows (TMA. 2021).

IV. Compensation for Damages of Healthcare Professionals during the Pandemic

It can be argued that the intensive working conditions imposed on healthcare workers were caused by the pandemic and the resulting public health crisis and that these measures were compatible with the necessities of the service provided and the public interest. As the circumstances are quite specific, the Council of State may not consider these measures to be a fault for which the administration is responsible. Nevertheless, it cannot be denied that healthcare professionals are placed in conditions that pose a risk to their health and, as this is encapsulated by the principle of professional risk, they should be eligible to receive compensation for damages from the administration, who would be held liable without fault.

The principle of professional risk is a subfield of the principle of risk, an area in which the administration is held liable without fault. There are two grounds for strict liability of the administration: the principle of risk and the principle of equality before public burdens. The principle of risk concerns third party damages and holds the administration accountable when there is a risk associated with a public service that is nevertheless necessary for the public interest. On the other hand, the principle of professional risk focuses on damages to public employees who work in risky situations to carry out a service of public interest.

The responsibility of the administration is conditioned on the existence of a causal link between the administrative activity and the damage suffered, whether the liability is for fault or without fault. Considering that it is virtually impossible to ascertain how someone contracted COVID-19, in the case of healthcare workers the recognition of the presumption that the transmission occurred in the workplace would be within reason, with studies showing that contact with COVID-19 patients automatically increases the risk of virus transmission (Iyengar et al. 2020) and that COVID-19 transmission is higher among healthcare workers than the general public (Nguyen et al. 2020). Physicians are expected to show as much diligence in their personal lives as in their professional environment; therefore. it can reasonably be assumed that those who contract the virus did so at work, unless there are findings to the contrary. In France, the presumption of such a link is provided by law for such cases as the transmission of HIV or hepatitis through a blood transfusion. Likewise, in Turkey, the Council of State does not seek to prove that a patient who received a transfusion was not infected by hepatitis in another manner. A similar arrangement can also be made for healthcare workers who contracted COVID-19, unless evidence to the contrary is presented.

The administration cannot claim that there is no causal link between the damages suffered by healthcare professionals and the restrictions they imposed on healthcare workers in order to guarantee the effective continuation of the health services. Placing doubt on the causality link by putting forth the possibility of household transmission is unacceptable. The appropriate causality theory is applied by first determining the contributing factors of the damage, and then by examining whether these factors caused or further increased the damage in question. The criterion for this eligibility assessment is the normal course of events in daily life. The possibility of household transmission is easy enough to verify by simply ascertaining whether a member of the same household was diagnosed with COVID-19 before the healthcare worker was. Moreover, in these cases, the direction of transmission is usually reversed, with transmission generally taking place from the healthcare workers to other family members. In fact, a study in the United Kingdom showed that hospitalization rates of healthcare professionals and their family members were 2 or even 3 times higher than other COVID-19 patients (Shah et al. 2020).

Healthcare professionals are not victims of the pandemic but of their fight against this global problem in substandard conditions. For physicians and other healthcare workers, the risks have increased exponentially because of decisions taken by the administration. In fact, the COVID-19 transmission rate among healthcare workers is 10 to 14 times higher than in the general public (TMA. 2021). It must be recognized that although other public and private sector employees also continued to work in pre-pandemic conditions, these statistics are unique to healthcare workers. Clearly, healthcare workers face great professional risk posed by the virus and at the very least a no-fault liability of administration for extraordinary damages must be accepted.

Conclusion

The COVID-19 pandemic has been a difficult and complicated period for virtually everyone around the world. Some have lost their jobs, some suffer from depression, and meanwhile millions have lost their lives. After more than a year, the world continues its struggle against the virus. During the pandemic, I became more aware than ever of the importance of healthcare as a public service. People have shown their gratitude to healthcare workers in a myriad of ways, from sending flowers to hospitals to applauding them en masse. In several countries, such as France, Germany, Belgium, Malaysia, and Norway, COVID-19 is now legally recognized as an occupational threat for healthcare workers (Sandal &Yıldız. 2021). In Turkey, in addition to no such legislation being drawn up, claims of household contamination have been used to create a false causal link.

Here, I have shown that healthcare workers have shouldered much of the burden of the COVID-19 pandemic, all the while having to work in difficult and dangerous conditions illegally imposed by the administration who showed a blatant disregard of their rights. Without question, the administration should be held liable for not taking the necessary precautions to preserve and protect the health of these employees, and if fault cannot be proven then, at the very least, damages should be awarded on the basis of professional risk.

References

Atay, E. E. (2018). İdare Hukuku. Ankara, Turkey: Turhan Kitabevi.

Circular of the President. n. 2020/4. Resmi Gazete, Retrieved from: https://www.resmigazete.gov.tr/eskiler/2020/03/20200322M1-1.pdf

Giritli, İ., Bilgen, P., & Akgüney, T. (2006). İdare Hukuku Dersleri, İstanbul, Turkey: Der Yayınları.

Gözler, K. (2019). İdare Hukuku Cilt:2. Bursa, Turkey: Ekin Yayınevi.

Gözler, K. (2020). Korona Virüs Salgınıyla Mücadele İçin Alınan Tedbirler Hukuka uygun mu? (2). Retrieved from https://www.anayasa.gen.tr/korona-2.htm

Gözübüyük, Ş., & Tan, T. (2019). İdare Hukuku: Genel Esaslar. Ankara, Turkey: Turhan Kitabevi.

Günday, M. (2011). İdare Hukuku. Ankara, Turkey: İmaj Yayınevi.

Iyengar K. P., Ish P., Upadhyaya G. K., Malhotra N., Vaishya R., & Jain V. K. (2020). COVID-19 and mortality in doctors. *Diabetes and Metabolic Syndrome: Clinical Research and Reviews*, 14(6), 1743–1746

Kalabalık, H. (2014). İdare Hukukunun Temel Kavram ve Kurumları. Konya, Turkey: Sayram Yayınları.

Karahanoğulları, O. (2004). Kamu Hizmeti: Kavramsal ve Hukuksal Rejim. Ankara, Turkey: Turhan Kitabevi.

Ministry of Health. (2020a). Retrieved from: https://shgm.saglik.gov.tr/Eklenti/36992/0/covid-19-salgini-suresince-personel-ayrilislaripdf.pdf

Ministry of Health. (2020b). Retrieved from: https://dosyamerkez.saglik.gov.tr/Eklenti/37462,covid-19-normallesmeustyazi5ebe9a5b-9c9a-4c93-888e-87f10ddb512apdf.pdf?0

Ministry of Health. (2020c). Retrieved from: https://ohsad.org/wp-content/uploads/2020/10/Personel-Islemleri.pdf

Ministry of Health. (2021a). Retrieved from: https://ohsad.org/wp-content/uploads/2021/01/SB_izin_emeklilik_19.01.2021.pdf

Ministry of Health. (2021b). Retrieved from: https://shgmadsdb.saglik.gov.tr/Eklenti/40314/0/covid-19-kapsaminda-covid-19-kapsaminda-kamu-kurum-ve-kuruluslarinda-normallesme-ve-alinacak-tedbirler-barkotpdf.pdf

Nguyen, L. H., Drew, D. A., Graham, M. S., Joshi, A. D., Guo, C. G., Ma, W., & Zhang, F. (2020). Risk of COVID-19 among Front-Line Health-Care Workers and the General Community: A Prospective Cohort Study. *The Lancet Public Health*, 5(9), 475–483. https://doi.org/10.1016/S2468-2667(20)30164-X

Sandal, A., & Yildiz, N. A. (2021). COVID-19 as a Recognized Work-Related Disease: The Current Situation Worldwide. *Safety and Health at Work*. ISSN 2093-7911. https://doi.org/10.1016/j.shaw.2021.01.001. (https://www.sciencedirect.com/science/article/pii/S2093791121000019)

Sevgili Gençay, F. D. (2020). Covid-19 Tedbirlerinin Kolluk Yetkisinin Sınırları Bakımından İncelenmesi. In B, Özcan Büyüktanır & B. Özpınar Gümrükçüoğlu (Ed.). *Pandemi ve Sağlık Hukuku: Disiplinlerarası Yaklaşımla* (pp. 297–318). Ankara, Turkey: Yetkin Yayınları.

Shah, A. S. V., Wood, R., Gribben, C., Caldwell, D., Bishop, J., Weir, A., et al. (2020). Risk of Hospital Admission with Coronavirus Disease 2019 in Healthcare Workers and Their Households: Nationwide Linkage Cohort Study. *BMJ*, 371, m3582 doi:10.1136/bmj.m3582.

Şahin, C. (2019). Devlet Memurları Kanununun 94. Maddesi Uyarınca «Çekilmiş Sayılma» İşleminin Nitelik ve Koşulları İle Öğretim Elemanları Bakımından Uygulanabilirliğine Yönelik Değerlendirmeler. *Ankara Hacı Bayram Veli Üniversitesi Hukuk Fakültesi Dergisi*, XXIII (4), 325–361.

Turkish Medical Association (TMA). (2020). Retrieved from: https://www.ttb.org.tr/haber_goster.php?Guid=70e89cf6-75a2-11ea-b329-aa051764b049

Turkish Medical Association (TMA). (2021). Retrieved from: https://www.ttb.org.tr/haber_goster.php?Guid=ae64240a-94a1-11eb-9b30-af7a56403e78

Ulusoy, A. D. (2020). Yeni Türk İdare Hukuku. Ankara, Turkey: Yetkin Yayınları.

Yıldırım, T., et al. (2018). İdare Hukuku. İstanbul, Turkey: Onikilevha.

Part VI Current Thematic Discussions in Health Studies

Kıvılcım Ceren Büken

Nüket Örnek Büken

Ethicolegal Aspects of the Right to Health and Bioethics

Introduction

Law and ethics are inextricably linked together. Human rights law, medical ethics and bioethics, inevitably, also coincide in many ways and look for answers to similar questions across a wide range of topics. While human rights law is – although largely based on a universal rights claim in an almost Kantian way – produced at the will of sovereign countries and in this way undeniably positivistic, bioethics and medical ethics remain free in their perceptions and reflections, encompassing a broader area of ethical responsibilities not only on the state or by law; but for the state, healthcare workers and other actors, including but not limited to legal documents (Peel, 2005). Ethics are there before the law, and while the law is in operation, encompassing the law itself and all that the law does not clearly regulate (Örnek Büken & Büken, 2004).

The right to health is therefore understood differently in human rights law, medical ethics and bioethics, while one holds states to account for fulfilling their obligations arising from international or regional human rights documents, the other encompasses a larger area of obligations and requires a larger number of subjects to abide by ethical norms and standards. It has been argued that the application of an ethical framework to the right to health would necessitate that not just states but non-state actors and individuals would have obligations to fulfil for the full realization of the right (Ruger, 2006).

With medical ethics and bioethics becoming more and more universal each decade, more attention has been being paid to how they relate to human rights law, it has been suggested by many scholars that these fields will develop together and become even more interlinked overtime (Ashcroft, 2010). It has repeatedly been questioned whether the normative framework of international human rights law may effectively be deployed in the solution of bioethical problems (Cochrane, 2012).

Attention has been drawn to the parallels between human rights and bio-ethics, they are, for two separate discourses, strikingly similar. Both conceived out of the horrors of the World Wars, they make claims of universality, but despite the similarities, they remain separate (Baker, 2014). It has been suggested that an international bioethics based on human rights could save humanity from endless disputes over whose principles are preferable since the preferable princi-ples are those that effectively protect human rights (Baker, 2014).

This chapter will explain the right to health the way it has been constructed in international human rights law, offer a medical ethics perspective to the right to health in international human rights law, then move on to explain how bio-ethics and international human rights law collide and the possible future aims of an emerging academic field, "biolaw", before briefly commenting on Turkey's current position regarding the subjects mentioned.

I. The Right to Health

A. Human Rights Framework on the Right to Health

The right of everyone to the enjoyment of the highest attainable standard of physical and mental health, has been codified in many human rights treaties, and enshrined in over 100 constitutions across the world (Hunt, 2006).

The Universal Declaration of Human Rights (1948). in its article 25, states that "everyone has a right to a standard of living adequate for the well-being of himself and of his family..." The Constitution of the World Health Organisation (1946) also states that right to benefit from the highest possible healthcare serv-ices of everyone without distinction is one of the fundamental rights of every human being.

The International Covenant on Economic, Social and Cultural Rights, which came into force in 1976, in its Article 12, states that States Parties to the Covenant recognize the right of everyone to the enjoyment of the highest attainable stan-dard of physical and mental health. The Article moves on to state that the full realization of the right to health by States Parties would require that steps be taken to provide for a reduction in stillbirth-rate and infant mortality, for the healthy development of the child, for the improvement of environmental and industrial hygiene, for the prevention, treatment and control of diseases and the creation of conditions which would assure medical service to all. The Committee on Economic, Social and Cultural Rights' General Comment No. 14 (2000) on the right to the highest attainable standard of health further elaborates the obligations this right brings to States parties.

As can be inferred from Article 12 of the Covenant, the right to health is inevitably very closely related to other human rights, since health is affected by many factors in human life. The right to life, the right to privacy, the right to equality and the right to freedom from torture are prominent among the many other rights, which may be tied to the right to health so tightly that the realization of state obligations regarding the right to health may never be fully achieved without the realization of state obligations regarding these other rights (CESCR, 2000, para. 3). The Committee on Economic, Social and Cultural rights also stipulates that the underlying determinants of health include access to safe drinking water and adequate sanitation, access to safe food, adequate nutrition and housing, healthy working conditions as well as healthy environmental conditions, adequate health-related education and gender equality (OHCHR, 2008).

The Declaration of Alma-Ata of 1978 has confirmed that health, which is a state of complete physical, mental and social well being, is a fundamental right and that the realization of the highest possible level of health is dependent upon the actions of many other social and economic sectors, in addition to the health sector. The Declaration draws attention to the gross inequalities in the health status of people in developed and developing countries and also to the inequalities which exist within countries, and firmly states that economic and social development is of utmost importance for the realization of the right to health. The declaration calls for a fuller and better use of the world's resources, a considerable amount of which is spent on armament and military conflict, for social and economic development of which healthcare is an essential part.

When it comes to economic, social and cultural rights, the aim is for "progressive realization", which means that the obligation for States parties arising from such rights is to ensure the "highest attainable standard of health". The inability of the state to realize the right to health completely therefore does not amount to a violation of Article 12 of the ICESCR, however it is important to distinguish inability from unwillingness of a State to comply with its obligations. The state is under an obligation to use all available resources as its disposal. It has been argued that progressive realization, along with problems of justiciability and indeterminacy that it brings, presents roadblocks to the goal of codifying and implementing an international right to health. (Smith, 2005) What "progressive realization" means in the end, is that instead of an absurd demand to construct a comprehensive and integrated health system overnight, the right to health is realistic in its goals, demanding more from States with high incomes than others with low incomes, and implementation is subject to resource availability (Hunt & Backman, 2008). States must have a comprehensive national plan which encompasses the public and private sectors for the development of a health system which includes appropriate indicators and benchmarks through which the improvement in the system can be monitored (Hunt & Backman, 2008). "Progressive realization" also carries a strong presumption that measures which lower the present enjoyment of the right to health may not be taken (Hunt & Backman, 2008). Finally, States must adopt the most effective measures to progress the enjoyment of the right to health and not just any measures which reflect some degree of progress, taking into account resource availability and other human rights considerations (Hunt & Backman, 2008).

Even though the Covenant provides for progressive realization, it imposes on State parties some obligations with immediate effect, which are called the "core obligations" arising from the Covenant. General Comment no. 3 (1990) insists that States parties are under an obligation to ensure the satisfaction of minimum essential levels of each of the rights in the Covenant, including essential healthcare. Which obligations would this then entail for the right to health? To begin with, the preparation of a comprehensive national plan for the development of a health system is one of the core obligations. The non-discrimination clause, that the right to health must be exercised without discrimination of any kind, also a core obligation, requires that health services and facilities be ensured for all, especially for the vulnerable since traditionally marginalized groups and individuals often are affected by health problems disproportionately, due to the fundamental structural inequalities in society (OHCHR, 2008), (CESCR, 2000, para. 30). Last but not least, States have an obligation of immediate effect to establish effective, transparent, accessible and independent mechanisms of accountability in relation to their duties arising from the right to health (Hunt & Backman, 2008). It is crucial that while deciding where to use finite resources, the decision process is discreet, non-discriminatory and non-arbitrary, that resource allocation is conducted in accordance with human rights standards and that the measures taken are deliberately and concretely targeted towards the fulfilment of the right to health (Porter, 2015).

Healthcare must be available, which means functioning public health and healthcare facilities, goods and services must be available in a sufficient quantity, of course, depending on the State party's developmental level. This available healthcare must be accessible, which means everyone should be able to access healthcare without discrimination on any prohibited grounds. Physical accessibility and economic accessibility must also be ensured; healthcare facilities must be within safe physical reach for all sections of the population, especially the vulnerable or marginalized and persons with disabilities, they must also be affordable for all. Information accessibility is also an important element of accessibility, everyone has the right to seek and receive information concerning health issues. (CESCR, 2000, para. 12) Available and accessible healthcare must also be acceptable, which means all healthcare services must be respectful of medical ethics and respectful of the culture and preferences of individuals. Healthcare must also be of good quality, which requires skilled medical personnel and scientifically approved drugs and equipment and adequate sanitation. (CESCR, 2000, para. 12)

Stemming from the Covenant, States Parties have an obligation to respect, protect and fulfil the right to health. The obligation to respect, a negative obligation, requires that States parties refrain from interfering with the enjoyment of the right to health. The obligation to protect requires that states take measures to prevent third parties from interfering with such enjoyment, and the obligation to fulfil ensures that the States parties adopt appropriate legislative, administrative, budgetary, judicial and other measures towards the full realization of the right. (CESCR, 2000, para. 33)

Although this is still an idea in construction and more research is needed on the subject, developed states under international human rights law also have responsibilities towards the realization of the right to health in poor countries (Hunt 2006, 604). These responsibilities can be traced through the Charter of the United Nations and the Universal Declaration of Human Rights, several other treaties and conferences such as the Millennium Declaration and the Paris Declaration on Aid Effectiveness (2005). As a minimum, States have a responsibility to "do no harm" to their neighbours, high-income countries have a responsibility to provide international assistance and cooperation to low-income countries, and low-income countries must seek the said assistance in order to fulfil their own obligations to those under their jurisdiction (Hunt & Backman, 2008).

Other international conventions such as the 1989 Convention on the Rights of the Child, the 2006 Convention on the Rights of Persons with Disabilities, 1979 Convention on the Elimination of All Forms of Discrimination Against Women and the 1965 International Convention on the Elimination of All Forms of Racial Discrimination also bring obligations to the State concerning the Right to Health, which indicates special attention should be paid to the right to health of the vulnerable. In fact, vulnerable groups or individuals such as women, children, persons with disabilities, indigenous peoples, refugees and the internally displaced, persons living with HIV/AIDS face more difficulty in relation to their right to health, whether from socio-economic factors or discrimination and stigma. Seemingly neutral laws and policies regarding the right to health may perpetuate the inequalities caused by vulnerability, states must therefore pay special attention to tailor their health policies to assist those in need. (OHCHR, 2008)

The European Convention on Human Rights, a civil and political rights document which does not include a right to health, has been making decisions relating to the right to health under some of its Articles such as Article 2- the right to life, Article 3- the right to freedom from torture and Article 8- the right to private and family life. It should be beneficial here to present some examples of the Court's such judgements where Turkey is found to be in violation of the right to health as it relates to the rights enshrined in the European Convention. In Asiye Genc v. Turkey, where a newborn with respiratory problems died due to the unavailability of incubators even though he was repeatedly transferred to different hospitals with the promise that incubators would be available at the next hospital, the Court decided that the State had violated its obligation under Article 2 ensuring the right to life, by not making sure that enough incubators for newborns were present and functional at hospitals and by not ensuring effective communication between hospitals and thus giving way to the death of a premature newborn. In Mehmet and Bekir Şentürk v. Turkey, the applicant's pregnant wife was told at the hospital where she went with complaints of persistent pain, that the child she was carrying had died and that she required immediate surgery; however, she would be charged a fee for the operation and a deposit of approximately 1,000 Euros had to be paid for the operation to take place. She did not have the money, and died on the way while being transferred to another hospital. The Court in this case found a violation of the State obligation to protect the patient's physical integrity, since emergency treatment at the first hospital was dependent upon advance payment and this requirement had caused the patient to decline treatment, a decision which cannot be said to have been an informed one, the medical staff knew her life might be put to danger if she were to be transferred to another hospital and Turkey's laws were not capable of preventing the failure to give her the necessary emergency medical treatment. In Oyal v. Turkey, a blood transfusion following premature birth had infected the applicant's son with HIV. The Court found a violation of Article 2 in this case, too, since Turkish authorities had not taken the necessary measures to prevent the spread of HIV through blood transfusions and had not conducted an effective investigation after the occurance. It can be incurred from the cases presented that the ECtHR also makes decisions on the right to health, through other rights that the European Convention secures, and brings positive obligations to States along with negative obligations.

B. The Right to Health in the Context of COVID-19

The Committee on Economic, Social and Cultural Rights in its statement on the COVID-19 pandemic repeats that the pandemic has had profoundly negative impacts on the enjoyment of economic social and cultural rights, and especially the right to health of the most vulnerable groups in society. Highlighting that the pandemic has vividly illustrated the indivisibility and interdependence of human rights, mainly because civil and political rights such as the freedom of movement and others have been affected by it, the Committee insists that the measures adopted by States to combat the pandemic must be reasonable and proportionate to ensure the protection of all human rights. The statement draws attention to the fact that the elderly and the immunocompromised, those in residential care facilities, prisoners, persons in detention facilities faced especially dire contagion and health consequences, while certain categories of workers such as delivery workers and manual labourers were exposed to higher risk of infection. The statement also mentions that many healthcare workers were infected due to inadequacies in, or shortages of protective equipment and clothing. The Committee therefore insists that all States parties must adopt targeted measures to mitigate the impact of the pandemic on the vulnerable such as older persons, persons with disabilities, refugees and conflict-affected persons, as well as communities' subject to structural discrimination. All workers should be protected from the risks of contagion at work and until such measures are adopted workers cannot be obliged to work and should be protected from disciplinary or other penalties for refusing to work without adequate protection. The statement also insists that accurate and accessible information about the pandemic is crucial in reducing the risk of transmission of the virus and to protect the population against dangerous disinformation; and reverberates that the pandemic has highlighted the critical role of adequate investments in public health systems, social protection programs, decent work, housing, food, water and sanitation systems and institutions to advance gender equality (CESCR, 2020).

In his July 2020 Report, the Special Rapporteur on the right of everyone to the enjoyment of the highest attainable standard of physical and mental health, Dainius Puras has focused on COVID-19 which he deems the biggest global health emergency of the past 100 years, noting that the impact of the pandemic was determined more by public health policy, socioeconomic inequality and structural discrimination than by biological factors (Puras, 2020). A human rights based response to COVID-19, he urges, would require universal health coverage and strong health systems which can provide testing and treatment to everyone who needs them, but also since human rights are interdependent and indivisible, and the underlying social determinants of health extend beyond the healthcare sector, the prevention of public health emergencies could only be made possible where all human rights are embraced (Puras, 2020).

UNAIDS in their report "Rights in the time of Covid-19" where they talk about the lessons the world could take from their experiences with HIV also stress the importance of the frequent sharing of information, combatting all forms of stigma and discrimination, ensuring access to free and affordable testing and care for the most vulnerable, removing the barriers people face to protecting their own health or the health of their communities such as fear of unemployment, healthcare costs, misinformation and lack of sanitation, and add that restrictions to protect public health should be proportionate, necessary, evidence-based and reviewable by court (UNAIDS, 2020).

C. A Medical Ethics Approach to the Right to Health

Medical ethics tends to evaluate ethical problems and the solutions which have been found for them, through a number of different philosophical principles. In order to understand the right to health as it stands in international human rights law through the lens of medical ethics, it is important to explore the philosophical bases that might have influenced such decisions.

Utilitarianism has been a dominant analytical model of health economics, and utilitarian theories of healthcare endorse an allocation of resources which maximize net social utility. However, measures of utility omit freedom as a good in itself and focus on achievement alone, and even if a right to healthcare would increase net social utility, utilitarianism would not care about the discrepancies between the wealthy and the deprived as long as net social utility was maximized, therefore utilitarianism cannot be said to be the approach taken when it comes to the right to health in international human rights law (Ruger, 2006).

The libertarian perspective largely endorses civil and political rights which are largely negative rights wherein the state is required to restrain itself from infringing into the liberty of the people. Economic, Social and Cultural rights which are largely positive rights where the state is required to take action necessitates a redistribution of resources which the libertarian perspective opposes in general (Ruger, 2006). A libertarian perspective would then, insist that increased taxes would infringe on individual liberties and therefore deny any societal obligation to provide healthcare to all (Roger, 2006).

Rawls's Theory of Justice might better explain the right to health as an international human right, as Rawls' theory contends that rational agents standing behind a veil of ignorance about their personal circumstances would choose principles of justice that maximize the minimum level of primary goods that are rational to want (Ruger, 2006). An egalitarian rights based theory, an "equality of opportunity" might explain the right to health as it stands, since the first concern of the right to health and its core principle is that there be no discrimination in the realization of the right to health.

Ioanna Kuçuradi defines human rights as "rights that every human person possesses just by virtue of being human" and further deliberates that human rights are those objective circumstances that expand the capabilities, and allow for the flourishing of the human person. Human dignity according to Kuçuradi, is the defining characteristic of the human being. Kuçuradi has defined human dignity as the self-awareness of one's being human and the value inherent in this (Kuçuradi, 2016).

The philosophical theory of the right to health must then stand on a human capabilities approach, emphasizing a good life free of disease and promoting individual agency, encompassing prevention and treatment for all, with an ethical demand for equality in health in a Rawlsian way, complete with a more nuanced demand for other determinants of health; all with the eventual aim of enabling "human flourishing" (Ruger, 2006).

II. Human Rights and Bioethics

Although human rights and bioethics have developed as answers to the same horrifying world events and embody principles many of which parallel each other; bioethics have not necessarily adopted the universality claim of human rights law.

The Council of Europe and UNESCO have been among the pioneers of organizations which have taken steps to associate bioethics with human rights law (Andorno, 2013). The European Convention on Human Rights and Biomedicine (hereafter the Oviedo Convention) (1997) has a wide area of reach as it has been signed by many States and is the first and only legally binding document which considers biomedical innovations in the light of human rights law.

The Oviedo Convention includes articles on consent, private life and the right to information, the human genome, the impermissibility of sex-selection through medically assisted procreation, scientific research, research on embryos in vitro, organ and tissue removal from living donors for transplantation purposes, and the impermissibility of the human body to be subject to financial gain. Turkey has ratified this Convention in 2003.

There are four additional protocols to the Oviedo Convention, one on the prohibition of cloning human beings, one concerning the transplantation of organs and tissues of human origin, one concerning biomedical research and another concerning genetic testing for health purposes.

It can be said that the Oviedo Convention has been a success, having brought different countries with different cultural, social and legal backgrounds on the same page on biomedicine and having remained in force for longer than 20 years. On the other hand, several countries including the United Kingdom, Ireland, Germany have not signed or ratified the Oviedo Convention for a number of different reasons. The United Kingdom, for example, has argued that the Convention constitutes a barrier to research on the human embryo and to the use of technologies which allow modification of DNA. Germany, on the other hand has refused to sign the Convention on the grounds that it is "too liberal" (Raposo, 2016).

It is also possible to find several articles regarding general ethical principles on biomedicine in international legal documents such as the Universal Declaration of Human Rights, The International Covenant on Civil and Political Rights, and The International Covenant on Economic, Social and Cultural Rights.

The Universal Declaration of Human Rights forbids all kinds of discrimination and torture or cruel, inhuman or degrading punishment, guarantees the right to life and the right to health of everyone, and brings the right to private life. The ICCPR and the ICESCR repeat and widen the rights mentioned and this time make them legally binding for States parties. The ICCPR, in its Article 7, declares that "no one should be subjected without his free consent to medical or scientific experimentation", which is the first time consent for biomedical research has been mentioned in a legally binding international document. The European Convention on Human Rights guarantees the right to life, and the right to private life which are rights very closely related to biomedicine.

The Oviedo Convention regulates in a more specific way the bioethical issues that may already have been falling under the area of power of one of the articles of the European Convention on Human Rights. Human dignity sits at the centre of the Oviedo Convention, as is the case with many other human rights documents. The Oviedo Convention has aimed at widening the framework on biomedicine in international human rights law and has aimed at creating a document that is a minimum standards document, after the ratification of which States parties are allowed to take stricter measures of their own choosing. It has been articulated that this measure of flexibility has been adopted because the States parties differ in their cultures, religions and ethical understanding. In this sense, the Oviedo Convention, although a regional document, can be said to have a universal effect which cannot be ignored. The 2005 UNESCO Universal Declaration on Bioethics and Human Rights mentions the Oviedo Convention.

In fact, the UNESCO Universal Declaration on Bioethics and Human Rights (2005) is a document which does bring the two fields together, stating in its

Article 14 "the highest attainable standard of health is one of the fundamental rights of every human being without distinction of race, religion, political belief, economic or social condition.", and calling for "respect for human vulnerability and personal integrity" in its Article 8, clearly the Declaration is breaching the gap between bioethics and international human rights law, having the right to health, an economic, social and cultural right on the same page with the right to autonomy, a civil and political right, which is a bringing together of differently designed human rights under the roof of bioethics.

While the universal effect the Oviedo Convention has had cannot be ignored, cultural relativism remains prominent in bioethics and arguments that any universal ethical norms claimed today are the individualistic values of the Western world are common. This ancient and unsolvable battle between cultural relativism and universalism still makes it hard to make normative claims regarding bioethics (Gert, 2014).

It is necessary therefore for ethical standards to be codified into legal documents and appropriate mechanisms to be developed for ethical values to be effectively implemented. There is an emerging field titled "bio-law", a branch of international human rights law, working on the creation of a universal law of biomedicine. The following decades are expected to bring the following principles along, as law and bioethics coincide further and further and bio-law becomes a focal point of study:

- That human dignity be confirmed as the highest principle,
- That the human being be held to be the priority and that the interests of science and society are seen to be of secondary importance,
- That biomedical research does no harm to patients and to participants, and if possible, that clinical trials be beneficial for the treatment or diagnosis of the patient,
- That the autonomy of patients and participants to any study be respected and as a direct result of that, that informed consent be taken prior to any biomedical interference,
- That equitable access to appropriate healthcare and essential medication be guaranteed,
- That freedom to conduct scientific research be guaranteed as long as respect for human dignity and human rights are placed at the core of such freedom,
- That health data of identifiable persons be protected,
- That the right of persons to be informed, or not to be informed about the state of their health and their genetic information be respected,
- That specific measures be taken for the protection of the vulnerable,

- That there be no discrimination or stigma attached to the state of health or genetic information of persons,
- That the human body and its parts not be subjected to financial gain,
- That the human identity and bodily integrity be protected and especially that cloning for procreation and human germ-line intervention be prohibited,
- That diverse, multi-disciplinary and independent ethics committees be set up in order to evaluate the ethical, legal and social issues which arise from bio-medical activities,
- That equity be guaranteed and the divide between the developed and developing countries be breached when it comes to international biomedical research.

III. A Brief Evaluation on Turkey

Article 56 of the Constitution of the Republic of Turkey states that "everyone has a right to live in a healthy and balanced environment" and that the State shall ensure the planning and functioning of health services for everyone to lead a healthy life, physically and mentally.

The 2019 report of the Human Rights and Equality Institution of Turkey claims that the 2003 "Health Transformation Program" has worked wonders in infrastructure, personnel, medication and many other aspects of health service. The massive "city hospitals" which have been built on the outskirts of cities as campuses, according to the report, have changed the Turkish health system to the better (TIHEK, 2019).

The 2003 Health Transformation Program was in fact one conducted with consultancy by the World Bank (Erus & Hatipoğlu, 2017). The aim of the program was to increase efficiency and improve access to healthcare, but also signified a neoliberal transformation which, according to some, has accelerated the commodification of healthcare (Cebeci, 2014). It has been argued that the healthcare model brought about by the transformation programme has created a "health market" with the goal of profit in mind (Büken & Büken, 2004).

The OECD Reviews of Health Care Quality: Turkey of 2014 observes that Turkey's Health Transformation Programme has dramatically expanded access to healthcare, but suggest that government focus should move from quantity to quality in healthcare (OECD, 2014).

In the Context of COVID-19, since the announcement of the first confirmed case of COVID on March 10, 2020, Turkey has taken many measures such as nationwide curfews and lockdowns, some age-specific curfews imposed were seen as some to be discriminatory on the basis of age. It has been observed that the Ministry of Health has not collaborated with the Turkish Medical Association during the pandemic and has not always accurately and transparently informed the public of the situation, creating a state of distrust in citizens of government-sourced information regarding the pandemic (Örnek Büken, 2020).

Conclusion

The areas of interest of the right to health in international human rights law, medical ethics and bioethics are inextricably intertwined, and as the fields are at present already greatly nourished by each other, they will continue to influence and be influenced by one another in the decades to come. International human rights law could benefit from ethical discourse, and bioethics could benefit from adopting a more universal claim following the example of international human rights law, and the development of the field, biolaw, which might in the future facilitate the broader codification of bioethical principles.

References

Andorno, R. (2013). *Principles of International Biolaw*. Droit, Bioéthique et Societé.

Ashcroft, R. E. (2010). Could Human Rights Supersede Bioethics? *Human Rights Law Review*, 10(4), 639–660.

Baker, R. (2014). Bioethics and Human Rights: A Historical Perspective. In Teays, W., Gordon, J. S. & Renteln, A. D. (Eds.), *Global Bioethics and Human Rights Contemporary Issues*. Rowman & Littlefield.

Cebeci, A. (2014). Metalaşma Sürecinde Hukuk'un Etkisi: Türkiye'de Sağlık Alanının Metalaşması. In Ozdemir, A. M. & Ketizmen, M. (Eds.), *Türkiye'nin Hukuk Sisteminde Yapısal Dönüşüm*, İmge.

Cochrane, A. (2012). Evaluating 'Bioethical Approaches' to Human Rights. *Ethical Theory and Moral Practice*, 15(3), 309–322.

Council of Europe. (1997). *Convention for the Protection of Human Rights and Dignity of the Human Being with regard to the Application of Biology and Medicine: Convention on Human Rights and Biomedicine*.

ECHR *Asiye Genç v. Turkey* (app. 24109/07) (2015).

ECHR *Mehmet and Bekir Şentürk v. Turkey* (app. 13423/09) (2013).

ECHR *Oyal v. Turkey* (app. 4864/05) (2010).

Erus, B. & Hatipoğlu, O. (2017). Physician Payment Schemes and Physician Productivity: Analysis of Turkish Health reforms. *Health Policy,* 121(5), 553–557.

Gert, B. (2014). A Global Ethics Framework for Bioethics. In Teays, W., Gordon, J. S., & Renteln, A. D. (Eds.), *Global Bioethics and Human Rights Contemporary Issues.* Rowman & Littlefield.

Hunt, P. (2006). The Human Right to the Highest Attainable Standard of Health: New Opportunities and Challenges. *Transactions of the Royal Society of tropical Medicine and Hygiene* (100), 603–607.

Hunt, P. & Backman, G. (2008). Health Systems and the Right to the Highest Attainable Standard of Health, University of Essex Human Right Centre.

Kuçuradi, I. (2016). *İnsan Hakları: Kavramları ve Sorunları.* Türkiye Felsefe Kurumu.

OECD (2014). OECD Reviews of Health Care Quality, Turkey.

Örnek Büken, N. (2020a). COVID-19 Pandemic in Turkey. *Bioethical Voices Newsletter of UNESCO Chair in Bioethics, Haifa* 7(20), 33–42.

Örnek Büken, N. (2020b). COVID-19 Pandemisi ve Etik Konular. *Sağlık ve Toplum Özel Sayı,* 15–26.

Örnek Büken, N. & Büken, E. (2004a). Hukukta ve Etikte Hak Kavramı ve Yaptırım Sorunu, *Sendrom,* 64–72.

Örnek Büken, N. & Büken, E. (2004b). Emerging Health Sector Problems Affecting Patient Rights in Turkey. *Nursing Ethics,* 11(6), 610–624.

Peel, M. (2005). Human Rights and Medical Ethics. *Journal of the Royal Society of Medicine* (98), 171–173.

Porter, B. (2015). Rethinking Progessive Realization: How Should It be Implemented in Canada? *Social Rights Advocacy Center.*

Puras, D. (2020). Final report of the Special Rapporteur on the right of everyone to the enjoyment of the highest attainable standard of physical and mental health, United Nations General Assembly A/75/163.

Raposo, V. L. (2016). The Convention of Human Rights and Biomedicine Revisited: Critical Assessment. *The International Journal of Human Rights,* 20(8), 1277–1294.

Ruger, J. P. (2006). Toward a Theory of a Right to Health: Capability and Incompletely Theorized Agreements. *Yale Journal of Law & the Humanities,* 18(2), 273–326.

Smith, G. P. (2005). Human Rights and Bioethics: Formulating a Universal Right to Health, Health Care, or Health Protection? *Vanderbilt Journal of Transnational Law* (38), 1295–1321.

Türkiye İnsan Hakları ve Eşitlik Kurumu (2020). İnsan Haklarının Korunması ve Geliştirilmesi (TIHEK) 2020 Yılı Raporu, Ankara.

UN Committee on Economic, Social and Cultural Rights (CESCR). *General Comment No. 14: The Right to the Highest Attainable Standard of Health (Art. 12 of the Covenant)*, 11 August 2000, E/C.12/2000/4.

UN Committee on Economic, Social and Cultural Rights (CESCR). *General Comment No. 3: The Nature of States Parties' Obligations (Art. 2, Para. 1, of the Covenant)*, 14 December 1990, E/1991/23.

UN Committee on Economic, Social and Cultural Rights (CESCR). *Statement on the coronavirus disease (COVID-19) pandemic and economic, social and cultural rights*, 17 April 2020, E/C.12/2020/1.UN General Assembly, *International Covenant on Economic, Social and Cultural Rights*, 16 December 1966.

UN General Assembly, *Universal Declaration of Human Rights*, 10 December 1948.

UNAIDS (2020). *Rights in the Time of COVID-19, Lessons from HIV for an Effective, Community-led Response.*

UNESCO (2005). *Universal Declaration on Bioethics and Human Rights.*

WHO/UNESCO International Conference on Primary Health Care . (1978). *Declaration of Alma Ata.*

World Health Organization (1946). *Constitution of the World Health Organization.*

Gamze Yorgancıoğlu Tarcan

Electronic Knowledge Technologies: Using of Telemedicine and Mobile Health in Turkey

Introduction

Globalization, liberal economies, the change of the concept of knowledge and social structures play an important role in the development of technology. Conceptually, it contains many simple and complex elements from production techniques to microchips, from computers to the internet. Especially since the 1980s, one of the important capital of organizations and societies has started to be knowledge and communication technologies. Especially in areas such as communication, medicine, biomedical engineering, biology, electronic knowledge technology has become an important component in the stages of data collection, storage, analyses and sharing.

In this study, the importance of Telemedicine and Mobile Health, which forms the basis for knowledge sharing between health care providers and health care recipients, has been tried to be explained. In this context, in the first part, the basic dynamics that make up the technology are explained by giving conceptual definitions such as data, knowledge, e-health, telemedicine. In the next section, the use of Electronic Knowledge Technologies in hospitals and its areas of use are mentioned. In the next section, the basic policies developed for health information technologies in Turkey were tried to be explained. At the end of the chapter, the topic is concluded with conclusions and recommendations.

I. Conceptual Framework

Data are objective facts about events that differ from each other. It is not possible for them to have any meaning on their own. It just explains some parts of what's going on; there are no reviews with in and does not provide a basis for decision making. Does not give an idea of its importance or whether it will work. Data is important because it is an indispensable raw material for creating information (Davenport and Prusak, 2001). Therefore, it can be described as any material that a person acquires from the outside world as a result of measurement, observation, experiment or research. This material can sometimes be factual that most people agree with (age, marital status, gender, temperature, etc.) and in some cases it can be judgemental by being influenced by the views and thoughts of the researcher or observer (pessimistic, good-bad, exhausted, ugly or beautiful).

Knowledge can be regarded as a product that results from experience, learning or the result of some conscious processing of raw materials such as sound, image, number, symbol acquired from the environment. For these terms expressed in different terms as information or knowledge in English literature, only information term is used in Turkish. However, there is a hierarchical distinction between these concepts. While information is defined as data that has a certain meaning and importance for the users, knowledge is a product or content that comes out after a series of mental processes such as thinking, interpretation, observation, research. Blum (1986) explained information as interpreted, organized and structured data, and knowledge as a synthesis of defined and shaped relations. Similarly, the knowledge has been discussed by various researchers as any applicable data based on the experience of individuals (Davenport et al., 1998; Drucker, 2001) and the meaning derived from conventional rules used in information processing (Köksal, 1981). From an individual point of view, knowledge is a collection of what a person has learned and experiences in the past. Experience, judgement, values, beliefs and intuition are the components that produce knowledge (Barutçugil, 2002). Chen (2001) approached knowledge with a system and a managerial perspective in which an organization or society discovers, collects, manages, uses, analyses and shares information in order to increase performance. At the same time, knowledge can be considered as a new production factor as important as capital in institutions. On the other hand technology is an indispensable element of knowledge (Davenport ve Prusak, 2001).

A number of functions are needed to obtain, store, share and keep up-to-date information. At this point, the concept of knowledge management, which cannot be considered independent of data and information, comes up. Grey (1996) expresses knowledge management as the creation, registration, organization, access and use of the intellectual capital of enterprises with a collaborative and integrated approach. Knowledge management has been reported by Jennex and Croasdell (2007) that there are original journals, professional community and interest groups related to the field, an academic curriculum for the field, basic assumptions and academic discussions in the field, and it is related to the field, which has been supervised by professional colleagues. It is considered as a new discipline that meets the criteria for finding scientific studies.

Producing accurate, appropriate, timely, economical and complete information, sorting and analysing the produced information, keeping it ready and sharing it when necessary, as well as planning, correct use, continuity and control of all kinds of technology used in these stages, knowledge management processes. Sharing information is a part of the knowledge management process; It refers to a process in which information and knowledge obtained from different sources are transferred (Huber, 1991). It can occur consciously between two or more individuals, as well as in a conversation setting or during a meeting (Marouf, 2005).

Some technologies are needed for the processing and sharing of information including hardware, software and internet. Therefore, knowledge technology is a term used to describe technologies that enable effective and efficient operations such as recording and storing of data generating knowledge by passing it through a certain process, accessing this information, storing and transmitting information (Bensghir, 1996). In other words, it is any technology that includes electronics such as radio, television, telephone and computer related to obtaining, storing, processing and distributing data (Gregory, 2004).

In 2001, Electronic Health (eHealth) has been defined by Eysenbach (2001), who explained that the delivery of information to patients and stakeholders could be enriched by the intersection of medical informatics and public health business. In general, eHealth should be distinguished by medical informatics or the inclusion of computer and software in medical treatments and management, in order to improve care effectiveness: this discipline is way more "ancient" than eHealth; according to Mihalas and colleagues (2014), the history of medical informatics can be traced back before the 1970s, with pioneer work on signal analysis, modeling and simulation of biological processes, and the first attempts to develop decision support systems. It is around the 1980s that medical informatics acquired international recognition by means of funding, the development and sharing of methodologies, and the foundation of specialization schools (Pravettoni & Triberti, 2020).

Telemedicine is defined as an application of Information & Communication Technologies (ICT) to provide and support healthcare and exchange healthcare information when a distance separates the participants (Wootton et all., 2017) The word is a combination of two Greek words τήλε = tele - meaning "at a distance" and "medicina" or "ars medicina" meaning "healing" and its introduction is ascribed to Thomas Bird. In 1970s Bird had used this phrase in order to illustrate health care delivery, where physicians examine patients at a distance through the use of telecommunications technologies (Jordanova and Lievens, 2011).

Telemedicine is a broad term that encompasses a range of technologies from digital x-rays to telephone consultation, to the use of video conferencing to performing remote surgery. Telehealth is a remote access training network between citizens and healthcare professionals for the purpose of continuous improvement of healthcare services with the diagnosis, treatment and prevention of diseases used by all healthcare professionals. The definition of telehealth made by the World Health Organization (WHO); healthcare where distance is a critical factor is the continuous education of healthcare providers to improve the health of individuals and their communities, through the exchange of information applicable to the diagnosis, treatment and prevention of diseases and injuries, research and evaluation, by all healthcare professionals using information and communication technologies (World Health Organization, 2010). In this sense, telehealth is a broad concept that includes telemedicine applications. In telehealth applications, data which is collected and shared into four basic groups: Written text - written record (ECG, patient records, laboratory reports, radiology reports, prescriptions), image (body photographs, radiology records, still and moving images), video (video recordings of the patient's examination) and voice (breathing sounds, patient's speech). Telemedicine communication is done through copper wires, fiber optic cables, high frequency radio, VHF (very high frequency) and UHF (ultra high frequency) or satellite. The technological infrastructure (internet, telephone, satellite etc.) of the national communication network in a country determines the boundaries of tele-medicine applications.

Mobile Health spreads from simple short messages used to raise awareness of the society, to warn the them about epidemic diseases and to direct the society, to video tele consultation and tele visit applications, to making an appointment on a mobile phone, mobile application or website, to sending medical data from portable or wearable devices. Information technologies that find a wide range of applications from smartphone applications to self-color blindness test, to remote chronic disease management. (Tezcan, 2016). It is especially important for the remote monitoring of chronic diseases such as diabetes, Parkinson's, chronic obstructive pulmonary disease, kidney failure. The recent 2019 Coronavirus (COVID-19) outbreak has demonstrated yet another reason to use telemedicine and telehealth – protection from exposure. The World Health Organization (WHO) declared COVID-19 a pandemic on March 11, 2020. Due to the infectious nature of the virus, responding to the outbreak required patient isolation, monitoring of contacts, and quarantining. The efforts to control the virus consequently interrupted routine care for non-COVID-19 patients. As a result, the use of telemedicine and telehealth became a viable alternative to provide care to these patients while reducing the risk of transmission (George and Heitmann, 2021).

Health Information Management Systems (HIMS) is the planning, establishment and operation of the information system and architectural structure in hospitals, monitoring its development and compliance with the planned objectives (Winter et al., 2011). In addition to these, electronic knowledge technologies, allow access to comprehensive data and sharing of data, enabling the analysis of reports and consultations (Haux, 2010), reducing costs, communication, facilitating information storage, increasing quality, providing easy adaptation to changing customer demands, (Akyel & Bal, 2010), reducing the medical error rate (Meyer et al., 2007). In addition, it enables competitive advantages such as increasing operational efficiency, creating inter-organizational synergy, innovation and market advantage in terms of general business (Bakos & Treacy, 1986).

II. Use of Electronic Knowledge Technologies in Hospitals

With the establishment of Medicare and Medicaid programs in the United States in the 1960s, hospitals preferred the cost-based reimbursement method. This method revealed the need for financial reports on the hospital's service provision. In these years, information technologies started to be used at administrative and financial levels in large hospitals and academic medical centres. During the same period, few hospitals developed their main computers for administrative and financial services through leased programmers and analysts. In the same period, interest in clinical information systems to support patients and maintain clinical records is quite limited (Glandon et al., 2008). The widespread use of the Internet and computer networks in this period enabled remote interaction and data sharing between computers. Physicists working at the Swiss CERN Institute have developed a software called MOSAIC to easily access each other's research reports. The internet has become a platform that anyone can use easily. Firms such as Netscape and Microsoft have also started to launch software that helps to surf the internet (Yeloğlu & Sözen, 2010).

The 1970s and 1980s were a turning point for computers, computers became smaller and began to become a part of health care organizations. During this period, the focus of information technology applications in health services was to achieve better health management, income calculations, payments and other financial reports, while in the 1980s, the focus shifted to the patient and clinical systems that help improve diagnosis and treatment emerged. Also, during this period, digital technologies mainly showed themselves. Computers have moved to common use areas, and large amounts of data and image records have begun to be shared between physicians and other healthcare professionals via e-technologies (Tan et al., 2005).

The 1990s are the period of dramatic changes in the environment of health services. Clinical information systems and strategic decision support systems have attracted attention for service providers in achieving the balance between expenditure and quality service delivery. These changes have been supported by technologies such as notebook computers. Data collection tools, access to information from anywhere, rapid communication between service providers have increased the use of hardware technologies. At the same time, electronic data exchange and networks have supported institutional information systems by establishing links between health care organizations (Glandon et al., 2008). In the period from the 1990s to the end of the 2000s, computerized patient records, especially corporate activities and information systems oriented to inter-institutional patient information sharing, came to the fore (Vest, 2012).

Today, the application areas of information technologies and information systems have expanded considerably in health sector. Especially database technologies, internet and communication technologies have transformed health services. Portable devices, such as mobile phones and PDAs (Personal Digital Assistant), Universal Mobile Telecommunications System (UMTS), Digital Video Broadcasting (DVB-T) and internet technologies has become a routine communication channel between patient and health service providers. These modern developments in information technologies have encouraged many countries to have national eHealthlth records and applications such as e-health, e-prescription, and telemedicine. Based on developments in the field of health and technology, access to information by patients and their relatives, increasing opportunities for rapid and effective diagnosis and treatment, enables data sharing among insurance institutions, patients, healthcare institutions and other stakeholders.

In short, electronic knowledge technologies for hospitals like computer hardware, computer software, internet, intranet allow medical and personal data of patients or employees to be accurately and securely recorded and stored, and transferred to the relevant person in a safe, accurate, complete, timely manner to meet managerial needs. In the same time these are sub-systems that include human, legal regulation and financial resource components as well as physical elements such as database and communication technologies. Investments and management of these technologies require detailed decision-making and political processes.

III. Health Knowledge Technology Policy Implementation

The advantages of Industry 4.0 or the 4th Industrial Revolution, which was introduced at the Hannover Fair in Germany in 2011, on the internet, cyber systems, automation systems and data exchange opened the door to some innovations in the health sector and health services. Technologies such as sensors, artificial intelligence, robotic diagnosis and treatment applications, portals, blockchain and bitcoin have initiated the digitalization of healthcare institutions, making the data transfer between the service provider and the customer faster, easier and safer. In addition, fast and safe technological applications with low margin of error in screening, diagnosis, treatment, decision making, data management and analysis processes have become widespread.

Ever increasingly since the launch of the Lisbon Strategy (launched in March 2000 by the EU Heads of State and Government, it was aimed to make Europe *the most competitive and dynamic knowledge-based economy in the world, capable of sustainable economic growth with more and better jobs and greater social cohesion*) at the turn of the millennium, the European Union (EU) has targeted the acceleration of scientific and technological innovation as a key policy objective. Emphasized as one of the privileged means to steer the EU out of its current economic and political gridlock, the acceleration of innovation has also been envisaged as a prominent lever to relaunch the promise of the European project and to promote the further consolidation of the fragile European polity (Marelli and Testa, 2018).

According to the report of World Health Organization (WHO) in 2016, approximately half of the countries in the world have a specific national telehealth policy. The number of telehealth programs reported by the countries has increased from 138 in 2005 to 206 in 2010 and to 375 in 2015. The most reported program is tele-radiology. Approximately 3/4 of the countries in the world have own tele-radiology programs and policies. While the region reporting the most programs is Europe, the region notifying the least programs is Africa (WHO, 2016). Beyond the use of these increasingly important electronic knowledge technologies, the advantages and disadvantages of these technologies are more important. It is more important than the quality and quantity of technology to use it effectively, ethically and correctly at the appropriate place and time.

WHO, European Union (EU), International Telecommunication Union (ITU) and European Space Agency (ESA) - have officially adopted the denomination "eHealth". "eHealth refers to the use of modern information and communication technologies to meet the needs of citizens, patients, healthcare professionals, healthcare providers, as well as policy makers (EU, 2003). It is necessary to underline that "e" in the eHealth does not stand only and exclusively for electronic". It characterizes in details what eHealth is all about:

• Efficiency - one of the strategic promises of eHealth is to increase efficiency in health care, thereby decreasing costs; For example, telemedicine technology can have a cost-reducing effect if the patient does not come to the hospital during the epidemic period.

- Quality; It enables effective, efficient and low-cost methods and procedures for preventive and improving health services, diagnosis, treatment and rehabilitation.
- Empowerment of consumers and patients or patient-centred medicine: that centredness is widely regarded as a core indicator of quality care and critical component of care (LaNoue, & Roter, 2018). It alsa catalyzes encouragement of a true partnership between the patient and healthcare professionals.
- Education (continuing medical education) through online sources; may comprise a variety of interventions based on learning tools, theories, content, objectives, teaching methods, and setting of delivery. In terms of the type of learning technologies, digital education includes, but is not restricted to, online and offline computer-based learning, massive open online courses, virtual reality, virtual patient simulation, mobile learning, serious gaming and gamification, and psychomotor skills trainers (LaNoue, & Roter, 2018).
- Exchange of information; ensures that up-to-date, valid and accurate information is shared among the parties in the health system.
- Extending the health care beyond national boundaries; helps to achieve the goal of providing fair, equitable and widespread health service to everyone in need.
- Ethics: E-health brings a new form to the interaction between patient and physician. Online professional practices introduce new problems in ethical issues such as information, privacy, confidentiality and equality. The fact that health data is sensitive to privacy and confidentiality in all country practices. It has left the whole world alone with a number of ethical problems in information sharing. Privacy as a concept refers to an area where people can be alone, think, act, and decide on what limits they will communicate and communicate with other individuals (Yüksel, 2003). Data privacy is a process that includes determining who can access the data, in other words, authorization of those who can access the data. Confidentiality is one of the fundamental rights like human rights and is guaranteed by law. (Terstegge, 1998).

The property of data collected, stored, processed and shared by health institutions and organizations belongs to the patient and hospital management. All kinds of transactions to be made on this data, the use of the necessary permissions and authorizations for the sharing and destruction of the data are carried out within the framework of legal regulations. In this regard, to take measures to ensure information security in all information processes in Turkey the Information Security Policy Directive of the Ministry of Health, prepared by the Ministry of Health; to ensure that information is protected from all internal or external threats, whether intentionally or accidentally, by evaluating it within the scope of confidentiality, integrity and accessibility. It is to determine the procedures and principles that must be followed in terms of information security in order to be carried out quickly and safely. Similarly, the Law on the Protection of Personal Data, dated 07.04.2016 and numbered 9677 in the Official Gazette, protects the fundamental rights and freedoms of individuals, especially the privacy of private life, in the processing of personal data, and regulates the obligations of natural and legal persons who process personal data, and the procedures and principles to be followed. In (28.10.2017 dated) Official Gazette Number: 30224 With the Regulation on the Deletion, Destruction or Anonymization of Personal Data the procedures and principles regarding the deletion, destruction or anonymization of the processed personal data are specified in detail (Yönetmeklikler, 2017).

Beyond whether to use Telemedicine or Telehealth all over the world, the main controversial subject is when, where and how to use it for a cost-effective and quality health services. Especially in fields such as radiology and neurology, the transfer of images to virtual environment for remote interpretation is a common practice that is no longer perceived as telehealth. However, other medical fields also adapt to telehealth needs, and its use varies according to geographical regions and demographic segments (Olson & Thomas, 2017).

The first structure (Information Processing Department) related to health knowledge systems in Turkey was established within the Ministry of Health in 1995. Through the Telecommunications Authority of Turkey, The Ministry of Health, Turkey, requested Istanbul Technical University (ITU) to provide assistance in the implementation of Turkey's e-Health Project and support in their Health Transformation Project in 2003. This transformation project is an extensive and profound reform of the managerial and operational aspects of the health sector in Turkey, and includes a major re-organization of the delivery of medical services and of their finances through the social security and health insurance schemes. One of the key features of the transformation is the intended increased uses of ICT that support to the clinical, public health and managerial aspects of the health sector. Also Telemedicine Project was through tele-training and tele-medicine services practices, it is aimed to increase the quality, efficiency and effectiveness of the health services delivered regarding the areas on diagnosis, treatment, training, management, research, medical monitoring and treatment; and provide facilities for the specialization centres to consult each other. Telemedicine Project was formed considering the lack of sufficient specialist in the medicine sector, in order to meet the needs through consultation of a second opinion in complex cases, raising the patient satisfaction and for the implementation of right diagnosis and treatment. This will raise the opportunity for the implementation of tele-radiology and tele-pathology (tele-dermatology and tele-cardiology will be covered later). In 2011, with the Decree Law with the number of 663 about the Organization and Duties of the Ministry of Health and its Affiliated Organizations, General Directorate of Information Systems was established in order to spread eHealth technology use throughout the country and to monitor the development of these technologies in the world, and it officially became operational in 2012 (Mandi, 2004; Ministry of Health, 2018). The main duties of this department are to determine policies, strategies and standards, to carry out knowledge systems and technologies and to make and have all kinds of knowledge systems and projects that include personal health data, to follow international developments in the field of health knowledge systems and technologies, to share country practices and experiences, to cooperate with international organizations when necessary and to determine and implement the rules to be followed by public and private legal entities and real persons who will work in the field of health informatics and technology, to decide the suitability of their software and products when necessary, and to authorize their authors (Presidential Decree, 2018).

The Ministry of Health started the "Health Informatics Network" project in 2014. With this project, it is aimed to accelerate the health data in communication between individuals who receive health services all over the country and organizations that provide health services in a secure way and to make them more reliable. The most used electronic knowledge technology throughout the country is mHealth applications including e-pulse, filiation and isolation tracking application, 112 emergency help button, special children support system, disabled health communication system, national medical rescue team application, mental health support system, vaccine tracking system, obesity and diabetes clinic guide and central physician appointment system. Especially during epidemic periods, for example, *life fits into the home* (HES) application has been developed in order to inform and guide the citizen about Covid-19 pandemic and to minimize the risks related to the pandemic disease and prevent its spread. In this concept, isolated or infected people and the density of risky areas can be seen due to Covid 19. Also, information of the family (child and parents) and their risk status according to their regions can be displayed. The mobile applications unit under the General Directorate of Health Information Systems within the Ministry is responsible for publishing, tracking and updating mobile software, ensuring its security and controlling its functionality.

Moreover, Ministry of Health focuses on electronic knowledge actions to provide efficiency and effectiveness in health care supply, to make data management to ensure compliance with certain standards in informatics and to promote the use of health electronic knowledge technologies in the health care system. The importance of technologies such as electronic patient records, e-appointment systems, e-prescription, hospital information management and electronic patient files archive has been emphasized and efforts have gained momentum to spread automation systems. As of July 2019, 1855 health institution with Picture Archiving and Communication Systems (PACS) have been integrated and there are 184 million radiological images and 80 million radiology reports in the system (Ministry of Health, 2019). The National Health System (USS) and Decision Support System (DSS) have been developed to collect health-related data at national and international levels in a common database in order to increase the effectiveness and efficiency of health services and to improve health knowledge systems. The data obtained by these systems are actively used in determining health statistics and health policies, and are also securely shared with individual users through the E-Pulse portal. With the sharing of health data, it is possible for the citizens of the country to follow their own health records (diagnosis, treatment, report, prescription, etc.). In this way, repetitions of the procedure can be prevented and appointment, diagnosis and treatment procedures can be accelerated. At the same time, data such as blood pressure, heart rate, and calorie taken can be integrated into health-related wearable technologies and applications with the mobile application of the system. E-Pulse also includes e-government, hospital information management systems, core resource management system, public health, human papilloma virus (HPV) screening system, geographic information system, central physician appointment system, organ and tissue transplantation system, e-report, It can work integrated with e-prescription, Medula, mobile devices and death notification system.

Results and Recommendations

Mobile and wireless e-Health technologies, personalized medicine and interactive health services through social media applications related to electronic knowledge management will be three important mutation tools in health care systems (Eysenbach, 2001). The disparity between high-income countries and the rest of the world in telemedicine establishment may reflect the extent to which the implementation of, and capacity for telemedicine solutions are constrained by local resources and infrastructure. The most economically-developed countries generally have a sufficiently advanced information technology and communication infrastructure, greater freedom in their allocation of resources within the health care system, and more support for experimentation and research into new approaches to health care. This creates the capacity to develop and implement telemedicine solutions in a more formalized and systematic manner. In contrast, where countries outside of the high-income group do have telemedicine initiatives in place, they are more likely to be informal in nature (i.e., not part of a structured telemedicine program), such as connecting local health-care providers to specialists and consultative health care institutions (WHO, 2010).

Telemedicine or mHealth which is related with big data, has privacy about including individual data. This data set should not be damaged in any way, must not be accessed by unauthorized persons. In fact, while the health sector is digitalized on the other hand, it can also cause some problems in ethical areas such as privacy, information security, and confidentiality. The confidentiality of personal records should be guaranteed both ethically and legally. In this context, international documents such as the European Council Convention with the number of 108, the European Union Data Protection Directive, as well as international organizations such as the United Nations, the Organization for Economic Development and Cooperation (OECD) have regulations for the protection of personal data. The European Union General Data Protection Regulation (GDPR) numbered 679, which was adopted by the European Parliament on April 27, 2016 and became legally binding for all member countries in 2018, entered into force. In Turkey, mainly in the Constitution of the Republic of Turkey 1982, numbered 6698 dated March 24, 2016 Law on the Protection of Personal Data is situated along with a variety of regulations and circulars. Therefore, examinations and consultations, symptoms and examination findings, anamnesis and all kinds of health statistics related to the health status of a person are accepted as personal health data.

Standard guides such as Information Security Management System, which is based on ISO 27799 and ISO/IEC 27002 standards, can be applied to ensure information security in the health sector. Apart from this, policies to be developed by the management, data privacy agreements, in-service trainings, regular audits and administrative sanctions are within the scope of measures to ensure that individual users are sensitive about data security and privacy. Administration It should also establish strategy and implementation procedures that specify in detail which data will be shared with whom or with which institutions and organizations. Any data with privacy feature should be carefully and safely stored and protected against internal and external threats. The data controllers should be determined by the hospital administration within the framework of the legal and ethical regulations and practical orientation should be provided. In the hospitals such as polyclinics and examinations that everyone can easily see and hear, care should be taken by the administration to protect the information of the patients and to anonymize them if necessary. Team-working within a hospital or system would be best positioned to understand specific regional or national electronic knowledge systems about legal framework and cultural infrastructure. In addition to identifying national tele medicine advantages and disadvantages, these collaborations would also be important. Collaboration between hospital and health software supplier can play a key role. However, the applied and theoretical researches that will be done after evaluation and team work can guide decision-makers and field workers.

References

Akyel, R., & Bal, C. G. (2010). Bilişim ve bilişim teknolojileri. In A. Çelik, T. Akgemci (Ed.). Yönetim bilişim sistemleri. Ankara: Gazi Kitabevi.

Bakos, J. Y., & Treacy, M. E. (1986). Information technology and corporate strategy: A research perspective. *MIS Quarterly*, 107–119.

Barutçugil, İ. (2002). Bilgi yönetimi. İstanbul: Kariyer Yayıncılık.

Blum, B. I. (1986). Clinical information systems. *The Western Journal of Medicine*, 145(6), 791–797.

Davenport, T. H., De Long, D. W., & Beers, M. C. (1998). Successful knowledge management projects. *Sloan Management Review*, Winter, 43–57.

Davenport, T. H. & Prusak, L. G. (2001). İş dünyasında bilgi yönetimi. Günay, G. (Trans.) İstanbul: Rota Yayınları.

Drucker, P. (2001). *Management Challenges for the 21st Century*. New York: Harper Business Press.

European Union (2003). *Ministerial Declaration at Ministerial e-Health 2003 Conference*. Brüksel (Belgium).
    http://europa.eu.int/information_society/eeurope/ehealth/conference/2003/index_en.htm. Access Date 03.03.2021

European Union (2008). *"Regions 2020 - An Assessment of Future Challenges for EU Regions"*, SEC(2008), 2868 final, Brüksel (Belgium).

Eysenbach, G. (2001). What is e-health? *Journal of Medical Internet Research*, 3(2), e20.

Geena, G., & Heitmann, B. E. (2021). Legal and Regulatory Implications of Telemedicine. In *Principles, Strategies, Applications, and New Directions Rifat Latifi* (Eds Charles R. Doarn & Ronald C. Merrell). Springer, Switzerland.

Glandon, G. L., Smaltz, D. H., & Slovensky, D. J. (2008). *Information Systems for Healthcare Management*. (7th ed.). Chicago: Health Administration Press.

Gregory, S. (2004). *Dictionary of ICT* (4th ed.). Peter Collin Publishing.

Grey, D. (1996). What is knowledge management? The knowledge management forum. http://www.km-forum.org. 28.02.2021.

Haux, R. (2010). Medical informatics: Past, present, future. *International Journal of Medical Informatics*, 79, 599–610.

Huber, P. G. (1991). Organizational learning: The contributing process and the literatures. *Organizations Science*, 2(1), 88–115.

Jennex, M. E., & Croasdell, D. (2007). Knowledge management as a discipline. In *Knowledge Management in Modern Organizations* (pp. 10–17). IGI Global.

Jordanova, M., & Lievens, F. (2011, November). Global Telemedicine and eHealth (A Synopsis). In *2011 E-Health and Bioengineering Conference (EHB)* (pp. 1–6). IEEE.

Köksal, A. (1981). Bilişim Terimleri Sözlüğü. Türk Dil Kurumu Yayınları, No. 476, Ankara, 1981, s.84.

LaNoue, M. D., & Roter, D. L. (2018). Exploring patient-centeredness: The relationship between self-reported empathy and patient-centered communication in medical trainees. *Patient Education and Counseling*, 101(6).

Mandi, S. (2004). Turkey eHealth Strategy – Review & recommended improvements to. October 2004, Senior Expert Consultant to the ITU, Geneva.

Marelli, L., & Testa, G. (2018). Scrutinizing the EU general data protection regulation. *Science*, 360(6388).

Marouf, L. N. (2005). The role of business and social ties in organizational knowledge sharing: A case study of a financial institution (Doctoral dissertation, University of Pittsburgh).

Meyer, R., Degoulet, P. & Omnes, L. (2007). Impact of health care information technology on hospital productivity growth: A survey in 17 acute university hospitals. *Studies in Health Technology and Informatics*, 129(1), 203.

Ministry of Health (2019). Telemedicine and tele radiology department circular.

Olson, C. A., & Thomas, J. F. (2017). Telehealth: No longer an idea for the future. *Advances in Pediatrics*, 64(1).

Pravettoni, G., & Triberti, S. (2020). A "P5" approach to healthcare and health technology. In *P5 eHealth: An Agenda for the Health Technologies of the Future*. Springer, Cham.

Presidential Decree. (2018). Presidential Decree No.1 on the Presidential Organization. *Official Newspaper*, (1)30474.

Tan, J., Kifle, M., Mbarika, V., & Okoli, C. (2005). Diffusion of e-medicine. J. Tan (Ed.). *E-Health Care Information Systems.* Jossey Boss Publishing.

Terstegge, J. (1998). Milan Petkovi'c Willem Jonker (1998) (Eds.). *Security, Privacy, and Trust in Modern Data Management.* Springer.

Tezcan, C. (2016). *Sağlığa Yenilikçi Bir Bakış Açısı: Mobil Sağlık.* TÜSİAD. doi: TÜSİAD-T/2016–03/575.

Vest, J. R. (2012). *Health Information Exchange: National and International Approaches. Health Information Technology in the International Context.* Emerald Group Publishing Limited.

WHO. (2010). Telemedicine: Opportunities and developments in Member States: Report on the second global survey on eHealth 2009.

WHO. (2016). Global diffusion of eHealth: Making universal health coverage achievable, Report of the third global survey on eHealth: http://who.int/goe/publications/global_diffusion/en/. (11.03. 2020).

Winter, A., Haux, R., Ammenwerth, E., Brigl, B., Hellrung, N., & Jahn, F. (2011). *Health Information Systems Architectures and Strategies.* Springer.

Wootton, R., Craig, J., & Patterson, V. (2017). *Introduction to Telemedicine.* CRC Press.

Yeloğlu, O., Sözen, C. (2010). Bilgi toplumu ve teknoloji kullanımı. A. Çelik, T. Akgemci (Ed.). Yönetim bilişim sistemleri. Ankara: Gazi Kitabevi.

Yönetmelikler. (2017). Kişisel Verilerin Silinmesi, Yok Edilmesi Veya Anonim Hale Getirilmesi Hakkında Yönetmelikte Değişiklik Yapılmasına Dair Yönetmelik. Tarih: 28.10.2017. Sayı: 30224

Yüksel, M. (2003). Mahremiyet Hakkı ve Sosyo – Tarihsel Gelişimi. Ankara Üniversitesi SBF Dergisi, 58 (01).

Sibel Özcan

Health Tourism and Free Healthcare Zones

Introduction

Although there are much earlier examples, it is known that the improving middle class of 19th century Europe travelled to thermal springs because it was good for their health and the wealthy in less-developed countries travelled to developed countries for treatment in the 20th century. However, the mobility, which is today called health tourism, differs from these examples in terms of quality and quantity. Looking at today's and past examples, the first difference that stands out is that today this mobility is from developed countries to developing countries. Another difference is that many more people today are travelling to get health care (OECD, 2018: 6).

In recent years, news about health tourism has frequently appeared in the media and newspaper columns. Therefore, it would not be surprising that a larger proportion of the population travels abroad for medical reasons compared to the past. There are many reasons that support such an import or export. Technological advances in information systems and communication meet the needs of patients and the so-called third parties in healthcare to receive treatment in another country at lower costs. The improvements in social security systems or private health insurance market result in patients becoming mobile. This result is further increased by short movements between countries due to work or vacation (OECD, 2011: 5).

Approximately 100 million people in OECD countries are over the age of 65, and this number is expected to rise to 200 million by 2030. It is also estimated that nearly half of the health expenditures will be for this population. Therefore, it is important for those who need health care to obtain the service at a lower cost (Bookman & Bookman, 2007: 6).

The countries that export health tourism make many promotional efforts towards health tourism. The promotions aim to reduce the concerns of patients by emphasizing certain facts, for example, that the service providers get their medical education in developed countries, that they have high-quality medical facilities, there is no waiting time, the costs are affordable, and that both the quality and the quantity of treatment are adequate (Cook, 2008: 5). The countries compete to get a share from the growing health tourism industry through promotions. For this purpose, there is a race between countries for providing high-quality service at lower costs[1] (Sandberg, 2017: 281).

Thus, countries will have foreign exchange earnings, improved employment rate and infrastructure system thanks to the increasing number of tourists. Another expected benefit is that new technologies and treatment methods will increase the health standards for their own citizens. This improvement in healthcare sector standards will allow healthcare professionals who have gone abroad for work to return to their home countries (OECD, 2011: 17, 18).

However, in addition to the benefits, some downsides are likely to arise. For example, while providing low-quality healthcare to its own citizens, high-quality service for foreign patients may pose a risk. Similarly, it may be a risk factor for the countries to redirect the already scarce public resources to private sector service providers through tax exemptions or subsidies. Such a distinction between the private and the public sector will cause healthcare professionals to prefer working in the private sector and move from rural areas to cities. It would not be wrong to define this as a domestic brain drain (OECD, 2011: 17, 18).

I. Health Tourism and Related Definitions

Today, the USA and Western European countries are the leading countries that import healthcare services, while the countries that export such services have spread to all continents including Latin America, Eastern Europe, Africa, and Asia (World Tourism Organization and Travel Commission, 2018: 4). Before discussing the reasons for such global mobility, it would be best to explain the basic concepts.

The International Tourism Organization explains the concept of *health tourism* as an umbrella concept. *Wellness tourism* and *medical tourism* are the concepts covered by health tourism. According to Health Tourism Association, health tourism refers to people travelling abroad to obtain favourable but certainly not inferior medical treatment. The people travelling for this purpose aim to get the same quality or higher quality treatment services for more affordable prices.

While health tourism covers to all tourism activities related to health, medical tourism is preferred for the interventions within the scope of a specific treatment

---

1   Here, it should be noted that the main factor determining the low costs in preferred countries is low costs of labour. Furthermore, few to none malpractice cases and low costs of medications also support the preferability of these countries in terms of costs (Smith & Forgione, 2007: 25).

(Connell, 2006: 1094). Additionally, medical tourism includes medical treatment resources based on analysis and interventions that may or may not require surgical procedures. This definition includes diagnosis, treatment, prevention, and rehabilitation. Wellness tourism aims to ensure a physical, mental, emotional, intellectual and spiritual balance of the travellers.

Lastly, medical tourists are defined as people who demand to receive modern and high-quality health care at affordable prices and travel from their country of residence to another country for this purpose. The medical tourists do not show a homogeneous distribution as expected. This group may include women and men, elderly and young people, and tourists of various races (Bookman & Bookman, 2007: 46–48).

II. Factors and Decision-Making Process

Many people vote with their feet when it comes to access to health care. The shortcomings of health insurance in the country of residence are considered to be among the reasons why people seek their treatment abroad. In priority order, one of the examples of this is the long waiting times for the treatment of certain diseases. However, the most important reason that makes people seek treatment abroad is considered to be the fact that the treatment costs abroad are much lower compared to the expenses in their home country (OECD, 2011: 15; Connell, 2006: 1094).

Although almost all citizens in the European Union have access to healthcare services, there are also those who do not for various reasons. The participants of the income and living conditions survey conducted in the member states of the European Union were asked whether their healthcare needs were met when they needed them, and if not, the relevant reasons. The survey conducted with people over the age of 16 tried to determine the people who could not get examined by a doctor and who could not be treated in the last 12 months due to reasons such as long waiting lists, not being able to afford the service, or needing a certain transportation cost to get the treatment. While the percentage of people who stated that they could not access healthcare services due to the reasons stated above was %3.1 in the total population in 2010, which was the beginning of the data collection, this rate was 2 % for 2019 (OECD, 2018: 170; Eurostat, 2017: 53).

From a different angle, as well as the advantages arising from the exchange rate differences in favour of the developed countries, the widespread use of airway transportation, and the ageing of the baby-boomer generation that came after the war are also considered among the reasons why developing countries are preferred in medical tourism (Connell, 2006: 1094).

Although there are not enough studies on medical tourism, the process is divided into four stages from the emergence of this need. These stages are seeking treatment privately, making the decision to go abroad for treatment, determining the destination country, and determining the person or institution providing the treatment. It is also possible to use an intermediary institution in order to shorten these stages (Hanefeld, Lunt, Smith, & Horsfall, 2015: 362). Similarly, Smith and Forgione developed a two-stage model on the subject. In this model, firstly, the country is chosen, then comes the selection of the facility to get treated (Heung, Küçükusta, & Song, 2010: 240). The model identified the factors that influence the determination of, firstly, the countries from which healthcare services are to be received, then the facility to receive such services. In this two-stage model, neither of the acknowledged factors is considered to be superior to the other and both of them are important in the decision-making process. While the economic conditions, political climate and regulatory standards of the destination country are important in the country selection; costs, training of physicians, quality of the service provided and lastly, the accreditation of the facility are taken into consideration in the selection of the facility that will provide the service (Smith & Forgione, 2007:19).

Although this model identifies the factors that influence the decision-making process, it also has certain shortcomings. For example, the country and facility ranking vary based on the preference of the patient. In other words, it is not always necessary to choose the country first. In some cases, it is possible to first choose a physician or hospital with certain qualifications. Besides, although it is accepted that economic conditions, political climate and regulatory standards cannot be ignored in the country selection, additional factors such as geographical distance, how much the government supports the promotion of medical tourism, infrastructure and superstructure conditions, and the training of healthcare professionals should be included in the assessment. In addition to these, the reputation of the physicians or the facility is also important in the selection of the facility to be treated (Heung, Küçükusta, & Song, 2010: 242).

The medical tourism model suggested by Heung, Küçükusta, and Song addresses the decision-making process in terms of demand and supply. The demand part includes the selection of country, hospital, and physician. The selection of the destination country includes the country's characteristics, the distance and flight costs in addition to the economic and political conditions and regulatory standards acknowledged by Smith and Forgione, and the selection of hospital includes the reputation of the hospital instead of the quality of care. In the model, speciality, respectability and recommendations are important in the selection of the physician as well as the selection of country and hospital. The supply part includes the infrastructure and superstructure facilities, promotional efforts, quality assurance, and communication opportunities in the medical tourism industry offered by the private sector or the state (Heung, Küçükusta, & Song, 2010: 245, 246).

As stated before, accredited institutions can also factor in the decision-making process. Accreditation is considered to be one of the reasons to choose certain institutions not only for the patients travelling from abroad but also for the citizens in the country. Accreditation serves the goal of minimization of risk as well as the maximization of quality. USA Joint Commission International[2] and UK Quality Healthcare Advice Trent Accreditation monitor the institutions that provide healthcare services in many countries around the world (OECD, Medical Tourism: Treatments, Markets and Health System Implications: A Scoping Review, p. 28). Similarly, there are accreditation institutions such as the Canadian Council on Health Services Accreditation and the Australian Council on Healthcare Standards.

III. Health Tourism on a Global Scale

When considered together with globalization, the importance of the healthcare sector in international trade increases in the economies of both developed and developing countries. The advances in information, technology, and transportation have resulted in the mobility of both patients and healthcare providers.

Underdeveloped countries export their expertise and services in the healthcare sector to industrialized countries. Industrialized countries, which previously exported medical services to underdeveloped countries, are now importing healthcare services from these countries. This can be interpreted as a shift in the direction of mobility in international trade (Horowitz & Rosensweig, 2007: 26).

While the Northern America and Western Europe countries rank the first in the list of healthcare importer countries, the countries that provide and export services in this sector are actually located in all continents. Latin America, Eastern Europe, Africa, and Asia are included in these rankings with various countries in these continents.

Medical tourists travel all over the world for many reasons such as dental treatment, heart surgeries, organ and stem cell transplantation, gender reassignment surgeries, and in vitro fertilization (IVF) treatment. For example,

---

2   Joint Commission International, one of the aforementioned accreditation institutions, provides accreditation to 1007 healthcare facilities in 73 countries around the world, 30 of which are located in our country, Turkey (Joint Commision International, 2021).

while some countries in Central and South America have a reputation for cosmetic procedures, plastic surgeries and dental treatment; India, Singapore and Thailand, which are located in Asia, have shown success in orthopaedics and heart surgeries (Horowitz & Rosensweig, 2007: 26).

There are also European Union (EU) regulations on this matter. The resolution of the European Court of Justice in 1998 stated that healthcare services could not be considered in isolation from the other EU member states. Thus, cross-border healthcare services were included in the political agenda (OECD, 2011: 7). Later, in 2011, the scope was expanded through a regulation (*The European Parliament and Council Directive 2011/24/EU*) that allowed bilateral agreements with non-EU member states. With this arrangement, it is ruled that patients have the right to receive healthcare services abroad, including planned treatment services, and that they do not need prior permission for this.

Considering the increasing role of the service sector in economies, the World Trade Organization issued a general regulation on the trade of service provision. With the General Agreement on Trade in Services (GATS) of 1995, the service sector gained greater importance in international trade. The regulation on data collection is especially significant. GATS identified four cases for international service provision. In the first of these cases, the service is provided without the need for the customer or service provider to change locations. In terms of our subject matter, sending the test results to a physician abroad and taking their opinions is an example of this. In the second case, the consumer travels to the country where the service is provided. The activities on health tourism fall into this category. In the third case, the service provided in one country is provided by the legal representative of an institution operating in another country. In the last case, the service provider is temporarily in another country for this purpose (Bookman & Bookman, 2007: 27).

Although such a classification has been made in order to collect data, unfortunately, currently very few countries have been found to have data entry. Therefore, it should be noted that the global size of health tourism is based on forecasts and estimates, not objective data.

There is no definitive information on how many people receive services through health tourism. The reason for this is that some institutions that collect data do or do not include the number of people who get healthcare services when they travel to a country for business or leisure. Therefore, although it is predicted that the shared data cannot be verified, it is acknowledged that the number of participants of health tourism has increased over the years (Horowitz & Rosensweig, 2007: 24).

IV. Health Tourism in Turkey

Turkey is one of the countries that are preferred to receive healthcare services and this is due to sociological and economic reasons. The reasons include close relationships due to kinship ties, movement from countries with a large Turkish population to our country, the advantage of the infrastructure and qualified personnel, the lack of waiting time, and the advantageous treatment fees. However, the demand faced by our country for receiving healthcare services and therefore its share in the sector, unfortunately, falls short of its potential. Therefore, the significance deserved by the subject matter has been demonstrated by including health tourism in the Development Plans, which include long-term goals.

The 11th Development Plan covering the periods of 2019–2023 frequently mentions the concept of health tourism under the "Qualified People, Strong Society" section. The targets determined to achieve this goal are increasing the recognition and preference of our country in the field of health tourism and improving the health tourism service capacity in terms of quality and quantity; completing the legal arrangements for health tourism, strengthening the accreditation and inspection infrastructure; ensuring the integration of medical tourism with elderly and rehabilitation tourism as well as thermal tourism; carrying out the promotional and marketing activities of our country in health tourism sector, and lastly, strengthening the roles of service provider and payer in the healthcare system more effectively mainly in service quality, financial sustainability, audit and performance.

Although it is included in the development plans, the available data suggest that there has not been much progress towards the goals set in the development plans. Although the challenges faced in terms of data collection are not ignored, the data of the visitors departing based on the reason of arrival received from the Turkish Statistical Institute shows the low percentage of tourists prefer our country for health reasons when compared to other reasons. The data presented in a table in Appendix 1 is provided as a graph in Fig. 1. When we look at the reasons for the arrival of the tourists (foreign nationals and Turkish citizens living abroad) in our country, it is seen that very large proportion of the reasons are travel, leisure, visiting relatives, and shopping.

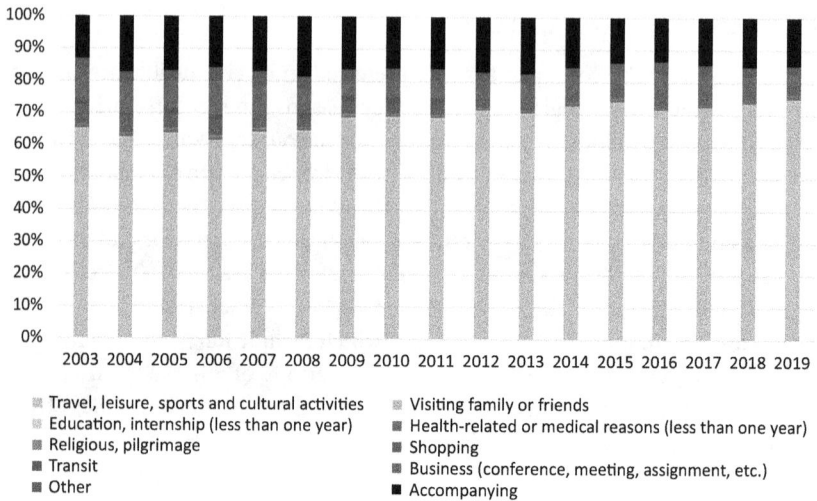

Fig. 1: Departing Visitors by Purpose of Visit
Source: TurkStat Departing Visitors Survey

Appendices 2 and 3 provides the reasons for the arrival of foreigners and citizens of the Republic of Turkey who live abroad. As the table shows, the percentage of foreign visitors who declared their reason for arrival as health and medical reasons increased from 0.75 % in 2003 to 1.25 % in 2019. Among our citizens living abroad, the percentage of those who came for health reasons was 1.41 % in 2003, however, as a result of the fluctuation over time, in 2019, it decreased to the starting level at the beginning of the period. In 2019, only 1.42 % of our citizens living abroad declared that they came to our country for health reasons. Considering both results together, it can be said that although there is an increase in the preference of our country by foreigners, we cannot convince our citizens living abroad about the healthcare service provided in our country.

V. Free Zones

According to the definition of the International Labour Organization, industrial zones which are composed of foreign manufacturing companies that produce in order to benefit from financial incentives, and are included in the customs and trade regime of a country called *export processing zone*, but the concept of *free trade zone* is often used instead of this definition (ILO, 1988: 4). Export processing zones or free trade zones are commonly used by governments to support trade and direct foreign investment. Free zones are common in countries that have transitioned from import-substitution policies to export-oriented growth policies[3] (Engman, Onodera, & Pinali, 2007: 8).

Foreign investors in free zones make more profits since they are exempt from local regulations. Furthermore, developing countries are known to provide various advantages to these zones, aiming to attract multinational companies to the country. For example, in Asia, these zones are established in regions suitable for international trade. They prefer regions that are suitable for sea and air transportation. The countries offer certain opportunities such as establishing the infrastructure of industrial facilities, supplying cheap energy and water resources, and providing short and long-term storage facilities. Of course, besides physical facilities, not being subject to import quotas and exchange rate regulations, and the tax exemptions provided are among the other facilities offered to these zones (Rondinelli, 1987: 91).

Due to these advantages, these free zones may be provided not only to the manufacturing sector but also to the service sector. Currently, many countries are implementing policies similar to free zones regarding the provision of goods and services for the foreign market (Engman, Onodera, & Pinali, 2007: 5).

Although not widespread, free healthcare zones are among the practices that can be preferred. Thus, it is aimed to attract foreign investors and tourists who want to receive treatment to the country. It is also aimed to revitalize the transportation and tourism sectors this way (Sedef, 2018: 138). The unique health free zone in the world was established in Dubai. Dubai Healthcare City (DHCC) aims to dominate the Middle East market and have a say in the Asian market.

---

3   However, the construction and operating costs of these zones are often high. This makes it challenging for developing countries to establish free trade zones. These zones create little workforce or management skills as well as very low domestic added value. There is a low rate of modern technology or know-how transfer and low connectivity with domestic manufacturers. Apart from all these, it is predicted that with the establishment of the free zones, there will be a domestic migration from the rural areas to the regions near the free zones or there will be a high dependence on the production of the companies owned by foreigners. These companies may move to another country or reduce their production due to changing fees, costs, or international trends. Although it varies from country to country, it should be noted that free zone practices may bring certain disadvantages (Rondinelli, 1987: 89, 90).

For this purpose, doctors who have done internship in Europe or America are generally employed (Connell, 2006: 1095).

A. Free Zones in Turkey

The resources of the Ministry of Trade lists the establishment purposes of free zones in our country as encouraging export-oriented investment and manufacture, accelerating foreign direct investments and technology entry, directing businesses to exports, and developing international trade. Our country has 18 free zones established for this purpose[4] (Republic of Turkey Ministry of Trade, 2021).

Free zones offer various advantages to businesses. The first is undoubtedly, that the businesses with production licenses are exempt from income and corporate tax on the gains they make from the sale of the products they manufacture. Another advantage is that the long-term operating licenses allow these businesses to make long-term plans. In connection with the facilities offered in trade, the companies in free zones do not pay Value Added Tax, since they are subject to the export regime for the goods they buy from Turkey. Payment for the activities carried out in free zones in foreign currencies also provides a realistic inflation accounting opportunity. Lastly, the reduction of bureaucratic procedures is also one of the advantages offered to companies operating in free zones (Republic of Turkey Ministry of Trade, 2021).

Specialized free zone practice has been implemented in recent years. Stating that the sectors that create high added value would be supported, the first sector in this field was determined to be the IT sector, and the Istanbul Specialized Free Zone was established. (Republic of Turkey Ministry of Trade, 2021)

---

4   A. Free Zones in Turkey
    The resources of the Ministry of Trade lists the establishment purposes of free zones in our country as encouraging export-oriented investment and manufacture, accelerating foreign direct investments and technology entry, directing businesses to exports, and developing international trade. Our country has 18 free zones established for this purpose (Republic of Turkey Ministry of Trade, 2021).
    A. Free Zones in Turkey
    The resources of the Ministry of Trade lists the establishment purposes of free zones in our country as encouraging export-oriented investment and manufacture, accelerating foreign direct investments and technology entry, directing businesses to exports, and developing international trade. Our country has 18 free zones established for this purpose (Republic of Turkey Ministry of Trade, 2021).

As noted earlier, apart from the free zones operating for export, the eleventh development plan included the concepts of health valley and healthcare technology development zones. The "Competitive Production and Efficiency" section of the Development Plan included pharmaceuticals and medical devices as the priority sectors in industrial policies. The policy targets set in this area aim to increase the competitive power in the global market. It is aimed to improve the R&D and production capacity by launching Health Valley as an integrated health ecosystem that includes all stakeholders of the sector such as universities, research centres, laboratories, technology firms, application centres, physicians, and engineers. In health technology development zones, it is envisaged to include pharmaceutical and medical device production areas, technological facilities, which established to serve common use, and support for clustering will be provided. Although healthcare free zones are planned in many provinces such as İstanbul, İzmir, Antalya and Diyarbakır in our country, unfortunately it has not yet been realized.

Evaluation and Suggestions

Our country is thought to have important advantages in health tourism, which addresses the concepts of both health and tourism. The geographical location of our country as well as our cultural and historical heritage, and its climate already attract millions of tourists, and the education and experience of our healthcare personnel also make our country preferable in the healthcare sector.

As discussed in detail before, there are many reasons for people to travel to another country for treatment. But perhaps the most prominent of these reasons is the high costs of treatment. The fact that the desired treatment is expensive in the country of residence leads people to seek treatment that is at least the same quality but at more affordable prices. Developing countries seek to offer healthcare services that are as quality as in developed countries at affordable prices in order to get a larger share from health tourism.

Preparing cultural programs open for the attendance of both patients and their relatives during the recovery period after the treatment, the cooperation of hotels and hospitals to not overly occupying the beds in the hospitals will be advantageous for both service users and service providers.

Therefore, it will be beneficial to direct the tourism advantages of our country to health tourism, which is preferred by people who seek healthcare services and vacation in another country. Giving priority to infrastructure investments in this field has been identified as a policy and has been included in development plans. While the development and production of high value-added products in the pharmaceuticals and medical devices field is an important goal in itself, establishing healthcare free zones compatible with health tourism subsequent to this goal will enable our country to attain the position it deserves in the health tourism field.

In recent years, since incentives for areas with high added value have been implemented with the establishment of new generation specialized free zones, a similar practice in healthcare can attract domestic and foreign investors to the zone. Thus, foreign currency inflow will be provided, new employment opportunities will be created, and the service quality and efficiency will increase in the healthcare sector due to the increasing competition. The improvement of health tourism is also expected to bring indirect contributions to the economy. The developments in health tourism will have a chain effect on many aspects, for example, airline companies will increase the number of domestic and international flights for the international visitors, the infrastructure investments will be improved, the number of companies operating as intermediary institutions will increase, and the construction sector will grow with the establishment of new facilities to meet the increasing demand. Of course, all these developments will provide positive results in terms of economic growth and development as a whole.

As of 2020, the pandemic that affected the entire world has shown us the importance of investing in the healthcare sector. For this reason, the duties of healthcare technology development zones and the health valleys have increased even more. Establishing free zones in healthcare service delivery in a way to complement the investments in this field will enable us to get a share from the globally growing market and strengthen our economy.

Any support provided in order to improve the technological and scientific infrastructure, contribute to lightening the burden of pandemic on countries. For this reason, the establishment of healthcare free zones as well as the health valley and healthcare technology development zones included in the development plans means the realization of a structure that complies with and fosters the development goals. In this way, gaining an advantage in the competition in the health tourism field can be made possible by offering the tourists the purpose of obtaining quality healthcare services under suitable conditions.

Appendix 1: Departing Visitors by Purpose of Visit, Total

Yıl	Total	Travel, entertainment, sportive or cultural activities	Visiting relatives and friends	Education, training (less than a year)	Health or medical reasons (less than a year)	Business (conferences, meetings, assignments etc.)
2003	16 302 048	8 445 416	2 101 732	79 021	139 971	1 604 905
2004	20 262 645	10 076 732	2 469 907	144 277	171 994	1 928 860
2005	24 124 504	12 024 521	3 281 111	99 957	220 338	2 068 954
2006	23 148 670	10 328 750	3 836 601	106 250	193 728	2 462 609
2007	27 214 986	13 002 599	4 319 515	149 430	198 554	2 347 545
2008	30 979 974	15 031 984	4 864 747	157 464	224 654	2 367 268
2009	31 972 377	16 407 366	5 380 786	217 665	201 222	1 577 508
2010	33 027 941	17 448 324	5 194 790	176 975	163 252	1 723 940
2011	36 151 327	18 602 663	6 058 787	240 583	187 363	2 134 624
2012	36 463 921	20 331 030	5 436 739	222 442	216 229	2 158 204
2013	39 226 226	21 680 347	5 757 757	190 272	267 461	2 333 144
2014	41 415 070	23 904 039	5 979 016	176 324	414 658	2 315 225
2015	41 617 530	24 215 399	6 403 696	144 093	360 180	2 212 327
2016	31 365 330	15 287 344	7 031 921	101 142	377 384	1 810 536
2017	38 620 346	19 389 968	8 436 850	104 904	433 292	1 780 820
2018	45 628 673	25 355 412	8 050 784	114 036	551 748	1 902 089
2019	51 860 042	29 965 670	8 712 806	135 930	662 087	1 850 208

Source: TurkStat Departing Visitors Survey, edited by the author.

Appendix 2: Departing Visitors by Pupose of Visit, Foreigner and Citizen (Resident abroad)

Year	Total		Travel, entertainment, sportive or cultural activities		Visiting relatives and friends		Education, training (less than a year)		Health or medical reasons (less than a year)		Business (conferences, meetings, assignments etc.)	
	Foreigner	Citizen (Resident abroad)	Foreigner	Citizen (Resident abroad)	Foreigner	Citizen (Resident abroad)	Foreigner	Citizen (Resident abroad)	Foreigner	Citizen (Resident abroad)	Foreigner	Citizen (Resident abroad)
2003	13 701 417	2 600 631	7 976 038	469 378	839 087	1 262 645	72 060	6 961	103 403	36 568	1 470 606	134 299
2004	17 202 997	3 059 648	9 546 933	529 799	1 044 575	1 425 332	125 061	19 216	133 722	38 272	1 772 296	156 564
2005	20 522 622	3 601 882	11 465 344	559 177	1 480 067	1 801 044	88 356	11 601	164 597	55 741	1 883 023	185 931
2006	19 275 951	3 872 719	9 717 820	610 930	1 929 800	1 906 801	94 400	11 850	153 894	39 834	2 221 420	241 189
2007	23 017 078	4 197 908	12 348 050	654 549	2 068 642	2 250 873	135 303	14 127	154 603	43 951	2 092 248	255 297
2008	26 431 121	4 548 853	14 424 326	607 658	2 411 765	2 452 982	145 779	11 685	162 484	62 170	2 148 497	218 771
2009	27 314 205	4 658 172	15 680 336	727 030	2 825 952	2 554 834	196 409	21 256	132 677	68 545	1 397 262	180 246
2010	28 510 848	4 517 093	16 726 843	721 481	2 761 521	2 433 269	159 959	17 016	115 222	48 030	1 539 647	184 293
2011	31 324 528	4 826 799	17 850 584	752 079	3 332 705	2 726 082	223 522	17 061	142 463	44 900	1 960 613	174 011
2012	31 342 464	5 121 457	19 453 393	877 637	2 624 016	2 812 723	202 011	20 431	153 520	62 709	1 918 178	240 026

2013	33 827 474	5 398 752	20 637 476	1 042 871	2 947 172	2 810 585	169 941	20 330	188 295	79 166	2 082 477	250 667
2014	35 850 286	5 564 784	22 801 498	1 102 540	3 022 614	2 956 401	158 820	17 504	328 647	86 011	2 051 273	263 952
2015	35 592 160	6 025 370	22 768 327	1 447 072	3 257 492	3 146 204	121 103	22 991	260 339	99 841	1 965 768	246 559
2016	25 265 406	6 099 924	13 980 138	1 307 206	3 671 526	3 360 396	83 964	17 178	251 809	125 574	1 545 808	264 728
2017	32 079 527	6 540 819	17 977 537	1 412 431	4 710 532	3 726 318	89 371	15 533	326 709	106 583	1 552 171	228 649
2018	38 951 902	6 676 771	23 567 646	1 787 766	4 688 850	3 361 934	100 424	13 611	437 925	113 822	1 681 825	220 265
2019	44 712 970	7 147 072	28 062 125	1 903 545	4 965 261	3 747 546	115 566	20 364	560 520	101 567	1 617 561	232 646

Source: TurkStat Departing Visitors Survey, edited by the author.

References

Bookman, M. Z., & Bookman, K. R. (2007). *Medical Tourism in Developing Countries*. New York: Palgrave Macmillan.

Connell, J. (2006). Mediacl Tourism: Sea, Sun, Sand and .... Surgery. *Tourism Management, 27*, 1093–1100.

Cook, P. S. (2008). What Is Health and Mediacl Tourism? *The Annual Conference of The Australian Sociological Association* (pp. 1–13). Victoria.

Engman, M., Onodera, O., & Pinali, E. (2007). *Export Processing Zones: Past and Future Role in Trade and Development*. Paris: ΘECD Publishing.

Eurostat. (2017). *Final Report of The Expert Group on Quality of Life Indicators*. Luxembourg: Publications Office of the European Union.

Hanefeld, J., Lunt, N., Smith, R., & Horsfall, D. (2015). Why Do Medical Tourists Travel to Where They Do? The Role of Networks in Determining Medical Travel. *Social Science & Medicine, 124*, 356–363.

Health Tourism Board. (2021, April 16). Sağlık Turizm Kurulu Web Sitesi: http://www.saturk.gov.tr/images/pdf/tyst/06.pdf adresinden alındı

Heung, V. C., Küçükusta, D., & Song, H. (2010). A Conceptual Model of Medical Tourism: Implications for Future Research. *Journal of Travel&Tourism Marketing*, 236–251.

Horowitz, M. D., & Rosensweig, J. A. (2007). Medical Tourism-Health Care in the Global Economy. *The Physician Executive*, 24–30.

ILO. (1988). *Economic and Social Effects of Multinational Enterprises in Export Processing Zones*. Geneva: International Labour Office.

Medical Tourism Association. (2021, January 18). *Medical Tourism FAQs*. https://www.medicaltourism.com/frequently-asked adresinden alındı

OECD. (2011). *Improving Estimates of Exports and Imports of Health Services and Goods Under The SHA Framework*. OECD.

OECD. (2018). *Health at a Glance: Europe 2018: State of Health in the EU Cycle*. Paris: OECD Publishing.

OECD. (2011). *Medical Tourism: Treatments, Markets and Health System Implications: A Scoping Review*. OECD.

Quality Healthcare Advice Trent Accreditation . (2021, 4 21). https://www.qha-trent.co.uk/medical-tourism-and-accreditation adresinden alındı

Republic of Turkey Ministry of Trade. (2021, January 21). https://ticaret.gov.tr/serbest-bolgeler. https://ticaret.gov.tr/data/5b9b61fc13b8761cc09f9b92/gene l_bilgi.pdf adresinden alındı

Republic of Turkey Ministry of Trade. (2021, April 15). *ticaret.gov.tr*. T.C. Ticaret Bakanlığı: https://ticaret.gov.tr/data/5b9b666013b8761cc09f9bad/Avantajlar. pdf adresinden alındı

Republic of Turkey Ministry of Trade. (2021, April 15). *ticaret.gov.tr*. T.C. Ticaret Bakanlığı: https://ticaret.gov.tr/haberler/bakan-pekcandan-ihtisas-serbest-bolgesi-yatirimcilarina-destek-aciklamasi adresinden alındı

Rondinelli, D. A. (1987). Export Processing Zones and Economic Development in Asia: A Review and Reassesment of a Means of Promoting Growth and Jobs. *The American Journal of Economics and Sociology*, 46(1), 89–105.

Sağlık Turizm Kurulu. (2021, April 16). Sağlık Turizm Kurulu Web Sitesi: http://www.saturk.gov.tr/images/pdf/tyst/04.pdf adresinden alındı

Sağlık Turizm Kurulu. (2021, April 15). Sağlık Turizm Kurulu Web Sitesi: http://www.saturk.gov.tr/images/pdf/tyst/02.pdf adresinden alındı

Sandberg, D. S. (2017). Medical Tourism: An Emerging Global Healthcare Industry. *International Journal of Healthcare Management*, 281–288.

Sedef, M. (2018). A Model Proposal for the Development of Health Tourism in Pamukkale:"Pamukkale Health Free Zone". *International Journal of Health Management and Tourism*, 3(3), 133–146.

Smith, P. C., & Forgione, D. A. (2007). Global Outsourcing of Healthcare: A Medical Tourism Decision Model. *Journal of Information Technology Case and Application Research*, 19–30.

World Tourism Organization and Travel Commission. (2018). *Exploring Health Tourism-Executive Summary*. Madrid: UNWTO.

Part VII Noticeable Issues in Health Law

Burcu G. Özcan Büyüktanır

Clinical Drug Trials in Children

Introduction

Clinical drug trials in children pose a challenging issue in terms of protecting children's health. Volunteering in clinical trials is an issue that should be carefully examined considering the priority of protecting children's health. The issue has ethical and legal aspects. This study discusses the legal aspect of the issue.

It is necessary to protect the best interests of children in clinical trials. Children are not miniature people. They differ from adults physiologically, psychologically, and developmentally. Therefore, drug trials in children may yield different results than the ones in adults. Moreover, the use of drugs, which are used in adults, in children may have different side effects on children. This indicates the importance of drug trials in children. Drug trials in children should be performed only when they are in their interests and following the legal and ethical processes.

The paper examines in detail the legal nature of the contract for clinical drug trials in children and the children's consent to the trial as clinical drug trials in children is a specific issue with legality conditions.

I. Clinical Drug Trials in General

Clinical drug trials investigate a drug's effect, side effect, absorption, distribution or metabolism excretion, and dose adjustment in humans in four phases, where physician specialized in the clinical research field informs the participants for each phase, and trials are applied in volunteers after their consents are obtained (Kara Kılıçarslan, 2011; Doğan&Ünal, 2009). Clinical trials have four phases. Phase I, II, III, and IV. Each phase of those trials is conducted in humans. Phase I includes a small number of healthy volunteers (20–100 people) and examines the effects, safety, and dose setting of the drug on the human body. Phase II examines the effect of drug dose, which is tolerated by healthy volunteers, on patients (100–300 patients). Although a trial has a therapeutic purpose, its scientific purpose outweighs it. Phase III (100–3000 patients) consists of two phases as pre-license phase and license application phase. The pre-license phase includes the trials to collect data and determine the efficacy and safety of the drug in a large patient population. In case of positive results, a license application is made. Phase III trials are performed by specialist physicians. In Phase IV, the efficacy and safety of a drug are examined while it is used for treating patients after it is licensed and put on the market. The trial is conducted with a wide range of patients. The effectiveness of the drug and the frequency of its side effects are investigated (Deutsch & Spickhoff, 2003; Doğan & Ünal, 2009; Kara Kılıçarslan 2011). As a result of the data obtained in this phase, the drug may be withdrawn from the market, or it may be necessary to revise the drug package insert, which is an essential tool for the drug manufacturer to fulfil its warning obligation. We think that it is important in Phase IV to inform the patient that the drug is in Phase IV trials as per the physician's obligation to inform the patient.

The relationship between researching and developing a drug and preserving life, health, and bodily integrity is important. The primary purpose of clinical drug trials is to preserve the life, health, and bodily integrity of the volunteer; otherwise, it constitutes a violation of personal rights (Hausheer &Aebi-Müller, 2012). It is inevitable to conduct drug trials in humans for advancing science and developing new drugs, but it is also crucial to protect the interest of the volunteer, whether healthy or not. In other words, on the one hand, it is necessary to conduct trials for advancing science and treat preserving or preventing diseases; on the other hand, it is necessary to preserve the life, health, and bodily integrity of the volunteer (Spickhoff, 2005). Drug trials in children have particular importance in terms of preserving the life, health, and bodily integrity of children.

In Turkey, the main regulation governing clinical drug trials is Article 17 of the Constitution. Other sources of regulation include the Declaration of Helsinki, the Convention for the Protection of Human Rights and Dignity of the Human Being with regard to the Application of Biology and Medicine: Convention on Human Rights and Biomedicine, the Statute of Medical Deontology, and the By-Law on Clinical Trials of Medicinal and Biological Products (Official Gazette Date: 13.04.2013, Number: 28617). These documents specify the legality conditions of clinical drug trials. In addition, Articles 23 and 24 of the Turkish Civil Code protect the person (child) in clinical drug trials based on the protection of human values. If the volunteer's life, health, and bodily integrity are violated, then contractual or tortious compensation obligations will arise for the pharmaceutical company, the sponsor of the trial, and the practicing physicians (Spickhoff, 2005). Similar to a treatment contract, the practicing physicians have a duty of care (Zuck & Gokel, 2018). They are obliged to act with due diligence and care during a trial (Kara Kılıçarslan, 2011).

II. Clinical Drug Trials in Children

Clinical drug trials can be performed for therapeutic or scientific purposes. Regardless of whether they are considered a medical intervention, they are ultimately drug trials conducted in volunteers and are just interventions aimed directly at bodily integrity. It should be noted that clinical drug trials in unhealthy volunteers are legally similar to medical interventions for therapeutic purposes (Ozanoğlu, 2008). Legality conditions must be met in order not to violate personal rights.

A. Legal Nature of the Contract between Parties in Clinical Drug Trials in Children

The nature of the legal relationship between parties will differ depending on whether clinical trials are for scientific or therapeutic purposes. There is a contractual relationship between the volunteer and the responsible party conducting the trial. In clinical trials for therapeutic purposes, the contract between the researcher, institution, and unhealthy volunteers is basically a treatment contract because the patient's primary goal is to be treated. In the treatment contract made with the physician, the physician does not owe the outcome of the treatment. In the contract made for a clinical trial, treatment is not owed. Turkish law generally accepts that a treatment contract is a proxy contract. In clinical trials for scientific purposes, the contract with a healthy volunteer is unique and atypical (Kara Kılıçarslan, 2011).

In clinical drug trials in children, the child is the volunteer and the legal representative makes the contract on behalf of the child. Therefore, the prerequisite of clinical trials in children is the presence of the best interests of children. The contract for clinical trials in children is an atypical contract benefiting a third party where the performance is made for the child. Since the purpose of the clinical trial is primarily the child's treatment, the provisions of the proxy contract are applied due to the consideration and necessity of the child's best interests.

B. Legality of Clinical Drug Trials in Children

To ensure the legality of clinical drug trials, trials must be performed first in a non-human in vitro environment or a sufficient number of test animals (Doğan&Ünal, 2009; Kara Kılıçarslan, 2011). Permission to conduct the trial must be obtained from authorized institutions, and the trial must be approved. In Turkey, the competent authority is the Ministry of Health. The purpose and scientific status of the trial should be supervised and analysed in terms of ethical considerations. Damage to the subjects involved in the trial should not be disproportionate to the data obtained in the trial, and the subjects involved in the trial should not suffer heavy damages (Article 5 of the By-Law on Clinical Trials of Medicinal and Biological Products). In clinical drug trials, informing and obtaining the consent of volunteers are also indispensable for ensuring the trial's legality and protecting the volunteers' interests (Spickhoff, 2005). Information and consent must be in writing (Doğan&Ünal, 2009). Information should be detailed and facilitate the volunteers' understanding. It is not sufficient to provide information only in writing. Information should be individualized for the volunteer. Detailed verbal information should be given to the volunteers; their questions should be answered, and it must be clear that they understand.

Besides the above-mentioned legality conditions, clinical trials in children should be based on the expectation that their results will have real and direct benefits for the children's health (Büken, 2017). Drug trials in children are performed in cases where the subject matter is directly related to children or is a condition that can be investigated solely in children, or when the results of drug trials in adults need to be verified in children (Nickel, 2005). To perform a drug trial in children, it must be mandatory to perform it. In addition, there should be a general medical opinion that the trial does not pose a risk for the child volunteer and that it benefits the volunteer (Fischer, 2005; Büken, 2017). A common medical view must exist that the investigational product or procedure carries no known risk to children (Article 6 of the By-Law on Clinical Trials of Medicinal and Biological Products).

The ethics committee is informed on the clinical, ethical, psychological, and social aspects of the trial by a pediatrician, and assesses the trial protocol accordingly (Article 6 of the By-Law on Clinical Trials of Medicinal and Biological Products). The ethics committee may not approve any clinical trial in children unless a favourable view for conducting it has been given by a pediatrician. If deemed necessary for these trials, the opinion of a pediatrician or a pediatric dentist holding a doctoral or medical residency degree in a field relevant to the subject matter of the trial is consulted, and the decision on whether or not to authorize the trial is based on such opinion (Article 6 of the By-Law on Clinical Trials of Medicinal and Biological Products). If the child is capable of weighing the information provided and reaching a sound decision, all relevant information regarding the trial is explained to the child using appropriate language. The positive opinion of the child, who has the mental competence to express an opinion on the subject, should be taken; the consent of the child who has the mental competence to give consent must be obtained; the written consent of the legal representative must be obtained in addition to the child's opinion/consent.

The child is removed from the trial if he or she wishes to withdraw from it or refuses to take part in it at any stage (Article 6 of the By-Law on Clinical Trials of Medicinal and Biological Products). The design of the trial should minimize pain, discomfort, fear, and any risks related to the patient's condition or age. The risk limit and the degree of discomfort must be both specifically defined and continuously monitored. During the information phase, the child volunteer and his/her legal representative should also be informed about the possible disturbances (Heil & Lützeler, 2010; Volkmer, 2016).

Trials in children must improve the children's health and sustain a level that benefits children as a group besides their therapeutic purpose (Büken, 2017).

Article 5 of the Declaration of Helsinki states that, in medical research on human subjects, considerations related to the well-being of the human subject should take precedence over the interests of science and society. In the same vein, Article 18 of the Declaration suggests that the benefit targeted with the medical research involving human subjects should outweigh s the inherent risks and burdens to the healthy volunteers. Article 16 of the Biomedicine Convention states that the risks which may be incurred by volunteers should not be disproportionate to the potential benefits of the trial.

The limit of information given by researchers and physicians to volunteers in clinical drug trials is of particular importance. In drug trials, detailed information should be given in a way that facilitates the volunteer's understanding; risks should be explained but the limit should be drawn well (Deutsch/Spickhoff, 2003; Spickhoff, 2005; Volkmer, 2016). The scope of information should cover how the clinical trial works, its importance, risks, and content (Nickel, 2005; Zuck/Gokel, 2018) and the volunteer should be informed that he or she can leave the trial at any stage (Nickel, 2005).

In clinical drug trials, preserving the child's life, health, and bodily integrity and protecting and realizing the child's right to self-determination are ensured by considering two principles in the trial: The trial's benefit is more than its harm to the volunteer and it does not contain excessive risks for the volunteer; and the participation of the child volunteer and obtaining the consent of his/her legal representative or obtaining the consent of the legal representative together with the child volunteer who has the mental competence (Fischer, 2005; Spickhoff, 2005) .

C. A Special Issue: Child's Consent to Clinical Trial as a Condition of Legality

There are no convincing gains in clinical trials. Medical trials in children do not achieve any convincing gains other than covering the trial's costs. The legal representative, who consents to the trial with the child or on behalf of the child lacking mental competence, will not be able to exercise the right of not knowing on behalf of the child. Clinical drug trials are carried out in four phases after animal tests. Since the licensed drug is given to patients in Phase IV drug trials, the physicians are obliged to inform them that the drug prescribed for their treatment is in Phase IV as per their informing obligation. While the information is more comprehensive in Phase I, it can be narrowed in Phase IV (Doğan & Ünal, 2009). This request of the patient, who wants to exercise his/her right to not know about drug risks in clinical drug trials for therapeutic purposes, is acceptable in Phase IV.

In drug trials in children lacking the capacity to act, the person consenting on behalf of the child is the parent, who has the right of custody, or the guardian (if the child is under guardianship). Information is given to the legal representative and the child who can give consent and the child who can give an opinion based on the presence of mental competence. However, in clinical drug trials in children, consent differs depending on whether the children have mental competence and whether the clinical trial is therapeutic. In clinical trials for therapeutic purposes, their consent should be obtained if they have mental competence in the context of the children's right to self-determination (Deutsch&Spickhoff, 2003) and participate in decisions about themselves (Article 6 of the By-Law on Clinical Trials of Medicinal and Biological Products). In this case, the consent of the parents and child must be obtained together. Although age is not specified for the presence of mental competence, the presence of the mental competence of a child is checked on a case basis. The child, who does not have mental competence but has a certain maturity, should also be informed and heard about the trial (Article 6 of the By-Law on Clinical Trials of Medicinal and Biological Products) (Nickel, 2005; Heil&Lützeler, 2010; Volkmer, 2016). Informing the child about the trial, even if he/she does not have mental competence, is also important in terms of ensuring the child's right to participate in the decisions about him/herself. The information should be given to the child in a way that facilitates his/her understanding by taking into account his/her age, and be instructive about how the trial is performed, its potential risks, and benefits (Volkmer, 2016). Consent to the clinical trial for therapeutic purposes must be given by the parents together, who have the right of custody, on behalf of the child who lacks mental competence. The consent of the guardian is required if the child is under guardianship. In all cases, consent must be given in writing. The works of guardianship and supervisory authorities do not include giving consent to clinical trials. However, in terms of what should happen, it is necessary to include the approval of consents for the clinical trial in the works of the

Civil Court of First Instance, which is the supervisory authority, with an amendment to be made in Article 463 of the Turkish Civil Code.

We think that the best interests of children are important in obtaining their consent, in clinical trials for scientific purposes, whether they have mental competence or not; clinical trials for scientific purposes should not be conducted in children, at least in children who lack mental competence, due to the necessity of protecting children. The children should not volunteer with the consent of other people in a matter that directly concerns their health, as they do not yet have the competence for self-determination, even if these people are their parents. However, according to the current legal regulations, it is possible to perform clinical trials for scientific purposes with the written consent of the legal representatives if the children have mental competence. For those who lack mental competence, only the written consent of their legal representatives is sufficient.

In clinical drug trials with child volunteers, the most sensitive issues are supervision and not abusing custody rights. In case of contrary situations, the provisions of the Turkish Civil Code regarding the protection of the children in the custody relationship will be applicable.

Anyone under the age of 18 is a child. Parents who have the right of custody should not allow the children to be subjects in clinical trials for scientific purposes for a certain fee. Otherwise, they will be abusing their right of custody. Clinical trials with child volunteers should be the clinical trials, which solely aim at treating the child and in which the child's interest outweigh. This is a requirement of protecting the interests of children as well. The use of unlicensed drugs is very frequent in pediatric drugs because clinical drug trials are very limited in children. Conducting drug trials in healthy children is contrary to their best interests. This is also against the Convention on the Rights of the Children. In addition, according to Article 6 of the By-Law on Clinical Trials of Medicinal and Biological Products, the starting point can be the general medical opinion that the clinical trial in children directly benefits the child. However, according to the Biomedicine Convention, to which we are a party, drug trials in children are allowed provided that it benefits the child or the same age group and poses minimum harm and danger to the child (Biomedicine Convention, Articles 6, 16, and 17).

Conclusion

Protecting the interest of the child is the most important issue for clinical trials in children. The UN Convention on the Rights of the Children acknowledges the principle of the interest of the children as the basic principle. At the same time, the children have the right to express their opinion on matters related to their own lives. Clinical trials are necessary for applying effective and safe treatments for children. Keeping all these in mind, clinical trials should be carried out with the child's consent based on the presence of mental competence together with the opinion of the child and the parent or guardian considering the child's best interests as a priority.

Consent must always be informed consent. The information should be detailed and the child should be informed in a way that he/she can comprehend. The balance of risk and benefit must be acceptable for the child in the trial. It should be possible to withdraw the child from the trial without giving any reason.

Considering the emotional effects of the trial on children, the child's interest should become a priority in all practices. The results of the trial and its effects on the child should be assessed from a physiological, psychological, and mental perspective. This multi-dimensional assessment should also be taken into account in protecting the child's interests.

Special conditions are required for trials in children. Since children cannot directly decide on their own lives and bodies, there must be other conditions besides the special conditions listed above. The trial should also be beneficial for other children. The trial should be solely performable in children.

As a result, the trial should be assessed meticulously considering the priority of the child's best interests.

References

Büken, N. (2017). Klinik Araştırmanın Katılımcısı Olarak Çocuklar, *Journal of Pediatr Inf*, 11(2), 87–93.

Deutsch, E. & Spickhoff, A. (2003). *Medizinrecht* (5th ed.). Springer.

Doğan, M. & Ünal, A. (2009). İnsanlar Üzerinde İlaç Deneyleri ve Ortaya Çıkan Hukuki Sorunlar, *Erciyes Üniversitesi Hukuk Fakültesi, İlaç Hukuku, I. Sağlık Hukuku Sempozyumu*, Cilt/Sayı, s. 151–168.

Fischer, G. (2005). Die Prinzipien der Europäischen Richtlinie zur Prüfung von Arzneimitteln. In Deutsch, E. et al. (Eds.) *Die klinische Prüfung in der Medizin, Europäische Regelungswerke auf dem Prüfstand*, Springer.

Hausheer/ Aebi-Müller (2012), Das Personenrecht des Schweizerischen Zivilgesetzbuches, Dritte Auflage, Bern.

Heil, M. & Lützeler, C. (2010). § 4 Klinische Prüfung. In Dieners, P. & Reese, U. (Eds.), *Handbuch des Pharmarechts, Grundlagen und Praxis*, N. 204–212, C. H. Beck.

Kara Kılıçarslan, S. (2011). Klinik İlaç Araştırmalarından Doğan Sorumluluk, *Gazi Üniversitesi Hukuk Fakültesi Dergisi*, XV (3), 285–310.

Nickel, L. C. (2005). Überlegungen für die Umsetzung der Richtlinie 2001/20/EG (GCP-Richtlinie) in deutsches Recht. In Deutsch, E. et al. (Eds.), *Die klinische Prüfung in der Medizin, Europäische Regelungswerke auf dem Prüfstand*, Springer.

Ozanoğlu, H. S. (2008). Hasta ve Gönüllü Hakları Açısından İlaç Araştırmalarında Hukuki Sorumluluk, *Ankara Barosu II. Sağlık Hukuku Kurultayı 7–8 Kasım 2008*, s. 379–386.

Spickhoff, A. (2005). Freiheit und Grenzen der medizinischen Forschung. In Deutsch, E. et al. (Eds.), *Die klinische Prüfung in der Medizin, Europäische Regelungswerke auf dem Prüfstand*. Springer.

Volkmer, M. (2016). In Körner, H. H. & Patzak, J. (Eds.), *Betäubungsmittelgesetz (Arzneimittelgesetz Grundstoffüberwachungsgesetz) Kurz Kommentare, Band 37*, N.188–193, C. H. Beck.

Zuck, R. & Gokel, J. M. (2018). In Quaas, M. et al. (Eds.), Nationales Recht, Klinische Prüfung, *Medizinrecht* (4. Auflage), n. 10–14, Verlag C. H. Beck.

Dila Okyar

Orhan Emre Konuralp

The Critical Analysis of the Consumer Status of Patients Under Turkish Law

Introduction

The historical development of Turkish consumer law dates back to 1995, when the first Consumer Protection Act, no.4077 (Official Gazette Date: 08.03.1995, Number: 22221) has entered into force. This Act was prepared within the framework of the customs union between Turkey and the European Union ("EU") with the purpose of harmonization. This legislation was important in terms of collecting the scattered provisions of that time on consumer protection under a single act (Akipek Öcal, 2018). Although the Act was revised in 2003, consumer law has made great progress over time and thus, it became highly necessary to enact a new law. Accordingly, with the aim of ensuring full harmonization of Turkish national law with the EU legislation on consumer protection, the New Consumer Protection Act ("CPA") no. 6502 (Official Gazette Date: 28.11.2013, Number: 28835) has entered into force on 29.05.2014.

The most striking feature of the CPA, with respect to our study, is the expansion of its material scope of application. In this regard, the new definition of "consumer transaction" is of utmost importance. It is the fundamental concept at which the heart of consumer law, so to speak, beats at. The current CPA defines consumer transaction in an extremely wide manner, especially to eliminate hesitations in the judicial practice during the application of the former CPA. The similar approach is also seen in the concept of "services", which is broadly defined to include all kinds of activities other than providing goods. Thus, all contracts that consist of an obligation of intangible nature, in which one party is the consumer and the other is the provider, are qualified as consumer contracts.

In the field of health law, the significant impact of bringing the consumer law to such a wide area of application is seen in the qualification of contracts between patients and private healthcare providers as consumer contracts. This especially manifests itself in the legal regime applicable to medical malpractice cases. In our study, the consequences of the consumer status of patients and qualification of medical malpractice cases as consumer disputes will be evaluated, in terms of both substantive and procedural law.

Consumer law, which started to develop as a sub-branch of the law of obligations, by declaring its independence over time, has become a separate branch of law. However, due to its multi-disciplinary nature, it has relations with many branches of public and private law. Since consumer contracts constitute the main subject of consumer law, its relationship with the law of obligations has a special weight. Art. 83/1 CPA which reads as *"general provisions apply in the absence of an applicable provision in this act"* is a clear indication of its inevitable "umbilical bond" with the law of obligations. In the light of this fact, while presenting our evaluations with respect to substantive law, provisions of the CPA will be comparatively evaluated with the provisions of the Turkish Code of Obligations ("TCO"), no. 6098 (Official Gazette Date: 04.02.2011, Number: 27836), the Turkish Civil Code ("TCC"), no. 4721 (Official Gazette Date: 08.12.2001, Number: 24607) and related provisions of Turkish health legislation.

I. Overview of the Material Scope of Application of the Consumer Act

The material scope of application of the CPA is considerably extensive (Aydoğdu, 2015). The Act covers both consumer transactions and consumer-oriented applications (art. 2 CPA).

A. The Backbone Concept of Consumer Law: Consumer Transaction

The concept of "consumer transaction" is defined under art. 3/1-L CPA:

> including contract of work, transportation, brokerage, insurance, agency contract, banking and similar contracts established between real or legal persons acting for commercial or professional purposes, including public legal entities in the goods or services markets, or acting on their behalf or account, and consumers, all kinds of contracts and legal transactions

Two main requirements need to be satisfied in order to qualify as a consumer transaction: party and subject matter.

1. Requirement as to Parties

The Turkish legislator has defined the concept of consumer transaction in a radical broadness. Accordingly, any contract concluded between consumer and seller or service provider constitutes a consumer transaction. The Turkish legislator has adopted the subjective system in the CPA since the concept of consumer is taken as basis (Kara, 2021). "Consumer" refers to *any natural or legal person acting for non-commercial or non-professional purposes*" (art. 3/1-K CPA). Provider means *"any real or legal person, including public law entities, who provides services to the consumer for commercial or professional purposes*" (art. 3/1-I CPA). Thus, it is the opposite purposes of the parties that leads to the qualification as a consumer transaction. The provider may be a real person merchant, tradesman, self-employed person or a public[1] or private law legal person (Havutçu, 2014). The provider is the person who carries out the activity of providing services subject to the contract in a continuous manner for the purpose of gaining profit. The expression "for commercial or professional purposes" in the definition of seller/provider is too broad for the purpose of the law, as it includes the person who sells goods occasionally. Thus, in accordance with the expression "in the course of this trade" of art. 1/2-c of 1999/44/EC, it should be read as "within the scope of commercial and professional activities" (Gümüş, 2014). Interesting to note that, when defining the consumer, the CPA preferred the expression of "non-commercial or non-professional purpose" instead of the expression of "special purpose", which was used in the former CPA. This expression is understood, in terms of real person consumers as "the purpose of meeting personal or family needs" and in terms of legal person consumers as "meeting the needs other than the commercial or professional activity of the legal person" (Aydoğdu, 2015).

Also, in the definition of consumer, unlike the definition of provider, the expression "including public legal entities" is not included. Thus, the law implicitly denies the consumer status of public legal entities, since they cannot pursue any personal purpose (Gümüş, 2014). Private law legal persons, on the other hand, can enjoy the consumer status only to the extent that they act within the framework of their ideal purpose (Gümüş, 2014). The person who claims to be a consumer is under the burden of proof (art. 6 TCC).

2. Requirement as to Subject Matter

The provision of goods and/or services constitutes the subject of a consumer transaction. The provision of both goods and services can possibly coexist in the same contractual structure (Akipek Öcal, 2018; Gümüş, 2014). The term "goods"

---

1   The public legal person is to be understood as public legal entities (e.g. state-owned enterprises or local public institutions such as Istanbul Water and Sewerage Administration) operating exclusively under the private law provisions.

includes movable items subject to shopping (art. 3/1-H CPA) and the term "services" refers to "any subject matter of consumer transaction other than providing goods that are made or promised to be made in return for a fee or benefit" (art. 3/1-D CPA). Based on the expressions of "subject to shopping" and "in return for a fee or benefit", consumer transaction is required to be onerous (Aydoğdu, 2015; Özel, 2019; Kara, 2021). Providing money or benefits other than money to the other party is sufficient to satisfy this requirement (Havutçu, 2014). The concept of service is also defined quite broadly. Since there is no restriction as to the type of service, all kinds of services such as accommodation, education, health, cleaning, financial services, transportation, insurance, tourism and communication may constitute the subject of a consumer transaction (Havutçu, 2014; Aydoğdu, 2015).

3. Other Distinguishing Features of Consumer Transaction

In the definition of consumer transaction, explicit mention of some types of contracts by name is remarkable. The underlying reason of the Turkish legislator is to eliminate the previous jurisprudence, which highly restricted the material scope of the consumer law (Havutçu, 2014; Sirmen, 2014; Kara, 2021). In fact, the consumer transaction definition of the former CPA was sufficiently broad to cover all types of contracts, since it describes it as "all kinds of legal transactions between the consumer and the seller/provider in the goods or service markets" (art. 3/1-h). However, despite the wording, the judicial practice has left some types of contracts outside the scope of the law by subjecting the concept of consumer transaction to a narrow interpretation. The disputes arising from contract of work related to the goods to be manufactured and (due to being regarded as absolute commercial cases) the contracts regulated in the Turkish Commercial Code, such as transportation and insurance were regarded as falling outside the scope of the former CPA (Havutçu, 2014).

The expression of *"and similar contracts"* indicates that this enumeration is not limited; only (Gümüş, 2014; Akipek Öcal, 2018). Important to note that, only the mention of these contracts by name is not sufficient to qualify as a consumer contract; in each concrete case, whether the contract in question also meets the requirement as to parties is to be evaluated. (Akipek Öcal, 2018). The CPA, in its fourth part, also specifically regulates some types of consumer contracts. Consumer transactions are not limited to these contract types as well. Also, innominate contracts, concluded within the framework of the principle of freedom of contract, can qualify as consumer transactions (Gümüş, 2014). The term "consumer contract" is a supreme concept including both nominate and innominate contracts (Havutçu, 2014). Pursuant to art. 83/2 CPA:

> the fact that a transaction, to which consumer is a party to, is regulated in other laws does not prevent this transaction from being considered as a consumer transaction and the implementation of the provisions of this Act regarding jurisdiction and territorial jurisdiction

The expression of "*contract and legal transaction*" is also remarkable. As known, legal transaction is a supreme concept which covers both unilateral and bilateral transactions. A consumer transaction often appears as a consumer contract. This wording is interpreted as the legislator's intent to emphasize the unilateral legal transactions which the consumers may conclude in relation with a consumer contract (Havutçu, 2014).

B. Consumer-Oriented Applications

This concept, newly introduced by the CPA, is not defined in the text but explained in the explanatory statement as applications of the seller/provider before, during and after the conclusion of a consumer contract. Followingly, after-sales services and unfair commercial practices not based on a consumer contract are given as examples. With respect to our study, the importance of this new concept manifests itself in providing a legal basis for *culpa in contrahendo* liability (Özel, 2019). Accordingly, the compensation claims of the consumers for damages suffered due to faulty behaviour of the seller/provider even in the pre-contractual phase are accepted to fall within the scope of the CPA. In fact, disputes arising from such compensation claims were already considered within the scope of the former CPA as the decision of General Civil Chamber of Turkish Court of Cassation dated 01.12.2010 sets a good example (registration no. 2010/13-593, decision no. 2010/623).

II. Consumer Disputes Arising from Health Law

A. The Determination of the Consumer Status of Patients

Health law is a branch of law that regulates mainly the legal relations of people receiving health services with institutions providing health services and the legal relations of such institutions with the State. The "patient", as the basic concept of health law, refers to "*any real person who needs to benefit from health services*" (Art. 4/b of Regulation on Patient Rights). It does not refer only to persons whose health is impaired. It is interpreted widely as to cover persons who receive health service relating to, for example, aesthetic intervention for beautification, circumcision, check-up and voluntary termination of pregnancy without any medical necessity. In cases where the provision of health service includes a medical intervention, patient is regarded as the passive subject of the medical intervention. "Medical intervention" means all kinds of medical activities performed on the human body by professional persons (physicians and other health personnel) authorized by law to perform the medical profession for the purposes (diagnosis, treatment, protection and increasing the health welfare of the person) stipulated in the law.

According to the Turkish Constitution, *"everyone has the right to live in a healthy and balanced environment [...] The state fulfils this task by utilizing and supervising the health and social institutions in the public and private sectors"* (art. 56). The legal qualification of the healthcare institution where the faulty medical intervention has taken place is decisive in determining the legal regime applicable to medical malpractice cases. A patient can apply either to a private medical clinic of a self-employed physician or to an official or private healthcare institution. Official healthcare institutions are hospitals affiliated to the Ministry of Health within the state legal entity (state hospital, city hospital), university hospitals affiliated to the university rectorship within the university legal entity (state and non-profit private university hospitals) and family practice centres. General Civil Chamber of Turkish Court of Cassation has decided that malpractice disputes arising from medical interventions carried out at non-profit private university hospitals shall be included in the jurisdiction of the administrative judiciary (case registration no. 2014/566, decision no. 2015/1339, decision date. 13.05.2015). Liability for damages incurred due to faulty medical intervention performed at official healthcare institutions fall outside the CPA and thus, the medical liability cases shall be brought before the administrative courts.

With respect to our study, the consumer disputes arise in cases where the patient applies to a private healthcare provider (self-employed physician or a private healthcare institution such private hospital, medical centre, polyclinic) to receive health services under a contractual relationship. In most of the cases, the patients enjoy the status of consumer as they receive healthcare services for personal purposes. However, there may be exceptional situations where the patient acts with a professional purpose. An example would be an actress having a breast augmentation surgery for a movie project (Gözpınar Karan, 2018). The contract for medical treatment of the minor concluded by the parents is regarded as a "contract for the benefit of the third person" (Çilenti Konuralp, 2020). In such cases, the third party who benefits from the service is accepted to hold the consumer status (Gözpınar Karan, 2018). Also, Patient Rights Boards are established in 2014 to evaluate the applications with the violation claim of patient rights that could not be resolved on-site by the health institution. Among the members of these Boards is "a representative from the consumer associations, if not from the patient rights associations". This fact is considered as another indication of the consumer status of the patients (Akipek Öcal, 2018). However, applications regarding medical malpractice claims fall out of the scope of these Boards. Private healthcare providers qualify as "providers" since they act with commercial/professional purposes. Accordingly, the contract between these parties for the provision of healthcare services qualify as consumer contracts (Gümüş, 2014; Akipek Öcal, 2018).

In this acceptance, two features of the CPA are influential. First, within the framework of full harmonization, the preparatory studies of the CPA make mention of the 2011/83/EU Directive on Consumer Rights and states that it was transposed to Turkish law. This Directive explicitly excludes contracts for healthcare from its scope as it mentions that "*healthcare requires special regulations because of its technical complexity, its importance as a service of general interest as well as its extensive public funding [...] The provisions of this Directive are not appropriate to healthcare which should be therefore excluded from its scope*" (N.30) whereas the CPA does not provide for such an exception. Secondly, as a result of wide scope of application of the CPA, the judicial hesitation during the former CPA as to whether the agency contracts qualify as consumer contracts was eliminated. This is of importance since, as will be explained below, contracts concluded with private healthcare institutions and self-employed physicians are subject to provisions on agency contract.

The validity of informed consent forms, which are in principle required to ensure the legality of the medical intervention, is another important legal aspect in health law disputes. These constitute the typical example of a unilateral transaction under consumer law, concluded in connection with a consumer contract. Accordingly, the provisions of informed consent forms are to be subject to the protective provisions of the CPA on unfair terms (Havutçu, 2014).

B. Main Types and Legal Nature of Health Law Contracts

1. Contract for Medical Treatment

Medical treatment contract is established between a self-employed physician and the patient where the physician is primarily obliged to provide medical treatment to the patient and the patient, as a rule.[2] is obliged to make a payment in

---

2   Since physicians perform their duty professionally, receiving fee is customary under art. 502/3 TCO.

return. Contract for medical treatment, in principle, is qualified as an agency contract, which is regulated under arts. 502-514 TCO (Şenocak, 1998). Thus, physicians perform their obligation without the risk of not obtaining the result. Since medical intervention is carried out over the human body, due to its nature, the result is not suitable for prior commitment. If the physician fulfils his duty of care, non-achievement of the desired healing does not result in the breach of contract. The voluntary guarantee of any result of healing will not be valid (Şenocak, 1998). On the other hand, contracts related to aesthetic surgery operations purely for beautification and dental practices such as prosthesis and aesthetic restoration are regarded as contracts for work. The decision of 15th Civil Chamber of Turkish Court of Cassation dated 30.09.2019 sets an example for such court practice (registration no. 2019/2716, decision no. 2019/3692). In the contract of work, the physician is in the position of the contractor and thus, undertakes the result. As a result of broad definition of the consumer transaction of the CPA, both types are accepted as consumer contracts (Kara, 2021).

2. Hospital Admission Contract

The contract concluded between the patient and the private hospital operator for the provision of an inpatient treatment is named as the hospital admission contract. Disputes arising out such contracts are accepted as consumer disputes as well. The decision of 3rd Civil Chamber of Turkish Court of Cassation dated 19.12.2019 sets an example for such court practice (registration no. 2016/24615, decision no. 2019/12860). The most common type of this contract is "the contract of full admission to hospital". In the full admission contract with the addition of a treatment contract, the private hospital undertakes the hospital care, while the medical treatment is undertaken by both the private hospital and the physician based on joint responsibility. In the divided hospital admission agreement, there are two separate contracts to which the patient is a party: the treatment agreement between the patient and the physician and the hospital admission agreement between the patient and the private hospital. Medical treatment is undertaken by the physician and the hospital care by the private hospital (Yılmaz, 2019). This innominate contract is a type of mixed contract where the private hospital undertakes all healthcare obligations (medical treatment, accommodation, food, medicine, cleaning and other hospital care services) and in return, the patient is obliged to pay the service fee. The dominant obligation of the private hospital is the medical treatment, which belongs to contract of agency. Accordingly, the legal provisions on contract of agency are applied by analogy. The decision of General Civil Chamber of Turkish Court of

Cassation dated 21.10.2009 sets an example for such court practice (registration no. 2009/393, decision no. 2009/452). Another distinguishing feature of this type of contract is the contractual addressee of the patient. There is no contractual relation between the patient and the physician who performs the medical intervention. The patient is in a contractual relationship only with the private hospital operator. The private hospital performs through its own staff, who are in the position of auxiliary persons. Here, the obligations undertaken by the private hospital appear in a mixed structure, including both the provision of goods and services (Gümüş, 2014). The private hospital is liable for the acts of auxiliary persons (art. 116 TCO).

III. Research and Methods

This study examines both jurisprudence and relative doctrine. As it has already been stated, broad definitions of "consumer transaction" and "service" of the CPA requires analysis of both the doctrine and the approach of the courts. Since the scope of application of the CPA is broader than the 2011/83/EU Directive on Consumer Rights and other jurisdictions, the analysis is restricted to Turkish doctrine and jurisprudence. Another method used in this study is analysing statistics about consumer disputes in Turkey. These statistics are important to show the proportion of the consumer disputes and the significance of these disputes among all civil disputes.

The CPA has adopted a special dispute resolution method for the resolution of consumer disputes. Accordingly, disputes with a dispute value below 11.330 TL (1.000 €) are subject to mandatory arbitration (Ermenek, 2013; Taşpınar Ayvaz, 2016; Özsöker, 2019) and the parties must apply to consumer arbitration committees before applying to the court. If the value of the dispute is above this limit, the parties shall apply directly to the court. This limit is applied in 2021 and is updated every year regarding the inflation rate.

According to Judicial Statistics of 2019, 2.026.507 new civil cases were filed in Turkey, 59.589 of these cases were consumer cases. However, these statistics does not include statistics of consumer arbitration committees. This is because these committees are organized under the Ministry of Trade and the statistics are provided by this Ministry. According to these statistics, in 2019, 547.235 new consumer disputes were brought before consumer arbitration committees. It is seen that almost 1/4 of all civil cases are consumer cases (Konuralp, 2020).

Another interesting statistic about consumer disputes, which is directly related to our study, is about the legal nature of the disputes. Proportion of the defective service cases is in trend of increase year by year, as Tab. 1 shows:

Tab. 1: Percentage of the Cases Arising from Defective Service among All Disputes Before the Consumer Arbitral Committees

	2017	2018	2019
Number of Cases Arising from Defective Service	74.558	101.393	123.903
Total Number of Cases Before the Consumer Arbitral Committees	590.303	562.049	547.235
Percentage of the Cases Arising from Defective Service	12,6 %	18,0 %	22,6 %

Note: https://ticaret.gov.tr/data/5d774a6a13b876bdfcd7c332/7-T%C3%BCketici%20Hakem%20
Heyetlerine%20Ula%C5%9Fan%20T%C3%BCketici%20%C5%9Eikayeti%20%C4%B0statistikleri.pdf

VI. Critical Analysis of the Consumer Status of the Patients

A. Substantive Law Perspective

1. In General

On one hand, expansion of the concept of consumer transaction is favoured as it expands the protection area of consumer (Aydoğdu, 2014); on the other hand, such wide area of application is found to contradict with the "soul" of the consumer law. Even during the period of the former CPA, the following criticism was raised in Turkish doctrine: *"it is a ridiculous dream to apply consumer protection rules against dentists, auto repair shops, shoe shine halls, sculptors, heaters and taxi drivers"* (Serozan, 1996). Accordingly, the consumer status of the patients has also led to controversies. One view is in favour of the consumer status of patients on the ground that consumer protection provides additional protective measures (Akipek Öcal, 2018). The opposing views emphasize the incompatibility with the spirit of consumer law (Yılmaz, 2019) and raise the concerns as to commercialization of healthcare services (Gözpınar Karan, 2018) as well as the increase in the workload of consumer courts and the loss of significance of consumer courts as special courts (Tutumlu, 2014).

2. Main Legal Issues

a. Obligation to Contract

Due to professional autonomy, the health legislation grants the physicians, in principle, the right to conscientious objection (the right to refuse the patient), except in cases of emergencies. According to art. 18 of Regulation on Medical

Deontology, "the physician and dentist may refuse to provide care to the patient for professional or personal reasons, except in cases of emergency aid, or the performance of official or humanitarian duty". There is a similar provision for private hospitals under art. 32 of Act on Private Hospitals. However, the consumer law restricts the freedom of contract in favour of consumers. The provider cannot avoid providing service without a valid ground (art. 6/2 CPA).

b. Culpa in Contrahendo Liability

Starting from the moment of entrance of the patient in the domain of the health-care provider, the (potential) parties are mutually obliged to exercise duty of care in order to prevent damage to each other. Important to note that such obligation also expands to third parties (such as family member, friend or companion) who fall within the protection area due to their closeness to the performance. As explained above, such compensation claims are accepted to fall under the CPA. However, this is not a unique feature of the consumer law since *culpa in contrahendo* liability finds its roots in the rule of honesty (art. 2/1 TCC). Thus, a patient who slipped on the wet floor at the hospital entrance and injures his arm can bring the same compensation claims against the hospital under general provisions (Demir, 2010).

c. Liability for Faulty Medical Intervention

The malpractice liability brings into question the applicability of provisions on defective performance. In cases of defective services, the CPA provides consumers the following optional rights: right of re-performance, free repair, price reduction and withdrawal. However, the exercise of these rights mostly contradicts with the nature of defective medical services. In malpractice cases, the exercise of such right is either impossible, such as in the case where the patient dies or ineffective such as in the case of total loss/loss of function of an organ/limb or blood transfusion with hepatitis B virus (Gözpınar Karan, 2018; Yılmaz, 2019). The patients mostly claim compensation. Under art. 15/1 CPA, compensation claim is subject to provisions of TCO. Thus, the consumer status, in this regard, does not provide practical results to the injured patients.

d. The Validity of Non-liability Clauses

The CPA does not provide an explicit provision regarding the validity of non-liability clauses. It is argued that such clauses should be accepted as invalid due to mandatory nature of the CPA (Aydoğdu, 2015) as they also constitute an unfair term (Kara, 2021). The Regulation on Unfair Conditions in Consumer Contracts supports this view: such clauses are listed as an example of unfair term (Annex a-2). Unfair terms in consumer contracts are null and void (art. 5/2 CPA). However, the same result can also be reached under the general provisions of TCO. Since the medical profession requires expertise and can be carried out only with official permission, non-liability clauses are null and void under art. 115/ 3 TCO. Similarly, contractual terms limiting the liability of the private health-care institutions for the acts of auxiliary persons is null and void under art. 116/ 3 TCO.

3. Problematic Situations

The consumer status of the patients creates problems as to the jurisdiction of consumer courts especially in the following two situations. First is the lack of consumer status of the plaintiff who claims compensation for loss of support in case of death of the patient due to faulty medical intervention. Second is where the debt relationship between the patient and the healthcare provider originates from a source other than a contract. In cases of contract of full admission to hospital, since the only contractual addressee of the patient is the private hospital, the patient shall invoke the personal liability of the physician based on tort.

B. Procedural Law Perspective

1. In General

According to Turkish law, one of the most important consequences of qualifying a transaction as a consumer transaction is about the dispute resolution. As it has already been explained above, two kinds of dispute resolution methods are available for consumers: consumer arbitral committees and consumer courts. There are some differences between these dispute resolution methods that the parties of a consumer dispute will apply. First, according to art. 73/a of the CPA cases that fall under the jurisdiction of the consumer court are subject to compulsory mediation (Atalı et al., 2020). In other words, the parties must apply to a mediator before filing a lawsuit. If a lawsuit is filed without fulfilling the requirements of this obligation, the case is denied on procedural grounds. On the other hand, there is no compulsory mediation for the cases that consumer arbitration committees have jurisdiction on.

2. Ineffectiveness of Consumer Arbitration Committees in Health Law

Under Turkish law, although they make binding decisions on the parties, consumer arbitration committees cannot be described as a court since they are not a part of judicial organization but are organized under the Ministry of Trade (Konuralp, 2020). In addition, these delegations work as five-person boards consisting of one member each to be elected by the ministry of commerce, municipalities, bar associations, trade associations, and consumer organizations (Konuralp, 2020). Hence, their organization is kind of an administrative authority rather than a court. It is described as "kind of" because the decisions of the committees are not accepted as administrative decisions (Ermenek, 2013). As a matter of fact, these boards are not qualified as courts in Turkish law (Decision of Turkish Constitutional Court, registration no: 2007/53 decision no: 2007/61, decision date: 27 December 2007; Ermenek, 2013; Taşpınar Ayvaz, 2016). Consumer arbitration committees carry out their dispute resolution duty through a written procedure thus, in principle, there is no hearing that the parties can attend before reaching a conclusion (Özsöker, 2019). However, consumer courts, like other ordinary courts, are a part of the judicial organization and practise as a court (Atalı, 2020). Thus, consumer courts make a judgement according to the Code of Civil Procedure, they must hold a hearing and listen to the parties in any case.

It should be stated that since the value of disputes arising health law is significantly higher than other consumer disputes in average, for those consumer courts mostly have jurisdiction. Thus, consumer arbitration committees lose their effectiveness in dispute settlement in health law.

3. Consequences of Qualifying Patients as Consumers in Procedural Law

One consequence in this respect is the difference of the trial procedure. Turkish civil procedure has two kinds of procedure for civil courts. One is written trial procedure that is applied in general first instance courts, commercial courts and family courts. The other one is simple trial procedure. According to the CPA, consumer courts apply simple procedure, with the aim of completing consumer cases quickly (Baş Süzel & Erişir, 2018). However, this way is not always advantageous for the parties, because according to this procedure, each party has only one petition right. If the parties want to amend or extend their claim or defence, they need to use their amendment right which can be used once. In addition, despite the application of this method, consumer cases in consumer courts cannot be resolved quickly. According to the latest statistics,[3] this period is 425 days on average in consumer courts, while a civil case is concluded in an

---

3   https://adlisicil.adalet.gov.tr/Resimler/SayfaDokuman/1092020162733adalet_ist-2019.pdf

average of 280 days in Turkey. This also shows that average length doubled since 2015 (Baş Süzel & Erişir, 2018). Therefore, the application of the simple trial procedure does not provide benefit to the parties whereas this procedure limits the right of petition of the parties.

4. Direct Benefits That Consumer Can Enjoy

a. Waiver from Courts Fee

In the lawsuits to be filed by the consumers, there are two regulations in their direct favour. First, consumers are exempt from all charges when filing a lawsuit (Baş Süzel & Erişir, 2018). Under Turkish law plaintiffs shall pay two kinds of fee. One is fee for application to a court and the second one is deposit for court expanses such as notification cost. This waiver covers only the application fee (art. 73/2 CPA) thus, consumers shall pay the deposit even for consumer cases as well (Atalı et al., 2020). This fact is criticized as it limits the right of the consumers to access to justice (Atalı et al., 2020).

b. Territorial Jurisdiction of Consumer Courts

Another regulation in direct favour of consumers is about the territorial jurisdiction of the courts. In principle, the territorial jurisdiction of Turkish civil courts is determined according to the place of residence of the defendant and the place performance in cases arising from the contract (Pekcanıtez et al., 2017). However, according to the CPA, consumers have opportunity to file a lawsuit in their own place of settlements (Pekcanıtez et al., 2017).

As can be seen, although a special trial procedure has been applied for the consumers for dispute resolution, both the legislation and the implementation cannot provide significant benefit for consumers. In this respect, there is no crucial difference between ordinary cases and consumer cases.

Conclusion

The underlying aim for revising the Turkish consumer law and enacting a new code of consumer protection was to ensure full harmonization with the EU legislation. The preparatory studies of the CPA mention the transpose of 2011/83/EU Directive on Consumer Rights to Turkish law. The Directive explicitly excludes healthcare services from its scope. The CPA does not explicitly mention the consumer status of the patients. However, due to the broad definition of "consumer transaction" and "services", the patients qualify as consumers. This result is criticized by some of the authors, whereas in jurisprudence, the medical malpractice cases based on faulty medical interventions carried out at private law healthcare institutions are accepted to fall under the jurisdiction of the consumer courts. The examinations in this study indicate that qualifying patients as consumers does not bring vital advantages for patients. This fact is valid both for substantial and procedural issues. If the Turkish legislator decides not to describe patients as consumers, this would not bring significant difference than the current situation.

References

Akipek Öcal, Ş (2018). Hasta Tüketici Midir?. In Yücel, Ö. & Sert, G. (Eds.), *Sağlık ve Tıp Hukukunda Sorumluluk ve İnsan Hakları* (1st ed., pp. 251–262). Seçkin.

Atali, M. Et al. (2020). *Medeni Usul Hukuku* (3rd ed.). Yetkin.

Aydoğdu, M. (2015). *Tüketici Hukuku Dersleri* (1st ed.). Adalet.

Baş Süzel, E. & Erişir, E. (2018) Enforcement and Effectiveness of Consumer Law in Turkey. In Micklitz, H.-W. & Saumier, G. (Eds.), *Enforcement and Effectiveness of Consumer Law* (1st ed., pp. 645–671). Springer.

Çilenti Konuralp, A (2020). *Üçüncü Kişi Yararına Sözleşme.* (1st ed.). On İki Levha.

Demir, M. (2010). *Tıbbi Organizasyon Kusuru Açısından Hastanelerin Hukuksal Sorumluluğu*, (1st ed.). Turhan.

Ermenek, İ. (2013). Yargı Kararları Işığında Tüketici Sorunları Hakem Heyetleri ve Bu Alanda Ortaya Çıkan Sorunlara İlişkin Çözüm Önerileri. *Gazi Üniversitesi Hukuk Fakültesi Dergisi*, 17(1–2), 563–630.

Gözpınar Karan, G. (2018). Hastaya Sunulan Ayıplı Hizmetten Sorumluluk, *Terazi Hukuk Dergisi*, 13(143), 112–122.

Gümüş, M. A. (2014). *6502 Sayılı Tüketicinin Korunması Hakkında Kanun, Cilt I* (1st ed.). Vedat.

Havutçu, A. (2014). 6502 Sayılı Tüketicinin Korunması Hakkında Kanun'un Konu Bakımından Uygulama Alanı: Özellikle, Tüketici İşlemleri Bakımından Kanun'un Kapsamı. *Terazi Hukuk Dergisi*, 9 (Special Issue), 8–19.

Kara, İ. (2021). *Tüketici Hukuku* (2nd ed.). Yetkin.

Konuralp, O. E. (2020). Role of Mandatory Arbitration in Monetary Claims Against Consumers Under Turkish Law. In Wei, D: et al. (Eds.) *Innovation and the Transformation of Consumer Law* (1st ed., pp. 243–256). Springer.

Özel, Ç. (2019). *Tüketicinin Korunması Hukuku* (5th ed.). Yetkin.

Özsöker, G. (2019). *Tüketici Hakem Heyetleri* (1st ed.) Yetkin.

Pekcanıtez, H. (2017). *Medeni Usul Hukuku, Cilt 1* (15th ed.). On İki Levha.

Serozan, R. (1996). Tüketiciyi Koruma Yasasının Sözleşme Hukuku Alanındaki Düzenlemesinin Eleştirisi. *Yasa Hukuk İçtihat ve Mevzuat Dergisi,* 15(173/4), 579–598.

Sirmen, L. (2014). Yeni Tüketicinin Korunması Hakkında Kanunun Genel Olarak Değerlendirilmesi. *Terazi Hukuk Dergisi, 9* (Special Issue), 156–162.

Şenocak, Z. (1998). *Özel Hukukta Hekimin Sorumluluğu,* (1st ed.). Ankara Üniversitesi.

Taşpınar Ayvaz, S. (2016). Tüketici Hakem Heyetlerinin İşleyişi ve Sorunlar. In Aksoy, H. C. (Ed.), *Tüketici Hukuku Konferansı* (1st ed., pp. 283–306). Yetkin.

Tutumlu, M. A. (2014). Özel Hastanede Yanlış Teşhisten ve Tedaviden Kaynaklanan Tazminat Davasında Görevli Mahkeme Sorunu. *Terazi Hukuk Dergisi,* 9(93), 172–175.

Yılmaz, Y. (2019). *Özel Hastane İşleticisinin Hastaneye Kabul Sözleşmesi Çerçevesinde Yürütülen Tıbbi Müdahaleden Kaynaklanan Sorumluluğu,* (1st ed.). On İki Levha.

E. Neval Yilmaz

Selin Özden Merhaci

Deniz Odabaş

Medical Malparactice in Comparative Law: A Swot Analysis

Introduction

Medical malpractice is an increasingly important issue both in Turkey and all over the world. This concept becomes more and more complex and multidimensional with the involvement of medical ethics, law, economics and many other disciplines, and the intense coverage of the issue by the press. According to the World Medical Association's (WMA, 2005) statement on medical malpractice published in 1992 and rearranged in 2005, medical malpractice involves the physician's failure to conform to the standard of care for treatment of the patient's condition, or a lack of skill, or negligence in providing care to the patient, which is the direct cause of an injury to the patient (WMA, 2005). On the other hand, the physician should not bear any liability for an injury which occurs in the course of medical treatment which could not be foreseen and was not the result of any lack of skill or knowledge on the part of the treating physician.

In different legal systems, different methods are foreseen for determining the liability of the physician arising from medical malpractice or the compensation of the damage which has been given as a result of medical procedures. Each system and method have its own advantages and disadvantages. In this review, methods of different legal systems will be examined using the methods of comparative law and the SWOT analysis.

I. Literature Review/Findings

In the literature review the implementations of some of the countries were investigated and it is found out that the methods used in determining the liability of the physicians arising from malpractice are;

– Cases evaluated by the judiciary,

- Systems that are not based on fault, in which only the patient's damage is compensated by proving the existence of causation, and decided by the boards specially created for this,
- Methods such as "the strict liability of the state" or "alternative solutions/mediation".

A. Turkey

In Turkey, cases related to alleged malpractice should be filed in the general courts. Cases related to civil liability are heard in civil courts, cases related to criminal liability in criminal courts, cases related to the liability of the state in administrative courts, and cases related to the liability of private hospitals in consumer courts within the framework of the procedural law. There are no specialized health courts or a specific legislation in a special area of health law in Turkey. Courts decide in the light of expert reports, reports prepared as a result of the examination of the Forensic Medicine Institute and the reports given by the High Health Council (until 2016, after which the High Health Council was dismissed).

In Turkey, the assessment of liability arising from the physician's malpractice is done according to the principles of agency contract, contract of work, torts, strict liability of the state or tortious liability of the agency without authority according to the characteristics of the case.

When different studies on the cases related to malpractice claims are reviewed, it is seen that 997 cases were reported to the High Health Council between 1993 and 1998 with malpractice claims, and in 47.7 % of these cases, it was decided that the physicians were liable (Gündoğmuş et al., 2005). The most common causes of malpractice are negligence, wrong treatment and inadequate diagnosis. In the study, which examined 330 cases with medical malpractice claim to the General Assembly of the Ministry of Justice Forensic Medicine Institution between 2000 and 2011, it was found that there was "medical malpractice" in 33.3 % of 330 cases (Yazıcı et al., 2015). In a retrospective study of 112 cases examined by the High Health Council between 2000 and 2004, including emergency treatment services, it was decided that 57 cases (50.9 %) had no malpractice, and 55 (49.1 %) cases had medical malpractice (Türkan & Tuğcu, 2004).

While there were 696 files related to malpractice applied to the Forensic Medicine Institute between 1991 and 2000, and 525 files between 2001 and 2005, this number increased significantly after 2005. The First Forensic Specialization Board of the Forensic Medicine Institute, which is the council that examines the cases resulting in death, detected malpractice in 1060 cases in 2013, 1320 cases in 2014, and 1148 cases in 2015. There is no study examining the penalties and compensations paid in all these malpractice cases collectively (Yılmaz, 2019).

In Turkey, cases pending before the courts continue for years. Especially malpractice cases are concluded in periods of up to 8–10 years due to the need for expert examination. The long duration of the lawsuits has caused our country to be convicted many times on the grounds that it constitutes a violation of the right to a fair trial by the European Court of Human Rights (Şekerci Vs Turkey, Application No. 9961/08, 01.07 2014). The length of trial periods can be explained by various factors such as the insufficient number of judges and prosecutors, the high workloads, the cumbersome and complex processes in the judicial activities, the slow functioning of institutions such as the Forensic Medicine Institute, the fact that conciliation and mediation activities have not been sufficiently developed until today.

B. France

In France, which constitutes the main legal order of the Romanistic legal family (Zweigert & Kötz, 1998), in the Patient Rights Law dated March 4, 2002 and numbered 2002–303, regardless of who the relevant actors are (private or public institutions), the rules and rights and responsibilities related to medical rights violations are defined (G'Sell-Macrez, 2011). This law defines patients' rights and lays down general principles regarding the responsibility of health professionals and health institutions. Although medical malpractice rules are determined in general terms, malpractice cases can be brought before administrative or civil courts, depending on whether the disputes occur in private institutions or public institutions or in a private practice. In cases where there is a crime in terms of criminal law, a lawsuit can be filed against the health worker in criminal courts. In addition, physicians are evaluated by disciplinary committees in case of violation of ethical rules.

The Patient Rights Act not only regulates the resolution of disputes between patients and healthcare professionals, but also provides for compensation for injuries that cannot be attributed to any negligence. In case that a harm occurs as a result of preventive medicine, diagnosis or treatment activities, the patient can apply to the "National Medical Accidents Compensation Fund" (*Office National d'Indemnisation des Accidents Medicaux [ONIAM]*). In addition, ONIAM is responsible for compensating victims who cannot be compensated by the health worker or their insurer, even if the liability rules apply. In such cases, it is accepted that the compensation of the damage from the fund is based on the principle of "national solidarity" (Helleringer, 2011).

The Patient Rights Act has provided a new procedure for the benefit of victims to provide simple and rapid compensation. Victims who have been harmed by medical intervention have two options: (1) To apply to a mediation commission with their allegations, or (2) to file a lawsuit against a healthcare professional. The Patient Rights Act and the Law on Medical Malpractice of 30 December 2002 contain regulations on regional reconciliation and compensation commissions in each region: (*"Commission Regionale de Conciliation et d'Indemnisation des accidents medicaux, affections iatrognes et infections nosocomiales"* [CRCI]) (The Regional Reconciliation and Compensation Commission for Medical Accidents, Inflammatory Conditions and Nosocomial Infections). This new organization aims to provide new ways to resolve disputes amicably and assist victims to obtain rapid compensation. CRCI's are led by a judge and consist of twenty people, divided into six main categories representing patients, health-care professionals, hospital practitioners, healthcare institutions and facilities, ONIAM and insurers. The mission of CRCI's is twofold. First, medical malpractice to mediate the resolution of disputes arising from job claims. The second function of CRCI's is to ensure that victims of medical malpractice with serious injuries can easily receive compensation. The commission must answer the application within 6 months. Two solutions are possible at this stage. The application will be denied if the damage is not due to medical care or negligence and the damage is not an abnormal result for the patient's initial state. The second possibility is that the commission decides to compensate the patient for his damage. The notification is forwarded to the institutions responsible for the payment of the compensation. If the compensation to be paid can be based on the rules of compensation liability, while the compensation is paid by the health worker's insurance, in cases where no liability can be determined, but there is a loss, ONIAM pays compensation in accordance with the principle of public interest and "national solidarity" (G'Sell-Macrez, 2011).

The personal liability of the physician is not taken for the damage suffered by a patient of a public hospital. This situation, in the absence of a personal fault, is deemed to be the administration's service fault, and the damage is compensated by the administration. In France, the strict liability of the state is accepted, especially in cases where the doctor provides health products and hospital-acquired infections (G'Sell-Macrez, 2011).

C. Germany

In Germany, mediation services of health institutions or liability insurers often have a role in solving malpractice claims. Most of all malpractice claims are resolved at the mediation or insurance stage, with only 8 % of cases being sued (Palmer, 2009). Most of the damages caused by personal injuries in Germany are covered by the social security system (Kesgin, 2018). The compensation for damages and losses incurred in medical malpractice cases are determined according to the provisions of the German Civil Code. Similar to Turkish law, material damages are fully compensated and no punitive damages are given. In medical malpractice cases and in cases of personal injury in general, treatment, rehabilitation and long-term care expenses are ordered, as well as compensation for lost earnings and non-pecuniary compensation. After a major legislative change in 2002, the award of non-pecuniary damage was facilitated, resulting in a significant increase in malpractice cases (Cioffi, 2002).

In Germany, the malpractice victim directs the claim for compensation to the insurance of the physician or hospital. If the victim is not satisfied at this level, they can go to court or use the services of a mediation centre. Mediation services are free of charge, however, if filed with a court, if the claimant loses the case, he or she has to pay the costs of the case and the other party's costs and attorneys' fees, thereby indirectly encouraging the use of mediation services and the settlement of disputes through mediation (Weidinger, 2006).

If the mediation centre is of the opinion that there is a damage for which the health worker is responsible, the victim can apply to the insurance company again. In 85 % of such cases, the mediation centre's opinion is the basis for a final solution. In the remaining 15 % of cases, the plaintiff goes to court, and the court's decision mostly parallels that of the mediation centre. In practice, the vast majority of malpractice claims are resolved out of court immediately or after consultation with a mediation centre. Mediation centres are run by official medical professional associations, but they are independent organizations whose independent judgement is highly respected. Lawyers and physicians work in the centres and evaluations are generally carried out by volunteer physicians free of charge. In addition to advising malpractice victims on their claims, the centres also keep statistics on the claims presented to them, and these statistics are audited annually by the Federal Medical Association (Katzenmeyer et al., 2016).

D. United Kingdom

The medical liability of workers employed by the National Health Service (NHS) in the UK is handled according to the liability principle of tort law. When allegations of NHS staff negligence arise, the Clinical Negligence Scheme for Trusts / CNST comes into play (Feikert, 2009). The goal is to provide a resource for NHS organizations to finance the cost of malpractice claims. All healthcare institutions in England are included in this program (Nair & Chandraharan, 2010).

In England and Wales, courts reviewed the malpractice claims under tort law. Claims are brought against the National Health Service Institutions rather than individuals. As part of this practice, National Health Service Institutions are responsible for the misconduct and negligence of their employees, including physicians and nurses. This responsibility stems from the duty of care that the National Health Service Institutions owe to their patients. As a result of this responsibility, a state policy has been developed and "NHS medical indemnity system" has emerged. If harm occurs to a patient or volunteer due to misconduct or negligence of an NHS employee during his or her tenure, this must be compensated by the NHS (Feikert, 2009). When the NHS is liable for the health worker's fault, it accepts full financial responsibility and does not recourse the costs to the health worker in question. When faced with a malpractice claim, the NHS assumes legal and administrative costs, tries to reach a compromise where possible, pays the amount which is determined as a result of a court order or mediation action (British Medical Association, NHS Indemnity).

The NHS Litigation Department follows a policy to resolve disputes using alternative methods, avoiding litigation wherever possible. 96 % of the applications are resolved "out of court" using the "alternative dispute resolution" method, and of all the applications made in the last 10 years, 41 % were left without follow-up by the complainant, 41 % were resolved through alternative dispute resolution methods out of court, 4 %. of them were settled by conciliation at court stage (in this group the previously reached compromise was approved by court decision) and only 14 % of them were tried. The number of malpractice claims made in courts annually is less than fifty (Feikert, 2009).

E. United States of America

In the United States, malpractice claims are resolved by courts. Malpractice cases are a relatively common occurrence in the United States. The legal system is designed to encourage extensive exploration and negotiations between the parties before going to jury trial. Many conflicts are resolved by reaching a consensus at the negotiation stage. The injured patient should demonstrate that the physician's negligence in care and that negligence has caused the injury. The compensation paid usually takes into account both economic losses and moral damages (Bal, 2009).

The malpractice assessment system in the United States has two main purposes: to compensate patients harmed by the negligence of healthcare providers and to discourage providers from behaviours that cause malpractice. However, in practice, the system runs slowly and is very costly. The system has been criticized for both its inability to compensate patients suffering from malpractice, and for causing new damages due to the payment of compensation to those who do not actually need to be compensated (Seabury et al., 2014). The failures of the liability system and the high cost of health care in the United States have led to a significant debate on tort policy (Kessler, 2011).

In addition, in the 1970s and 2000s, very high compensation put insurance companies and indirectly physicians in a difficult situation, and for this reason, "malpractice crises" were mentioned. Although these crises are tried to be solved with a number of judicial reforms, malpractice cases continue to be a serious problem (Randall, 2000).

F. Nordic Countries

Within the Scandinavian Model, the patient insurance system differs between countries. Sweden is the first Scandinavian country to develop a patient insurance system. The first patient insurance program came into effect in 1975. Subsequently, the development in Sweden became widespread, with the "Patient Insurance Laws" and "Patient Injuries Laws" were adopted in Finland in 1984, Norway in 1988 and Denmark in 1992 (Von Eyben, 2001). Although all these reforms differ among themselves, they are all inspired by the Swedish plan.

In Sweden, patients are compensated for damages arising from the interventions of healthcare professionals as a result of the examination of the applications made to LÖF (*Landstingens Ömsesidiga Försäkringsbolag*), which we can translate as "National Mutual Insurance Institution". In this system, which has been in effect since 1975, patients can demand financial compensation for their damages or the negative effects of treatment. Insurance covers both material and immaterial damages. For this, it is necessary to prove that there is a causal link between the damage complained of and the intervention performed and that the damage is preventable (Hafström et al., 2011). In determining compensation, it does not matter whether there is a negligence or a fault. For this reason, the compensation mechanism in this model is called "no-fault systems".

Complaints made to the LÖF institution in Sweden are examined and resolved by consulting specialist physicians. These physicians work for LÖF for a few hours a week, and they can generally be physicians who either work full time in hospitals or have recently retired. The selection criterion is to have a reputable place and experience in the specialty (Essinger, 2009). It is noteworthy that as a result of the complaints made to the LÖF in Sweden, only 30 % of the examinations made in the Malpractice Disciplinary Board (HSAN) were punished, although compensation was paid in 90 % of the applications until the 2000s. This inconsistency is explained by the different objectives of the two institutions. For LÖF to pay compensation, only the existence of a causal link and the fact that the damage cannot be prevented is sufficient, HSAN gives disciplinary penalties only if the intervention is not based on scientific and up-to-date evidence. LÖF institution does not aim to punish physicians and other healthcare professionals (Hafström et al., 2011).

In Sweden, the person who claims to be harmed due to a medical intervention must file a complaint within 3 years after learning about the damage and within 10 years from the occurrence of the damage. Applications are finalized within 3–6 months. 70 % of these compensations are paid within 6 months of the application, and 80 % within 8 months (Essinger, 2009).

All Scandinavian legal systems, with the exception of the Danish system, allow the application of tort Law provisions as an alternative to no fault compensation systems. Therefore, the patient has the right to claim compensation based on both the right to compensation according to the private insurance program and tort law. Under Swedish law, in cases where court proceedings are applied, patient insurance comes into play as liability insurance. By filing a lawsuit, the burden of proving the conditions on which the claim is based passes to the plaintiff. In this case, the plaintiff must prove his harm, the causal link and fault, if any. Therefore, using the right to complain within the scope of patient insurance instead of filing a lawsuit is significantly more advantageous for the plaintiff (Essinger, 2009).

II. Research and Methods

This study is conducted in accordance with the methods of comparative law. It is a theoretical, descriptive, and qualitative review study, and the different methods used in determining the physician's liability arising from malpractice will be examined by comparative methodology.

Comparative law is the comparison of the different legal systems by using its own method called functionality, to determine the differences and similarities between the nations . This comparison takes place by comparing the institutions, which fulfils the same function, and making a critical judgement at the end of the research (Zweigert & Kötz, 1998; Oğuz, 2021).

In a comparative study written laws, customary rules, case law, doctrine, contracts, general terms and conditions and commercial practices should be investigated (Oğuz, 2021). For this reason, the material of this study includes all kinds of written and unwritten legal sources of the countries included in the study, as well as information materials prepared by the relevant institutions and organizations of various states and the documents prepared by international institutions and organizations such as the World Health Organization and the World Bank.

In the light of the findings of the literature review, it was decided to analyse the findings by using a technique called SWOT analysis. The SWOT framework is created by Albert Humphrey, who developed the approach at the Stanford Research Institute back in the 1960s and early 1970s.[1] SWOT (Strengths and Weaknesses, Opportunities and Threats) analysis is a method of comparison that is made to follow and interpret the developments in or around a certain organization, institution or organization and consists of systematic evaluation of certain factors (Songur et al. 2013). While, by definition, opportunities (O) and threats (T) are essentially considered as external factors over which there is no complete control, while internal factors that may have some control over strengths (S) and weaknesses (W). With this method, the current situation of the institution/concept is analysed and the strategies to be implemented are determined. In SWOT analysis, the characteristics of the examined institution are classified as strengths, weaknesses, opportunities and threats. Strengths, features that make the organization work well, weaknesses, characteristics that negatively affect the performance of the organization, opportunities are the issues that the institution will benefit from, and threats are forces beyond the control of the organization (Baraz, 2012).

Although "SWOT analysis" is not used in comparative law, in accordance with the principle of functionality, the aim is to analyse the results and to evaluate the research results and to present the most appropriate solution by indicating the weak and strong aspects of the implementations of the different legal systems. For this reason, it is thought that the evaluation of the results using SWOT analysis in our study will not damage the scientific quality of the study and will contribute to the point of setting an objective evaluation criterion for the comparison. Since the aim of the study is "the examination of the methods used in determining the malpractice of physicians in different legal systems", the

---

1   The British Library, https://www.bl.uk/business-and-ip-centre/articles/what-is-swot-analysis#.

strengths and weaknesses of these methods, the opportunities they provide and the negative aspects they cause could be discussed based on objective criteria as a result of the comparison of these methods using SWOT analysis.

Due to the fact that there are details regarding insurance companies and some public institutions among the methods used in determining the liability of physicians arising from malpractice in countries belonging to different legal systems, it is predicted that the SWOT analysis will facilitate the adaptation of the results of these companies and institutions to daily life.

III. Discussion and Evaluation

The legal systems that conduct the determination of liability arising from medical malpractice to the judicial organs, the systems that use no-fault compensation procedures and the application of the strict liability of the state are compared and contrasted by SWOT analysis and the results are given in the Tables 1–3 (Yılmaz, 2019).

The issue of evaluation and/or litigation of malpractice claims has become an issue that is discussed and sought solutions all over the world due to the increasing number of cases. Physicians complain about working under the threat of lawsuits and try to protect themselves to some extent with defensive medicine practices. In recent years, it is observed that the interest in branches such as Gynecology and Obstetrics, General Surgery, etc., which were very popular in Turkey, has decreased rapidly due to the high number of lawsuits in these branches. The long-term consequences of this situation, unfortunately, are not sufficiently evaluated, and no action has been taken to take precautions yet. Considering the current developments, it is certain that we are facing the threat of not being able to find surgeons to perform high-risk surgeries in the coming years. Before the problem reaches this level, urgent measures must be taken.

In addition to the increasing malpractice cases, the slow functioning of the legal system in Turkey constitutes an important problem that has been discussed for many years. A civil lawsuit takes an average of 2–3 years at the first instance and in cases where more than one expert review is required. With the additional time spent by Court of Appeal and the Court of Cassation in reviewing the final decision of the first instance, this period get much longer, sometimes reaches a level that violates the "right to a fair trial". In a study examining 30 malpractice cases that were proceeded between 1978 and 2006 (28 damages, 2 criminal cases), it was found that 16 files (53.3 %) were finalized by the Court of Cassation under 5 years, 10 files (33.3 %) between 5 and 10 years and 4 files (13.3 %) in longer than 10 years (Can et al., 2011). In its decision numbered 2014/14189 and dated 25.10.2017, the Constitutional Court of Turkey ruled that *"the right to trial within a reasonable time was violated"* in a malpractice case that lasted for 7 years.

It can be advocated that the trials made in courts have a deterrent aspect. A possible threat of lawsuit can push medical professionals to be more attentive and careful. One of the most important arguments of the authors who oppose no-fault compensation systems is that in cases where compensation payments are made without proving or evaluating the fault, healthcare professionals and institutions will work more carelessly with the idea that "I will not be given a liability anyway" (Kass & Rose, 2016). In addition, the deterrence function of the courts may be harmed, as the vast majority of complaints will be resolved before a lawsuit is filed. According to Howell, the main weakness of flawless compensation systems is that it cannot be guaranteed that people who could potentially cause damage, healthcare workers and institutions, in the context of our topic, will fulfil their responsibilities at the highest level with the removal of their legal responsibilities and the risk of compensation (Howell et al., 2002). There is also a concern that healthcare professionals and organizations, who will not have to be held accountable for adverse events once the concept of fault disappears, will not take the trouble to learn from adverse events by examining them. There are even concerns that in the long run, no explanation will be given to the patients and even no apologize will be done for the damage caused.

It is thought that in good medical practice within the framework of ethical rules will be fulfilled by the obligation of diligence and these concerns will be unfounded if the rules of medical ethics are followed. On the other hand, with the withdrawal of the concept of fault from the scene, costly and unnecessary defensive medicine practices will decrease, and economic gains will emerge as a result. The deterrent role of the judicial remedy can already be met by disciplinary investigations and, in some cases, the sanctions available under the criminal law and occupational health and safety legislation (Yılmaz, 2019).

The most important purposes in the implementation of no-fault compensation systems are shortening the compensation payment process, reducing the threat of litigation and litigation costs, increasing the service quality and increasing patient safety as a result of the easier reporting of medical faults (Gostin, 2000). Against these advantages, there are concerns that, in case of a mistake, the lack of an adequate legal "deterrence" from the early stages of legislation will encourage implementation below current medical standards (Hiatt et al., 1989). The general impression is that no-fault compensation systems in the Scandinavian countries are working well. The general purpose of these systems is to make it easier for patients to receive compensation. In this context, no-fault compensation systems have certainly been successful. Another aim is to provide a model that will be more economical than litigation. In this context, systems are perhaps less successful. There are studies showing that administrative costs are quite high in the operation of these systems (Ulfbeck et al., 2012). It should also be remembered that a very common and functional insurance system and strong financial resources must be available for this system to function well.

Luntz and Hambly, on the other hand, take a different view of the deterrent function of the courts. According to these authors, almost everyone nowadays purchases insurance to provide financial protection against adverse events. In fact, these insurances have been made compulsory for some professional groups such as physicians. The availability of insurance can take away the deterrent function of the courts, as individuals will be more comfortable not paying their own compensation (Luntz & Hambly, 2002). However, it should be noted that we do not agree with this view. In the period since the 1970s, insurance premiums have increased tremendously in all countries, especially in the United States, and physicians have been forced to leave their profession from time to time due to high premiums or the refusal of insurance companies to insure. In Turkey, professional liability insurance has been implemented for physicians since 2012 and has a shorter history compared to other countries. However, considering the rapidly increasing malpractice cases and high compensations, it is certain that similar problems will also be experienced in Turkey. Therefore, we are of the opinion that the deterrence function of the courts will always continue.

When the different legal systems that evaluate malpractice claims in courts are examined, it is seen that alternative remedies have an important place in this issue. Although there is no specific regulation on alternative remedies for malpractice cases in the United States, the legal system is designed to encourage extensive exploration and negotiations between the parties before going to jury trial. An extremely important part of the disputes is resolved at this stage. However, this system can sometimes lead to unfair results due to the bargaining capabilities of the parties. In this context, sometimes malpractice victim patients are not sufficiently compensated, and sometimes compensation can be paid to people who do not actually need to be compensated (Seabury et al., 2014).

France, which has institutionalized the alternative solution for evaluating malpractice claims, is a good example. In France, victims who suffer harm as a result of preventive medicine, diagnosis or treatment activities have two options. Victims can apply to a mediation commission called the "Regional Compromise and Compensation Commission (CRCI) for Medical Accidents, Inflammatory Conditions and Nosocomial Infections" or file a lawsuit against the healthcare professional. CRCIs, which have been operating since 2002, have been established to resolve disputes amicably and help victims receive fast compensation and constitute an alternative to courts (Helleringer, 2011). In Germany, the malpractice victim starts the process of demanding compensation with the application to be made by the doctor or the hospital to the insurance company, and if he is not satisfied at this level, he can go to the court or use the services of a mediation centre. The fact that mediation services are free of charge paves the way for people to apply this method first. In Germany, 85 % of malpractice claims are resolved as a result of mediation activities, and only 15 % of cases go to court (Weidinger, 2006).

Problems regarding the establishment of causal link in Anglo-American law and the determination of the concepts of fault and liability result in making contradictory decisions in trials. In the United Kingdom, the settlement of malpractice claims through alternative solutions is encouraged, and a special fund has been established for compensation payments financed by the participation fee paid by the health institutions. According to the NHS Trial Chamber Report, 96 % of the applications are resolved "out of court" using "alternative dispute resolution" method. It is reported that the number of malpractice claims filed in courts in a year in the United Kingdom is less than fifty (Feikert, 2009).

Although the litigation is a good method in terms of exercising the right to litigation, the fact that this method lasts for years, the high costs for both states and parties, especially in Anglo-American law, the difficulties in establishing a causal link and in determining the fault and separating intent, negligence and perfect liability. There are many weaknesses, such as the victim who lost the case having to pay the costs of the trial, the victim's obligation to prove the fault or malpractice, and the rising costs due to defensive medicine practices. However, alternative solution methods to be applied in addition to litigation can be considered as an opportunity in this regard. The most important threats to the remedy are the violation of the right to a fair trial, the conflicting decisions made due to difficulties in establishing the causality link and the determination of the fault, the inability to compensate the victims, the compensation to the persons who do not actually need to be compensated, the absence of specific legal regulations on malpractice in many countries.

Conclusion

Lawsuits filed without a serious basis put physicians under great pressure. They work under the threat of lawsuits and bear the material and moral burden of compensation of these lawsuits that last for years. With the widespread use of defensive medical practices that emerged as a result of this, both the increased costs in healthcare services become inevitable and these practices lead to patient rights violations and become a ground for situations that may result in malpractice. An even greater danger will be that physicians, especially in some surgical branches, will begin to avoid performing some major and dangerous surgeries due to the threat of litigation. If this happens, within a few years, there will be no hospital or surgeon to do some major surgeries. This is not a utopian idea, but a reality that unfortunately threatens our near future.

For all these reasons, just like "Labor Courts", "Consumer Courts", "Intellectual and Industrial Rights Courts", "Health Courts" should be established and special legal regulations and special criteria should be introduced in the evaluation of malpractice claims. In addition, it should be ensured that the judges who will serve in these courts undergo a special training. In this way, it will be possible to make more fair and non-contradictory decisions by shortening the duration of the trial.

Tab. 1: Evaluation of the Systems That the Judicial Organs Determines the Liability Arising from Medical Malpractice by SWOT Analysis (Yilmaz, 2019)

STRENGTHS			WEAKNESSES
• Exercising the right to litigation • Option to resort to alternative remedies before filing a lawsuit (in some legal systems)	S	W	• The lawsuits last for years • High costs of cases for both states and parties • Difficulties in establishing causation and fault (especially in Anglo-American law) • Difficulties in distinguishing intent, negligence and strict liability (especially in Anglo-American law) • The victim who lost the case had to pay the legal costs • The victim's obligation to prove the elements of tort • Rising costs due to defensive medicine practices
OPPORTUNITIES			THREATS
• Encouraging alternative resolution methods before litigation.	O	T	• Violation of the right to a fair trial • Conflicting decisions due to difficulties in establishing causation and fault • Paying compensation to those who do not actually need to be compensated, while the victims receive inadequate compensation. • Lack of specific legal regulations regarding malpractice. • Absence of Health Courts

Tab. 2: Evaluation of No-Fault Compensation Systems in Medical Malpractice by SWOT Analysis (Yılmaz, 2019)

STRENGTHS			WEAKNESSES
• Paying compensation by establishing a causal link without seeking fault • Healthcare workers who are not concerned about the case to keep better records • Malpractice claims being directly examined by physicians • Victim only needs to prove the causal link • 51 % "sufficient evidence" • Finalization of the applications in a short time like a few months	S	W	• Applicable in countries with a high level of welfare and strong social state structure • Restricting people's right to litigation • People's removal of their right to litigation (Denmark, New Zealand) • Impunity for faulty healthcare workers • All compensation costs are covered by the health insurance • High rejection rates due to not meeting the application eligibility criteria
OPPORTUNITIES			**THREATS**
• Adverse events to be discussed more openly and honestly • Future mistakes become more preventable • Increased patient safety • Payment of compensations from general health insurance funds • No pressure on healthcare professionals • Preventing defensive medicine practices • Better rehabilitation • Improved relationships between patients and healthcare professionals	O	T	• With the disappearance of the concept of defect, the deterrence on healthcare workers disappears • In the long run, healthcare professionals stop giving explanation or apologizing • The development of a culture of living by receiving compensation • Tax burden that may arise from rising costs

Tab. 3: Evaluation of the Strict Liability of the State in Medical Malpractice by SWOT Analysis (Yılmaz, 2019)

STRENGTHS			WEAKNESSES
• Compensation for damages caused by the state without seeking fault • Providing an easy solution in the person's dispute with the state	S	W	• (In practice in Turkey) Before applying for the strict liability of the state, one must first apply for the tortious liability of the state • Failure to implement fully
OPPORTUNITIES			THREATS
• For some adverse events, strict liability situations can also be recognized for non-governmental organizations and healthcare workers. • Events that cause the strict liability of the state can be identified in advance and direct compensation can be provided when they occur.	O	T	• Developing the rules by means of "case law" since the rules are not specified in the law • Difficulty drawing the line between fault liability and strict liability

References

Bal, B. S. (2009). An Introduction to Medical Malpractice in the United States. *Clin Orthop Relat Res.* 467 (2), 339–347. https://doi.org/10.1007/s11999-008-0636-2, Access date 12.06.2021.

Baraz, B. (2012). Çevre Analizi, Stratejik Yönetim I, Anadolu Üniversitesi AÖF, Eskişehir Ed. Deniz, T., Ulukan, C., s. 80-104.

Can, İ. Ö., Özkara, E., & Can, M. (2011). Yargıtayda Karara Bağlanan Tıbbi Uygulama Hatası Dosyalarının Değerlendirilmesi. *DEÜ Tıp Fakültesi Dergisi,* 25 (2), 69–76.

Cioffi, J. W. (2002). Restructuring "Germany Inc.": The Politics of Company and Takeover Law Reform in Germany and the European Union. *Law & Policy.* 24(4), 355–402. https://doi.org/10.1111/j.0265-8240.2002.00161.x

Essinger K, The Swedish Medical Injury Insurance Report, 2009, https://docpla yer.net/16172272-The-swedish-medical-injury-insurance.html (*Access date 21.02.2021*)

Eyben, von B. (2001). Alternative Compensation Systems. In P. Wahlgreen (Ed.), Tort Liability and Insurance (pp. 194–233). Stockholm Institute for Scandinavian Law. https://scandinavianlaw.se/pdf/41-7.pdf

Feikert, C. (May, 2009). Medical Malpractice Liability: United Kingdom (England and Wales). https://www.loc.gov/law/help/medical-malpractice-liability/uk.php

Gostin, L. (2000). A Public Health Approach to Reducing Error: Medical Malpractice as a Barrier. *JAMA* 283 (13), 1742–1743. https://doi.org/10.1001/jama.283.13.1742. PMID: 10755503

G'Sell-Macrez, F. (2011). Medical Malpractice and Compensation in France: Part I: the French Rules of Medical Liability since the Patients' Rights Law of March 4, 2002. *Chi.-Kent. L. Rev.*, 86, 1093–1123.

Gündoğmuş, U. N., Erdoğan, M. S., Şehiralti, M., & Kurtaş, O. (2005). A Descriptive Study of Medical Malpractice Cases in Turkey. *Ann Saud Med.*, 25(5), 404–408. https://doi.org/10.5144/0256-4947.2005.404

Hafström, L., Johansson, H., & Ahlberg, J. (2011). Diagnostic Delay of Breast Cancer: An Analysis of Claims to Swedish Board of Malpractice (LÖF). *Breast*, 20 (6), 539–542. https://doi.org/10.1016/j.breast.2011.06.007

Helleringer, G. (2011). Medical Malpractice and Compensation in France, Part II: Compensation Based on National Solidarity. *Chi.-Kent L. Rev.*, 86, 1019–1127.

Hiatt, H. H., Barnes, B. A., Brennan, T. A., Laird M. N., Lawthers, A. G., Leape, L. L., Localio, A. R., Newhouse, J. P., Peterson, L. M., Thorpe, K. E., et. al. (1989). A Study of Medical Injury and Medical Malpractice. *N Engl J Med.*, 321(7), 480–484. https://doi.org/10.1056/NEJM198908173210725

Howell, B., Kavanagh, J., & Marriott, L. (2002) No-fault Public Liability Insurance: Evidence from New Zealand. *Agenda*, 9(2), 135–149.

Kass, J. S., & Rose, R. V. (2016). Medical Malpractice Reform – Historical Approaches, Alternative Models, and Communication and Resolution Programs. *American Medical Association Journal of Ethics.* 18 (3), 299–310. https://doi.org/10.1001/journalofethics.2017.18.3.pfor6-1603.

Katzenmeier C, & Jansen C, *Möglichkeiten der Krankenkassen, ihre Versicherten beim Verdacht eines Behandlungsfehlers zu unterstützen*, Köln, 2016; 319.

Kesgin, S. Almanya'da Sosyal Güvenlik Sistemi (2018). http://kisi.deu.edu.tr//kamil.tugen/Almanya%20sosyal%20g%C3%BCvenlik%20sistemi.pdf, Access date 20.10.2021.

Kessler, D. P. (2011) Evaluating the Medical Malpractice System and Options for Reform. *J Econ Perspect.* 25(2), 93–110. https://doi.org/10.1257/jep.25.2.93

Luntz, H., & Hambly, D. (2002). Torts: Cases and Commentary. Lexis Nexis Butterworths, Fifth edition.

Nair, V., & Chandraharan, E. (2010). Clinical Negligence Scheme for Trusts. *Obstetrics, Gynecology and Reproductive Medicine*. 20(4), 125–128. https://doi.org/10.1016/j.ogrm.2010.01.004

Oğuz, A. (2021). *Karşılaştırmalı Hukuk*. Yetkin Yayınevi

Palmer, E. (June, 2009). Medical Malpractice Liability: Germany. https://www.loc.gov/law/help/medical-malpractice-liability/germany.php

Seabury, S. A., Helland, E., & Jena, A. B. (2014). Medical Malpractice Reform: Noneconomic Damages Caps Reduced Payments 15 Percent, With Varied Effects By Specialty. *Health Affairs*, 33(11), 2048–2056. https://doi.org/10.1377/hlthaff.2014.0492.

Songur, C. Top, M., & Tekingündüz, S. (2013). Sağlık Sektöründe GZFT (Güçlü-Zayıf Yönler-Fırsatlar-Tehditler) Analizi. *Sağlıkta Performans ve Kalite Dergisi*, (5): 1 69-99, https://dergipark.gov.tr/download/article-file/303530, Access date 21.02.2021.

Türkan, H., & Tuğcu, H. (2004). 2000–2004 Yılları Arasında Yüksek Sağlık Şurası'nda Değerlendirilen Acil Servislerle İlgili Tıbbi Uygulama Hataları. *Gülhane Tıp Dergisi*. 46 (3), 226 - 231.

Ulfbeck, V., Hartlev, M., & Schultz, M. (2012) Malpractice in Scandinavia. *Chi.-Kent. L. Rev.*, 87, 111–129. https://scholarship.kentlaw.iit.edu/cklawreview/vol87/iss1/6/

Weidinger. P. (2006). Aus der Praxis der Haftpflichtversicherungfür Ärzte und Krankenhäuser – Statistik, neue Risiken und Qualitätsmanagement. *Medizinrecht*. 24(10), 571–580. https://doi.org/10.1007/s00350-006-1763-y

World Medical Association-WMA. (2005). Archived: The World Medical Association Statement on Medical Malpractice. https://www.wma.net/policies-post/world-medical-association-statement-on-medical-malpractice/

Yazıcı, Y. A., Şen, H., Aliustaoğlu, S., Sezer, Y., & İnce, C. H. (2015). Evaluation of the Medical Malpractice Cases Concluded in the General Assembly of Council of Forensic Medicine. *Ulus Travma Acil Cerrahi Dergisi*. 21(3), 204–208. https://doi.org/10.5505/tjtes.2015.24295

Yılmaz, E. N. (2019). *Karşılaştırmalı Hukukta Tıbbi Malpraktis ve Arabuluculuk Uygulamaları*. Yetkin Yayınevi.

Zweigert, K., Kötz, H. (1998). Introduction to Comparative Law (T. Weir transl.). Clarendon Press.